Textbook of

Prevention Practice and Community Physiotherapy

Textbook of
Prevention Practice and Community Physiotherapy

Chief Editor

Dr Bharati Vijay Bellare

BSc (PT), PGCR, FIAP, PhD

Ex-Prof and HOD Physiotherapy

Lokmanya Tilak Municipal Medical College

Ex-Prof

MGM School of Physiotherapy, Navi Mumbai, Maharashtra, India

Sub-Editors

Pavithra Rajan

BPT (India), MSc (Canada)

PhD Candidate in Physiotherapy

Faculty of Health Sciences

University of Sydney, NSW, Australia

Dr Unnati Nikhil Pandit

MPTh (CVR), PhD

Prof-Director, Dept of Physiotherapy

Padmashree Dr DY Patil University, Nerul, Navi Mumbai, Maharashtra, India

JAYPEE *The Health Sciences Publisher*

New Delhi | London | Panama

JAYPEE **Jaypee Brothers Medical Publishers (P) Ltd**

Headquarters

Jaypee Brothers Medical Publishers (P) Ltd
4838/24, Ansari Road, Daryaganj
New Delhi 110 002, India
Phone: +91-11-43574357
Fax: +91-11-43574314
Email: jaypee@jaypeebrothers.com

Overseas Offices

J.P. Medical Ltd
83 Victoria Street, London
SW1H 0HW (UK)
Phone: +44 20 3170 8910
Fax: +44 (0)20 3008 6180
Email: info@jpmedpub.com

Jaypee-Highlights Medical Publishers Inc
City of Knowledge, Bld. 235, 2nd Floor, Clayton
Panama City, Panama
Phone: +1 507-301-0496
Fax: +1 507-301-0499
Email: cservice@jphmedical.com

Jaypee Brothers Medical Publishers (P) Ltd
17/1-B Babar Road, Block-B, Shaymali
Mohammadpur, Dhaka-1207
Bangladesh
Mobile: +08801912003485
Email: jaypeedhaka@gmail.com

Jaypee Brothers Medical Publishers (P) Ltd
Bhotahity, Kathmandu
Nepal
Phone: +977-9741283608
Email: kathmandu@jaypeebrothers.com

Website: www.jaypeebrothers.com
Website: www.jaypeedigital.com

Inquiries for bulk sales may be solicited at: jaypee@jaypeebrothers.com

Textbook of Prevention Practice and Community Physiotherapy

First Edition: **2018**

ISBN: 978-93-5270-325-8

Printed at Sanat Printers

Tribute

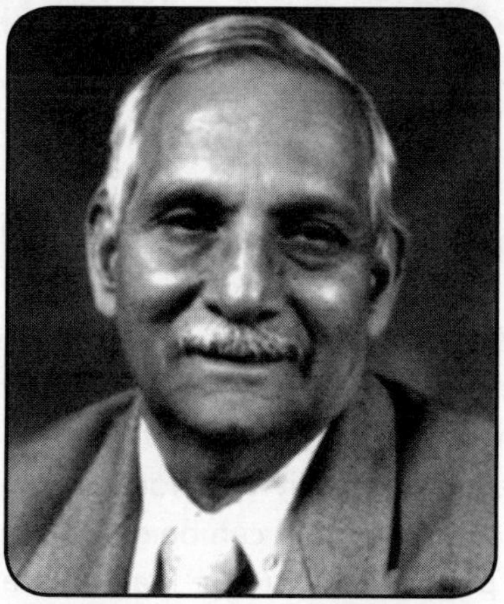

Late Dr Madhav G Mokashi

Look, my finger is pointing to the Moon,
Keep learning, keep growing, humility is a boon,
Let wisdom guide you, with simplicity be in tune,
Care, Compassion, Cheerfulness will dispel patients gloom,
Ennoble yourself with qualities of Head and Heart,
Enrich your Students, your Profession, Patients, Families, Caregivers,
Patience, Passion, Perseverance, Positivity makes everyone bloom,
Poise, Wonder, Empathy, Humor, Healing with words-deeds-and silence,
Laboring, keep sowing, nurture and groom, righteousness, mindfulness, upholding Ethics,
Inquiring, Questioning, Power Position Pomp in life should have no room,
Truth Awareness Happiness above all, all else will pass soon,
Madhav Mokashi Sir you touched so many lives,
Your giving sharing has ennobled enriched our Life,
We too are looking at the Moon, Sun, Stars and Galaxies,
But still rooted-treading your path, with a gratitude overwhelmed is this Heart,
You lead us to a Spring that knows no Summer an endless Inner Monsoon.

Dhruv Mehta

A Tribute

Psychophilosophy of Yoga and its Remedial Value

Yoga is a spiritual science to uplift human beings. Human birth is considered as a gift and a Jiva experiences-Bhoga and is supposed to move in direction of liberation from sorrows, i.e. *Apavarga*. It aims at union of Aatma in bound state with Prakruti (Nature) with Paramaatma while Prakruti remains active since binding other Jivas. It is multifaceted and at multiple levels. Life is full of miseries, is a statement of facts as observed and not a pessimistism. Actually it is assured that there is a permanent way out, by Yoga for liberation. Kleshas arising from Avidya-ignorance form the root cause of sorrows and can be cut off by sword of knowledge. Whereas Atma is the senescent inactive principle, the active Prakruti makes Jivas misconceive that it is the knower. Other Kleshas Asmita-ego, Sukh-Duhkha and Abhinivesh built-in desire for life, arise out of it. Abhinivesh is a very strong feeling in people of all kind and they simply cling to life at any cost. Sukh-Duhkha should be faced respectfully, as sources of knowledge which is perceiving in Aklishta manner; Klishta way of perception is on emotional channel especially desirous of something in possession or to get materialized. Else a cycle of new kleshas would be added. If aim of Yoga is Samadhi, Vyadhis consist of psychophysical disturbances. Vikshepas are obstacles to come in way along with the Sahabhuvas their associates and they are listed 9 as Vighnas. It may be recalled that God Ganesha is Vighna-hartaa remover of such Antaraayas–obstacles. They are Vyaadhi-diseases due to imbalance in Dhaatus causing Doshas-Vaata, Pitta, kapha. Psychosomatic disturbances/disorders are also included. Other consists of Styana-mental lethargy, Sanshaya means conflict to have faith to accept this or that, Pramaada-non alertness regarding Yogic remedies, Aalasya-lack of tendency towards Yoga due to physical idleness owing to Dhaatu-dosha as well inertia of mind dominant with Tam Guna, Avirati is strong desire towards sensual pleasures, Bhranti-darshana is deluded mind having false knowledge. Alabdha-bhoomikatva is not getting any footing in Yoga despite efforts, an 'avasthitatva' is even if there is some achievement on the path mind but mind is unstable. All such Antaraayas-internal obstacles act as Kleshas and make mind unstable hence come in way of Yoga hence termed as Antaraayas. If they are absent modifications in mind, any mentation is also absent.

An 8-step progression from Bahiranga external-Yama, Niyama, Aasan, Praanaayaama, Pratyaahaara to Aantaranga internal-Dhaarana, Dhyaana and samaadhi; Yoga prescribed is known as Ashtaang Yoga. Some schools exclude 'dos and don'ts'. Yamas are preparatory social dos and don'ts: Ahimsa-non-injury to others is rather for co-existence. There should be no hazard to surroundings. Place should be conducive to undertake Yoga in natural atmosphere.

Place should be with a raised platform. Trees having birds and lake, well of water or seashore are favorable. It should not be too windy and for 4 forearm distance free from fire, water, etc. to offer comfort. For a hut, place should be isolated and quiet and it should be fenced to avoid menace from wild animals. One must bear in mind that unless destined, if other practitioners around, it is encouraging.

Some schools exclude preparatory Yamas and the Niyamas. Yamas are social observances. Ahimsaa is no-harm or no-violence towards others. Satya is perceived facts by sensory organs so it is direct evidence as in science. Asteya is attitude of non-stealing. Brahmacharya is celibacy in student days after thread ceremony, a Sanskara. For family-holders, it is controlled sex. Aparigraha is no desire for other's possessions. Niyamas are personal observances: Shauh is from body to mind purification. It aims at Sattva-shuddhi. It rightly should be concerned with preventing pollution of air, sound, water, and the surroundings. The concept of ecology should be enclosed as of today. Santosh means self-satisfaction and faith that it is an internal quality and does not come by meeting the greed outside. Other 3 Niyamas: Tapa-austerity, Svaadhyaaya-study and performing sacred acts as advised in scriptures and Ishvara-Pranidhaana dedication to God and surrendering fruits of actions to Him form Kriyayoga.

Aasana is 3rd step and for preparing the body physique, though mind is on the performance to experience it. Asana is a total body posture and not for just any of the body segments. This feature distinguishes it from any local exercise. Mainly, spine is the key segment. There are many safety valves to protect body from injury. Most important is the respiratory and care should be taken that Valsalva maneuver does not take place. Weight of a body segment is used as resistance and spine the heaviest. It would not do harm to proximal and intermediate joint of limbs but if any digit comes under it, then a practitioner alone should owe the responsibility of fault. Next, there are head-low positions and there should be serial progression to poses like Shirshasana. Rush won't serve any purpose. Initially, Supta-Vajrasana or Matsyasana-touching head to ground from kneel-sitting Padmasana lotus pose should be practised. In other words, head-low position without loading head by body weight in a topsy-turvy pose is good enough. Such discretion is a must in general but absolutely essential in therapy. Neck segment of spine is most mobile and under loading vulnerable to neural injury since cervical vertebrae are slender and neural canal is packed with the ascending and descending tracts. Atlanto-axial joint is most mobile segment and if loaded directly by carrying luggage on it or vertically loaded as in Shirshasana, there are chances of natural glide. In Sarvangasana, the body weight is well distributed over arms and hands supporting the pelvis the neck flexion to 90°, is a weak point for possible injuries. However, the load of spine and lower limbs above is well aligned so that the primary and the secondary natural curvatures of spine are maintained and neutralize each other. Cervical spine is unlike lumbosacral spine which has less chances of it, since lumbar vertebrae are massive and there is more empty space in neural canal; while ligamentous and musculofascial injuries are common. Surgery—radiating pain is another red signal which should be respected. Asanas demand terminal range movements at various joints simultaneously. Therefore the mental scan must be on continuously to detect changes in neural comfort, which should be all the time of performance conceding that tolerance level of different patients is different. If there is previous sensory impairment, therapist has to be more attentive and be guided by his clinical acumen.

Use of VAS during performance pays but it is a subjective test after all. We (Gaurang Baxi and Mokashi MG; PhD thesis Dr DY Patil University Pimpri, Pune) found no incidence of injuries reported in case of 128 nerves with radiating pain subjected to Yogasanas program in nerves of upper and lower limbs and compared with Butler's neurodynamic nerve tension tests and mobilization. Yoga program was administered as a package wherein only one or two Asanas were specific to stretch that particular nerve. Yogasanas were comparable in effect as a test as well as a mobilizing technique.

Another significant feature of Aasanas is de-fatigability, rather one feels fresh after a session is over. If lactic acid level is raised in blood, there would be automatic rise in pulse rate (PR). However, this is not the case; PR is found to be raised. Granting recovery time of 3 minutes after any antigravity performance of an Asana, or at the end of session prior to Shavasana, PR is restored to the normal/the starting level. If someone wants to resort to Yoga with problem of high resting pulse, Pranaayaama is a better proposition to start; as for Aasanas, antigravity performance be avoided. Either moving in or out of it shall be against gravity. A better strategy is to allow them in horizontal plane, as in case of muscle power 2 on MMT. As the effort is lesser, it does work. Along with PR rise, there will be change in breathing pattern. Either it is faster or inspiratory time would be prolonged.

Yogis watched nature. Names of many Aasanas are of animals-Bhujanga-serpent, Matsya-fish, Ushtra-camel, Makara-crocodile, etc. It is described that Aasanas are as many as species which amount to 84 lakhs. They are known to God Shiva alone who on the weightage decided that 84 are representative. For meditation, Siddha, Padma, Sinha, Bhadra, Veera and Swastik Aasanas are important. Most of them are in sitting except Veera which is ½ Kneel-standing. Surprisingly, Vajraasana-adamant pose very stable is missing in this list. It was observed that animals like dogs while resting do panting. It could be their tried time-tested way to restore starting PR by hyperventilation. Accordingly, a method of Praanaayaama was introduced. Animals keep mouth open while breathing; is it way of cooling the system? They introduced Shitalee procedure with modification that mouth is closed like a beak and air is taken in through a small orifice only to get effective cooling.

It is emphasized that spine must be erect while meditating. Then there is Vruksha-tree, Parvat-mountain, from non-animals also. Sometimes breath is controlled in meditation but in patients, it is better to allow breathing to take its own course. Hatha-Pradipikaa is a work of much late origin but gives very minute technical details.

Praanaayaama is Gati-Vichheda control over movement of air in Shvaasa (Pooraka) and out Prashvaasa (Rechaka) while breathing. It is considered by Swami Vivekananda not as controlling physical air (Vaayu) element but control over consciousness and conscience. It is vital bioenergy. Air may move centrally from nostrils or touching medial/lateral surface and this way, its Desha-region can be described. Force of movement can be measured by placing cotton in front and gauge movement at 8, 12, 32 fingers distance away. Breathing is measured in Maatras time unit as 12, 24, 36. Time one-fourth of blinking is considered as kshana and can be expressed in physiological time unit. Breath in and out forms a cycle is Udghaata; likewise, it is expressed in numbers also. Thus it differs as Dirgha-depth and Sookshma-fineness. Third type is stopping breath for some time altogether; the column of air is Stabha-vrutti, i.e. still. It is comparable to preserve water in a Kumbha-pitcher and termed as Kumbhaka. It is performed either as Baahya as the air goes out or Antar as air enters in. In the fourth type, there is lack of breathing. Technically, there exists Gati-Vichheda but it is almost effortless; it removes impurities over sattva guna thus purifies it. There occurs Sattva-Shuddhi so Praanaayaama is a Shuddhi-Kriyaa. While practising it, the attention is on conscious physiological parameters hence it is a concrete thinking process. It is preparatory to meditation.

Ha and Tha point out the Sun and the Moon. In breathing through left nostril and left side passage is by Ida Naadi while right side is represented by the Pingalaa meaning the Sun. As known, Ida is feminine, emotions and represents mother while Pingala is opposite of it; centrally rises up Sushumnaa concerned with creativity and spirituality. Shiva-Svarodaya Shaastra is devoted to Praanas and Upa-Praanas-the subsidiary ones. God Shiva described to wife Devee Paarvati, 'Praana is the main remedy; none is more brotherly to survive and move towards liberation. It is the best friend'. Praanas are 5 and are referred as Pancha-vrutti due to different functions. Praana stays in heart and moves up; Apaana stays in anal region moves Arvaag, with both stays Vyaana is everywhere concerned with energy, up-moving is Udaana and stays around throat region, with all is Samaana and stays around umbilical region. It is believed that a Jiva's life span is fixed at birth and it is numbered in breathing cycles. Since in Praanaayaama the inward, outward or both movements of breath are prolonged, a Yogi's life is extended. Praanas function is Dhaarana-to preserve life and Indriyas have tendency to act as per Praana-Apaana drive; not only that but after end of life, they are responsible in carrying the Sookshma deha to its destined place. Of all 5 Praanas, the administrative Devataa is Vaayu hence all are referred as Praana. In Naabhi region-umbilical, Kanda is situated from which 72 thousand vessels arise for circulation of Praanas. Ida-flow is in Shukla paksha for 2 and ½ Ghatikas and sequence of Vaayu tatvas is in order of Vaayu, Agni, Bhumi, Jala and Aakaash for 3 days. Same way, Soorya-flow is in Krushna paksha for 3 days. It is advised that a light work should be started on moon-Svara and heavy work on Soorya-svara; devotional and spiritual actions be initiated when Sushumnaa is active. Shanmukhi mudraa is recommended for knowing which Svara is flowing-thumbs are placed over ears, middle fingers to close nostrils and fingers over eyes and mouth. A simple procedure reveals tatva flowing-exhale on a clean mirror: a square shaped figure-Pruthvi, half moon-Jala, tringle-Teja, circle–Vaayu and a dot-Aakaash.

As per Atharva veda in its Prashnopaishada, is described that Kundalini is situated like a serpent winded. Naadis carrying Praanas are 10; of these, Ida, Pingalaa and Sushumnaa are major. Of remaining 7, two supply eyes, 2 ears, 1 in each in mouth, reproductive organs and Moolasthaana. Upa-pranas 5 function as follows: Naaga-belching, Koorma-blinking, Krukal-sneezing, Devadatta-yawning; Dhananjaya occupies whole body and even after death it stays for some time.

Moolaadhaar Chakra is between anus and reproductive organs. It is lotus-shaped with 4 yellow petals. On the petals, there are Moola Akshars-letters in the form of Maatrukaas. Those letters are Vam, Sham, Shham and Sam. In the center is Lam Beeja. Kundalini Nadi faces downward and winds in 3½ turns with tail in its mouth asleep but when it is awakened, it faces upwards. Shad-ripus reside here which cause Yama-yaatanas. To awaken it is the ultimate aim of a Jiva. Devataa of this Chakra is Shri Ganesh. It represents earth. If achieved the beginning of spiritual progress starts; there are health, Vak-siddhi—the oratory, and memory of past lives. Next is Svadhishthana Chakra below umbilicus with lotus having 6 Saffron colored petals. On its petals, 6 rutus (seasons) and 5 Tattvas (reside). Maatrukaas are Bam-Shishira, Aakaash with desire for Brahma; Bham–Sharada, Jala tattva, mind is deluded; Mam-Henant, mastery destroys illusions; Yam-Vasanta, Vaayu Tattva, ruled by Daksha Prajaapati regarding procreation; Ram-Grishma, Agni; Lam-Prithvi, Varshaa, Devata-Indra and centrally is Beeja Vam. This Chakra is of Jala Tattva. God Brahma along with Devis Sarasvati and Raakini reside in it. If it is crossed, practitioner becomes devotional and egoless. On the whole, for a Yogi, it is Ishvara-Pranidhaana and self-surrender awards happiness independent of sensual pleasures. Third is Manipura Chakra with 10 petals. Devata is Maha-Vishnu and Mahalakshmi; Varuna and Devi Daakini also stay here. For Praanas-Upapranas, 10 Mahaa Vidyaas it is abode. On conquering it, Sookhma deha is endowed. All divine powers are received. Oja-Bala is gifted.

At the level of heart is Annahata Chakra, with lotus of 12 petals dark blue in color. It belongs to Vaayu Tattva and centrally, there exists a dark blue triangle in which exists a Baana-Linga. Devatas Shankar-Parvati reside and yam is the Beeja-akshara. Also Devi Kakani resides here. On petals, 12 letters are: gutturals ka, kha, ga, gha, yan, Moordhanya-Cha, chha, ja, za, an, and upper Taalavya-ta and thha. Anaahata sound without any objects struck is heard here. A Saadhaka would be gifted with prosperity, happiness, fortune, and Siddhis which he must humbly reject. This is abode of Jeevaatmaa who performs Ajapaajap along with So-ha dhvani while breathing. There is experience of overwhelming blue color due to presence of Neelavatee Devi an incarnation of mata Paarvati to kill Raktabeeja demon. Our self-incriminating and destructive emotions alike Kaama-Krodha get vanished along with ego and equanimity is felt.

Above Anaahata is Vishuddha Chakra with 16 white petals. Svaras numbered 16 reside on petals. Cente belongs to Aakash tattva. A, Aa, I, Ii, U, OO, Ru, Roo, Lru< lroo E, Ai, O, Ou, Am, Ah.

Science should not have any issues with God since there is no room for antagonism. Science deals with knowledge acquired from events perceived by sensory organs, i.e. from 'Sat'. From Darwinism anti-God stance entered in scientists. Darwin could only predict creation and provide laws of to reason out evolution. In fact Newton whose laws are so fundamental in physics saw His hand in universe everywhere. In a way scientists working for use of knowledge and skills in service of humanity are Gods agents. It makes no difference to God whether they are theist or not as long as they don't perform any unethical and criminal acts of injustice against the surrounding atmosphere, plant and animal life including human beings. A scientist is a human being and has right to hold any view; one who is theist or God-fearing need not feel as a stranger. Dedication to right work is a divine quality. Philosophy is considered to be the mother of sciences. Hence, scientists serve the mother, philosophy.

In Indology, philosophy is a way of life. Cultures like eastern versus western represent two different ways of thinking thereby living too. Religions are having great influence on people's thinking and sometimes the social mass thinking has a driving force that may come in way of individual's freedom of thought, expression and actions. Inter-caste or Inter-religion marriages is one of its examples. Likewise, there exist political, social, economical philosophies; how communism and the Nazi thinking influenced the world affairs is well known. Socialism and capitalism present other example. Personal thinking of Hitler, Gandhiji changed world history and subsequently geography also. Lokmanya Tilak expressed his thoughts boldly in early twentieth century, through an editorial weekly Kesari. He boldly stated, 'Independence is my birthright and I will regain it. Thirst for independence cannot be satisfied by good governance.' It evoked flame of new, bold thought against then ruling British who considered him as traitor—a court case was filed, found guilty and sentenced 6 years imprisonment. His remarks to the Court are typical of his unique personality 'There exists a Higher Court, and God will justify my actions'. He was sent to Mandale prison in Burma. However, his Mantra provoked a national spirit in minds of Indian population, Hindu and Muslims alike and also activated the extremists who equipped themselves to answer injustice by gunfire. Same Tilak wrote Commentary on Bhagvad Geeta and propagated view that Geeta is Nishkam Karma-Yoga-selfless action from detachment. Later on Gandhiji also in commentary of Geeta expressed view that it Bhakti-Yoga. Tilak had staunch faith in Hinduism but he did not mix it up with his political aim to get Swarajya. He maintained them apart. There are personal philosophies also which are rather in justification of their actions and behavior or rationalizations.

There exists philosophy of sportsman spirit; Late Vijay Merchant India's stylish opening batsman and captain in 1950s had a motto on letterhead, 'Play the Game'! He was an industrialist and worked for the cause of the disabled. Even the underworld seems to have some unwritten philosophy–more of working rules on how to deal internationally among themselves and with others. Philosophy survives because there are its followers. Ethics is an important feature of any philosophy aimed at humanitarian value. One part is the guiding principles; other part is freedom to implement them in life. Right to survive, for choosing livelihood, equality, justice for all, right for health, education, freedom of thought and its expression become such guiding principles included in the Constitution of many democratic nations. Swami Vivekanand Institute of Yoga is operated from Kanyakumari and taken over the rock island and constructed a memorial and a meditation hall. Yoga has been systematically investigated by Swami Shivanand who was a surgeon. He started Divine Yoga Institute in Rushikesh. Swami Kuvalayananda established Kaivalyadham in Lonavala while Yogendraji established Yoga Institute in Santacruz Mumbai. Yogi Mahesh runs research in some international centers. Yoga has evoked interest all over the world and different aspects of Ashtanga Yoga–8 steps of Yoga ladder are studied. Yoga with advents in information technology, the global thinking is emerged and a concern of justice to all. The walls of nationalism collapse and there is awakening. Yoga is an example of this kind. It has pierced the walls of religions smoothly. It is no more a Hindu property; it has gained the proprietary status. Yoga with Naturopathy is accepted as a Health discipline and is included under the Indigenous system of medicine under AYUSH Council. Morarji Desai National Institute of Yoga is established in New Delhi. Yoga Biomedical Trust in UK systematically maintains records of scientific papers published on Yoga. In the wake of this millennium, a Yoga University is constituted in Bangalore. Though in USA, Yoga is considered as a system of Alternate and Complementary Medicine, by the practitioners of modern medicine, i.e. Allopaths and declared it as not scientific, under the clout of evidence-based medicine (EBM) and so influenced the Government Agencies. About 28% of American citizens have turned to Yoga practices voluntarily (Barnes PM, et al., children and adults entry and Complementary and Alternate medicine use among children and adults; USA Statistics 2007). The United Nations has declared 21st June as the International Day of Yoga. The General Assembly recognized that Yoga provides holistic approach-health and well-being and that dissemination of information about benefits of practicing Yoga would be beneficial for the health of the world population. It must be realized that this has increased the responsibility of the scientists world over and on Indian health scientists in particular since the resolution in UN Assembly was moved by India. I am sure Indian Physiotherapists shall equip themselves to meet this challenge squarely. Philosophy is considered to be the mother of sciences.

I turned into Yoga in 1970, on health grounds following MI at the age of 33 years. My health was otherwise good—no hypertension, diabetes mellitus, headache, etc. That particular day, my brother and myself had been to market. It was late morning time and while returning I had a violent sneeze which caused chest pain. I felt heavy perspiration but not heart pain. As we came home, my wife, a medical officer, with central railway came to know of history and rushed me to headquarter hospital at Byculla. I was subjected to investigations and promptly hospitalized. Next day, Dr KK Datey eminent cardiologist of Bombay who was Honorary consultant, stamped it as atypical heart attack and my hospitalization continued. After a sneeze Christians say, 'God bless you'. Anyway, I was blessed to survive. What exercise to do? Cardiologists used to advise 'walk slow to fast but walk'. Today the same Mantra is chanted but a treadmill is harnessed so that desired speed is imposed. Physiologists prefer that no handgrip be used since it could cause Valsalva maneuver and lower diastolic BP. However, today the exercisers have BP sensors that detect BP from fingertips. The Yoga package was ready. Early that year, Dr Tulpule, Emeritus Professor of cardiology, from Grant Medical College and JJ Hospital, Mumbai wanted to present a paper in early 1970 and approached us at AIIPMR, Mumbai, with proposal to get some evidence that the ligaments get strengthened following Yoga training. We had no method in vivo to do so. Instead we offered whether nerve conduction velocities improved. Thus study was undertaken on a risk group for heart attack in the middle aged volunteers. Thus I was involved with both the studies. After MI, the program was readymade for me. As my pathological lab reports were normal, my mobilization was permitted as indoor patient. The stage was set for me since what to do was not a problem. Yoga program was ready for me. I self-volunteered and used to perform it, after ward rounds. Only thing I was a stage ahead in time or intensity of exercise. Yoga has some built-in precautions. Angamejayatva means tremors during performance. Tremors are incidental if fatigue occurs. One should actually feel fresh after Yoga. Tremor not attributable to fatigue is to be taken as pathological either of Parkinsonian type or cerebellar. Occasionally it could be iatrogenic. Another caution is Shvasa-Prashvasa meaning dyspnea-exhalatory type as in asthma while inspiratory is due to work more than lung capacity at that time. I used to take my pulse rate and monitor it. I realized that if it is to be imported in PT, a Physiotherapist must be trained in it. After discharge I joined class at Kaivalyadham Mumbai and completed 6-week program for the beginners. I would not bother how well my batch mate next to me is doing; it is not a competition. One must experience one's performance. Eventually within 6 months of MI, I could visit our family goddess temple of Ekaveera devi at karla which on hills near Lonavala. In 1973, I also joined Yoga teachers training at Kaivalyadhama Lonavala. Side by side, I could also spend some fruitful time at their research lab and hospital too. I could also undertake some investigative studies with Dr Bhole, MD in the lab. Since 1970, the concept invaded my mind that Yoga can be the ideal home program.

Further, I propose that in Yoga we find the roots of advanced exercise therapy. It does not require any equipment. The weight of body segment usually spine can be used in total-body postures to provide resistance. A patient or caregiver, mostly a family member could be trained in checking any faults in performance. A therapist can plan progression from simple to difficult postures. It is better to practice simpler postures in the beginning. It helps in re-establishing possible role of planning the task; job to be accomplished must be conceived in mind like a gestalt, i.e. in totality. Accordingly placing demand on motor centers for job-performance also be as a whole first. Emphasis should be on proximal fixation, distal to proximal sequence of movements, separation of voluntary components in the task, absorbing clues provided by therapist and use them in correction. Coordinated movement is smooth and recruits power or speed of performance in ramped fashion. After all speed is a function of power. Initially the performance be captured as a whole, without accuracy. From gross to finer motor control can be practised on simpler postures first. In difficult postures only gross control be initiated.

Asana is third step to prepare of and is just not physical exercises. Swami Kuvalayananda of Lonavala classified them as—1. Meditational 2. Relaxing mind-body and 3. For physical culture. However, it must be noted that any step on path of Yoga is psychophysical as mind being associated with performance. Hence mind is in experiencing mode. This step is used in therapeutics also and it is preferable that a health professional proficient in Yoga be responsible in planning, executing and teaching 'Dos and Don'ts' for success. With Lonavala Ashram Dr Vinekar was associated and they wrote a book on Asanas, Pranayam and Yoga Therapy in joint authorship. Dr Shivananda was an ophthalmic surgeon and established Divine Yoga institute at Rushikesh. Another pioneering exponent was Yogendraji of Yoga Institute Santacruz Mumbai. Those institutions carried out training of instructors as well published journals, books and carried out literary and scientific research too. Swami Bhaktivedanta at the age of 69 migrated to USA and established Hare Ram Hare Krishna movement. Yogi Ram offered himself to Yogic research. Geigi Pharmaceuticals published a pamphlet in late 1960s on the feats he achieved. While he was meditating he could change temperature of skin of forearm a proof of control over autonomic nervous system (ANS). Afterward he could recall conversation between the people in adjacent room at the time he was meditating. A cardiologist saw ECG of period of meditation and observed flutter like changes who remarked, 'Yogi must have popped of'. To his surprise, he was informed by the investigators that he was taking a lecture in next room. Yogi Ram established an Institute in Rushikesh where I spent a week but only after his demise. They run a hospital and a medical college too. In 1970s, Dhirendra Brahmachari was given charge of national Yoga institute by then Government headed by Smt Indira Gandhi the PM. Recently, Baba Ramdev has created quite a wave to popularize Yogaasanas. Similarly, Yogi Mahesh carried out such work in international institutes. Physiologist Wallace was associated with it. In one paper published, he brought out that during meditation body functions at submetabolic rate.

In Kaivalyadham Dr Bhole, MD from AIIMS Delhi was Dy Director Research. We (Mokashi and Bhole 1973) collected some data on oxygen consumption using direct method by respirometer. In Sarvangasana top-down vertical posture, we found that O_2 utilization was just 1.4 as against sitting-1.2 for maintaining posture for 3 minutes. We attributed to alignment of body segments especially the spine. Base is provided by arms flexed at elbows, hands supporting the pelvis and shared by head via neck flexion. Thus condition of Sukha-no discomfort was not violated. After training it could be done at minimal effort and Prayatna shaithiya was satisfactory. Effect is quoted in Patanjala Yoga Darshan is Dvandva abhighat-conquering over antagonistic muscle work. If Pavan-Muktasana all flexion pose is given following it, there is no muscle fatigue. This Dvandva could be sukha-Dukha but we can take a broader concept pertaining to autonomic nervous system. Thus of sympathetic outflow and parasympathetic have no conflict. Actually, if parameters like HR, RR, salivation, have been scored with SNS scores on higher side and shown by scientists that the scores reduce. It may be inferred that behind relief of various complaints of patients, Yoga program is successful even in Yoga classes also, run by instructors, there is sound scientific ground. Then if this training is guided by qualified health professionals, will be more beneficial to the patient population. Yogic curriculum is of Bandhas-neuromuscular or anatomically positioned locks like Moola-bandha-contraction of anal sphincters during breathing throughout, while Jaladhar bandha is closing of glottis actively as well as passively by neck flexion. In Uddiyan bandha is end-expiratory maneuver-first in standing the hands are pressed on each knee. Air is exhaled forcefully and then glottis is closed so that no air can escape out. Then a mock inhalation is carried out. It results in increased intra-thoracic pressure while the abdomen is sucked in. If pressure on any one knee is increased, that side vertical abdominal muscle bulk stands out and if done alternately it is *Nauli kriya* a cleansing procedure for stomach. Pranayam with those 3 bandhas together is considered to be effective. While breathing in meditation, Moola bandha with contraction of transverse abdominus is advocated irrespective of inhalation or exhalation using transverse abdominal as the core muscle. Neti is performed using thread traditionally while a thin catheter also is used. Traditionally Dhauti is used for stomach wash using flexible pipe of banana or bamboo. A plastic pipe is alternative. A practitioner drinks salt water to aid the process. Basti is like enema of present day using water. It can be realized that Yoga offers so many procedures not just passive, for ANS cleansing. For example, in Dhauti, when pipe is being swallowed, one has to suppress the gag reflex responsible for vomiting. A physiotherapist has no such battery at disposal to train ANS.

We (Mokashi and Gole, 'Training of ANS by Yoga presented in International Conference on Yoga and Research, Bangalore, 1993) have investigated a group of 7 Yoga instructors with electromyography and found that a majority of them tended to abdominal muscles contraction, inadvertently. As shown the performance on oscilloscope monitor, they could reverse to correct procedure. Further, we (Munira and Mokashi, presented in IAP Conference in Calcutta, 1983) trained school girls who were beginners in Yoga, in uddiyan bandha. EMG monitor was not used in training. They were given just demonstrations as in a Yoga class. After training, they were tested on EMG monitor. They were doing it in correct manner. Thus in performing Yoga for patients, there is scope to use biofeedback. Patients are benefitted by feedback. After all Yoga is learning is change in behavior. Here it is physiological behavior. Mudras are also performed like Bandhas Sinha-Mudra is control over muscles around throat while tongue is outstretched actively.

We have systematically investigated effects of Yoga package in patients with neurological disorders. A theme of Yogasanas was developed at All India Institute of Physical Medicine and

Rehabilitation Mumbai. I presented in World Congress of Physical Therapists in Montreal in 1974 (Pub WCPT proceedings.) Initially group of CP was treated but soon, hemiplegics, cerebellar lesions were recruited in studies. Early evaluation was by photographic records. Soon grading per Asana was worked out. If a posture had to be passively forced on a spastic patient-grade 0 was scored. If it needed to be forced on some segment while other segments could be moved passively-score 1 given. If movement of those segments was active-score 2 was given. Actively moving into full posture with some assistance was scored-3. Other 3 grades were granted for refinement of control distal to proximal. Usually spinal movements guide to choice in a package. Flexion: Matsyasan-Towards gravity from Vajrasan, Pavan-muktasana: antigravity performance from supine lying, Hasta-padasan from standing in Surya Namaskar series can be tried out. Spinal extension is antigravity in Matsyasan to Vajrasan in sitting while final stage of Surya namaskar is extension in standing with ULs in flexion at shoulders and outstretched hands. Surya Namaskara series is like motor development from prone lying. Actual prone lying is not there but a posture called *Sashtanga* is in between. Touching points to ground surface are 2 forefeet, 2 knees, chest, 2 palms in weight bearing, i.e. due to work of elbow extensors and forehead. Side flexion of spine is in Trikonasan performed in standing traditionally. Spinal rotation is achieved in Matsyendrasana: the spinal twist in sitting. A therapist should assist in performance as necessary. Modifications should be entertained as the clinical manifestation prevails. If spastic equines do not permit Vajrasan it could be done on edge of bed with feet out and therapist's support. Air filled or sponge pillows in different shapes are handy. Triangular, sloping, circular, square, roller shapes are handy. Support of bars, chair, etc. can be of additional assistance to a patient. Long sitting is difficult due to hip-knee flexors spasticity. If a patient is made to sit in chest-knee position use of active extensors can be encouraged in stretching the postural deformities. Balance must be given top priority, before any antigravity erect postures, be it sitting or standing. Similarly use of ice bag can be made. Short time application 5 to 15 seconds over antagonist muscles has stimulating effect. A spastic muscle needs long time application for 5 or more minutes. Care should be taken to avoid burns. Whether a patient would report on anesthesia developed must be judged. Otherwise clinical acumen of therapist is the deciding factor. Likely, some medication to control spasticity is on and at certain timeframe, a patient may have spell of drowsiness. Such time is not good for concentration in learning control but decidedly risky in activities like gait training. Yoga is one way of therapy here but the clinical picture of a patient must be given due respect for success. Measures of success should be decided. It should be sensitive. More attention should be there on making a patient functional than making one grade shift from score 1 to 2 which is of academic interest but whether a therapist time should be assigned to such gain especially in Government run places is questionable. Even for a physiotherapist in private practice, it should be considered on the ground of ethics. It won't add to the reputation of a therapist. Like a therapist must get due remunerations for service offered, a patient also must get some observable improvement. Those should be balanced. A therapist must strive to update knowledge and skills as a professional obligation but time and money spent need not be recovered from pocket patient-family.

Further, quality of performance was measured by modifying Bobaths key to grade postures. It was for spastics and based on Reflex Inhibiting Postures (RIPs). Cephalo-caudal development was the basis and 0-6 grades were the score. Scapula-shoulder control carried score-3, Elbow-4, Forearm pronation-supination-5 and wrist-hand-6. Soon 4+ score had to be considered since biceps could perform this action independently. In lower limb (LL), there is no separation of movements as in upper limb (UL). Percentage scores of the whole segment could be obtained by total raw scores by 1.6 and 2.5 and advantage was in judging that if 50% score was arrived in UL, hand function would be absent since recovery could not cross elbow joint; whereas if it was in LL, a patient could be ambulatory with foot drop plus other characteristic gait deviations at hip and knee.

Finally I arrived at the idea of scoring isolated movement control and technique used was from Cabat-Knott-Voss Proprioceptive Neuromuscular Facilitation (PNF) techniques. 1. First an agonistic pattern of movements is selected in which test muscle is a component. Say if supination is to be tested, a flex-adduction pattern with internal or external rotation is selected. 2. Pattern is performed and in the best groove it is resisted to get on 'hold' contraction. 3. Then command 'let go' follows for test supination while all the rest of pattern remains on hold. 4. Whatever degree of relaxation achieved is active relaxation and graded as per 0–4 grades of voluntary control. Grade 3 is against gravity or with resistance in any plane. Full ROM is not to be expected. Sometimes 5 grades are acceptable. Thus problem of voluntary control grading was solved directly. Some people take spasticity for measurement and reverse is taken as voluntary control. However, it is playing with spinal stretch reflex and not acceptable. The pattern of spasticity also must be noted. It is never in a single muscle. It will be over one or more segments. Again it is not the same in different muscles. In deeper postural muscles, it is more as in flexor digitorum profundus it is more than muscle flexor digitorium sublimis. Our finding is that it is always maximum in rotators. To stretch a spastic pattern, if first derotation is employed it pays. The grip over the segment should be neutral, i.e. on the sides of the joints. A spastic muscle squeezed will be more stimulated. Again a jerky movement provokes spasticity. There are some key movements proximal to a segment, which influence spasticity. For UL, the neck is such an influencing proximal segment. It also influences upper trunk which in turn influences lower trunk and pelvis.

Thus quantitative scores enable us to assess individual movement/muscle control but from it, function may or may not be predicted. Hand function may be present with tenodesis action. Similarly gait deviations, is a solution found out by system of a patient to be functional at a minimal energy cost. The system is function-oriented and not deformity conscious. It would adapt to compensatory deviations and adopt them. Whenever correction is imposed on it, it would protest in a different way. For example, if gait training is started, some component of deviation would respond favorably but the gait may be slower; or there may be compensatory shift. High step gait is compensation to reduce effect of foot drop. Sometimes resorting to ankle foot orthosis is an effective solution than training for reduced high stepping. Other deficits also be taken into account such as sensory or perceptual dysfunction. Training in sensory integration should be supplemented. For coordination, sensory-motor function is the key. Speech defects and perceptual deficits have a say in good hand function. Patients having global aphasia or sensory deficit of speech function may not understand the task. Similarly, instructions of therapist regarding what to do may not be well understood. Here lies role of demonstration. In a group, such patients are benefitted to observe others and perform accordingly. Most essential is kinesthetic experience and its retention as well as the recall in learning. A therapist must decide how long a particular procedure is to be continued in time per session and total number of sessions too. As long as the proceeding act is better than the preceding one in some minute aspect, the learning is on. There should be adequate short-term memory. Otherwise feedback has a role to help. Somewhere, there would be a plateau, and learning stops. Some more practice for work hardening may be required but more attempt would not result in betterment. If we take a common example of handwriting, simply copying as per the specimen will not improve the writing. Somewhere the progress halts and so the practice too.

Is Yoga a safe practice is the question asked often. The Yogic dictum is that Asanas should be performed where the feel is that of Sukh-comfort. Tolerance level of different subjects varies. There are Vikshepas psychophysical obstructions. Some are associates with them. Vyadhi-disease is one of them. Styana-mental lethargy, while Alasya-is physical idleness are other. Charaka, the noted Ayurvedic physician of 100 BC wrote that Pranayam as one of the causes of chest pain. He also mentioned that anatomy and the physiology are common for Bheshajas-physicians and Yogis. It was realized then that foods and chronic diseases are related. Swami Digambarji who succeeded Kuvalayananda told his experience while I was in Teacher's course there. He was with organization from the beginning before they were given land in Lonavala for Yoga Ashram. While he was performing some pranayamic procedure, he got memory loss. When he started remembering again, he found he was in Lonavala ashram. He was interested in Yadna and used to perform those vidhis dedicatedly there. Best part was that his memorizing power recovered to that extent that he could remember the minute details of Karma-kanda. He used to recite Visnu-sahastra-nama daily. This incidence made Kuvalayananda to strike a note of caution-remark in his book that when you perform pranayam, you play with your nervous system. In Dhyana-bindu-upanishada of Atharvaveda, it is stated that Pranayama must be performed slowly else, there is likelihood of cough, breathlessness, etc. Yadnavalkya Sanhitaa insists that Pooraka1 time unit thru Ida: Kumbhaka 4 units: Rechaka 2 units thru Pingalaa thus if 12 Matraas: 48: 24 Maatras Udghaata–cycle is considered Kanishtha-lower type. Twice is medium while thrice is Uttam-higher type. A Matra is described as time for a blink, followed by a clap and utterance of a Laghu-soft alphabet. Vasishtha sanhita states that Pranayama with a mantra is Sagarbha-impregnated otherwise it is Agarbha. In Yoga-Chintaamani another time unit Vipala is mentioned-time taken for a Chutakee. Thus, 42 Vipalaas are equal to 12 Matras in Kanishthha type. Medium is of 84 Vipalaas= 24 Matraas while 126 Vipalas = 36 Matras, Uttama type. In Uttama state, Praan moves up from Kundalini to Brahma-randhra in head. It is specified that if Poorak is fast there is no hazard; it would be deeper breath. But Rechaka as a rule has to be slower. Dhyana-bindu-upanishad of Atharvaveda underlines that when there is sweating, Pranayama is of lower type; when body has tremors, it is medium type while if body is lifted up, it is higher type.

I came across two young athletes a male with paraparesis and a female with quadriparesis following yogasanas. But it was purely due to overdoing. The precautions are prescribed and if there is violation, penalty is imminent. A paper was presented in Western India Orthopedic conference in which I also presented on gait deviations in cerebral palsy. In 1970s, in one of the Western India Orthopedic Conferences, an orthopedic surgeon brought out a series of

25 patients with injury to ligamentum flava and the cause was ascribed to Yogasanas. It must not be forgotten that a disease has its own course and would manifest accordingly. Similarly, a disease has its prognosis. We had two middle-aged females having motor neuron disease coming for treatment during the same period. Both were put on Yoga program. Both were known to me as family friends. Sometimes, a disease has suppression. This must not be taken jubilantly in favor of success of Yoga; similarly exacerbation as failure of Yoga. Eventually both the patients died soon. I recall Dr Vinekar who co-authored book 'Yoga Therapy' with Swami Kuvalayananda. His son after MBBS had got a PG seat in Orthopedics but had some waiting period. He joined an orientation course at our Institute meanwhile. Unfortunately as he was having evening walk near Nanavati Hospital santacruz was dashed by a lorry and his head hit the footpath side-stone and had instantaneous death. I saw Dr Vinekar sitting silently alone in smashan bhumi. He grew in atmosphere surrounded by Yoga, rather breathed Yoga. What was he thinking? Would he take the personal catastrophe and digest the grief philosophically? Within 6 weeks, the father succumbed to death and we had to visit smashan bhumi again. Impact of sorrow can overpower philosophy. King Dashratha died of putra viyoga had putrashoka in the end, as Ramayan depicts. Even false news of death of son Ashvatthama made Guru Dronacharya to lay down the weapons and go in meditation to leave this abode, as Vyasa described.

Ayurvedic physician Charak (100 BC) advised that heavy foods like meats, too sweet and very spicy though delicious, should be eaten in a controlled manner especially by those who do not do more work while those doing heavy work have no such limit. Yogis should have light nutritious diet containing cereals, milk and fruits. He should have proper deep sleep (non-rapid eye movements type) uninterrupted by dreams while *ati-nidra* is an obstacle. Earlier days cooking used to be done in ghee which also is considered heavy with high calories now while spicy foods and some vegetable oil go together as restrictions. Low calorie oils are available like soya, sunflower, etc. but on the whole use of oil should be limited. Poverty does not permit eating high protein diet, both animal and the plant proteins are almost prohibitive cost wise, for enough Dal-roti or Dal-chaval. South Indian dish like idli-sambar is ideal diet. Dosa also can be made without using oil. Fruits are decidedly costly while green vegetables may be the only affordable item and even if eaten abundantly has no food value for survival with one-third of our population below poverty line. A therapist will have to be realistic while advising on foods.

Lastly we discuss stress. Since Hans Seyle published his findings on stress disorders. In British Medical Journal it invoked tremendous interest world over. He observed a trio of signs-inflammation of gastric mucosa, shrinkage of thymus gland and enlargement of adrenal cortex, to various stressful conditions. Such conditions included physical agents like painful electrical stimuli, psychological agents like fear, biological agents like injections of toxic substances, etc. but body response was the same. He named them as the stressors. He described General Adaptation Syndrome in three stages. First was stage of Resistance in which an animal had release of adrenaline in the system to counter effects of stress. Next, emerged Stage of Adaptation which necessitated animal to have adrenaline, as supplement. If stressor agent continued to act, animal had no resources to counteract and eventually animal succumbed to death. It must be noted that the word animal is used as Prof Seyle was Director of Experimental Medicine at University of Montreal. I happened to visit him and his office was spread as much as a secondary school lab.

He is described as a genius and use of hydrocortisones as anti-inflammatory agent is credited to his work. He introduced the term distress to signify pathological process though now stress is in connotation. An important term he used is *eustress* for stress as a challenge taken positively by the system as well as the persons stressed. I believe rehabilitation process itself is against stress physical, physiological and psychological. At times, patients themselves are motivated, sometimes they need to be. A therapist usually is good communicator. Stress should be diagnosed early since due to its widespread nature of signs and symptoms, its local manifestations are treated by different specialists but the generalized syndrome is missed. Psychologist's help also can be taken. It should be borne in mind that stress is a slow killer. It is considered as chronic non-communicable disease (NCD) and as in case of other its relation with diet is also recognized. Failing which, another stressor agent may be added.

As for Yoga, it is stress-combatant since neuro-enzymes in the system are present. Alike Yoga, positive stress is stimulating to deal/cope up with stress. Yoga is self-selected discipline towards positive changes if 'Dos and Don'ts' are followed in practice. Overdoing is cautioned but is ignored. An overdose does not bring recovery faster, rather is harmful. Warnings are displayed but not attended to. Thus, a fault is punishable, rule of Nature. Moving away from Nature is invitation to dysfunction and ill health. Stress affects multiple organs and systems. So multiple organs failure is common. Yoga also treats multiple systems; so for stress, Yoga is right antidote, but provided that stress is detected in time. Stage of resistance is the right point at which Yoga can be more effective. Here, I mean a full package of Yoga and not any singular procedure. Any procedure in Yoga has its own physiological and the therapeutic effects. But a package has much more to offer. Diabetes Mellitus is a metabolic disorder and while performing rocking movement in Dhanurasana local pressure on abdominal organs can be beneficial but it is not the full treatment. A person must be committed to observe protocol regarding food and nutrition. Yamas and Niyamas prepare one for observing self-discipline. It is so that body is like a pharmaceutical factory to produce necessary medicines. Yoga package gives impetus to the process.

Late Dr Madhav G Mokashi
PhD, DSc, Dip PT

NB: *This article is dedicated to (Late) Dr MG Mokashi as our tribute. Readers should note here that this text includes his own thoughts and perception about yoga as a science and its remedial application.*

Contributors

Akhoury Gourang Sinha
BPT, MSPT, PhD (Sports Medicine and Physiotherapy)
Dean Faculty of Medicine and
Professor, Department of Physiotherapy
Punjabi University, Patiala, Punjab, India

Amita Anil Mehta
MSc (PT) FAIMER Fellow
Prof and HOD School of Physiotherapy
Seth GS Medical College, Mumbai affiliated to Maharashtra University of Health Sciences (MUHS), guide for MPTh and PhD (MUHS)

Bharati Vijay Bellare
BSc (PT), PGCR, FIAP, PhD
Ex-Prof and HOD Physiotherapy
Lokmanya Tilak Municipal Medical College
Ex-Prof
MGM School of Physiotherapy
Navi Mumbai, Maharashtra, India

Bhavana Suhas Mhatre
MSc (PT) FAIMER Fellow
Associate Prof, School of Physiotherapy
Seth GS Medical College, Mumbai affiliated to Maharashtra University of Health Sciences (MUHS), guide for MPTh and PhD (MUHS)

Damodar Bachani
MBBS, MD, MPHM
Country Project Manager
Building Healthy Cities (India, Indonesia, Vietnam)
John Snow India Private Ltd, New Delhi
Ex-Deputy Commissioner (NCD)
Ministry of Health and Family Welfare, Government of India
Ex-Director Professor and HOD of Community Medicine
Lady Hardinge Medical College and Associated Hospitals, New Delhi
Ex-Director, Center for Environmental Health;
Public Health Foundation of India, Gurugram, Haryana, India

Lata Shroff Parmar
MSc (PT), PhD
Professor/Principal, College of Physiotherapy,
Sumandeep Vidyapeeth (Deemed University)
Vadodara, Gujarat, India

Mariya Prakash Jiandani
MSc (PT) FAIMER Fellow
Associate Prof, School of Physiotherapy
Seth GS Medical College, Mumbai affiliated to Maharashtra University of Health Sciences (MUHS), guide for MPTh and PhD (MUHS)

Megha Sandeep Sheth
BSc (PT), MPT (Rehab)
Lecturer
SBB College of Physiotherapy
Ahmedabad, Gujarat, India

Monal R Velangi
Clinical and Sports Nutritionist,
PhD Research Scholar, MS, CDE
Dietitian, KJ Somaiya Hospital and Research Centre
Consultant-Dietitian, KJ Somaiya Super Speciality Centre
Visiting Faculty, Nirmala Niketan College (Mumbai University), Maharashtra, India

N Venkatesh
PhD, FIAP
Professor and Course Chairman, Faculty of Physiotherapy
Sri Ramachandra University
Chennai, Tamil Nadu, India

Nalin Kumar
BPT, PGDT, MPH, Eunice Kennedy Shriver Fellowship (2008) Special Olympics International
State Consultant Maternal Health, National Health Mission, Jharkhand
Co-Founder, Synaptic Healthcare Solutions Pvt Ltd
Clinical Director, Special Olympics International (Fit Feet)

Neeta Jayprakash Vyas
BPT, PhD
Ex-Principal and Prof
SBB College of Physiotherapy
Ahmedabad, Gujarat, India

Odette M Gomes
Retired Prof and HOD Occupational Therapy
TN Medical College and BYL Nair Hospital
Mumbai, Maharashtra, India

Pavithra Rajan
BPT (India), MSc (Canada)
PhD Candidate in Physiotherapy, Faculty of Health Sciences, University of Sydney
NSW, Australia

Prakash Doke
MD, DNB, PhD, FIPHA
Professor, Dept of Community Medicine
Bharati Vidyapeeth University Medical College
Former Director of Health Services
Government of Maharashtra
Former Executive Director
State Health System Resource Center
Pune, Maharashtra, India

Sabir Shaikh
D Pharm Logistic Management Diploma in Yoga Therapy and Naturopathy MA in Yoga Shastra
Asst Prof in KJ Somaiya Bharatiya Sanskriti Peetham
Visiting Faculty in NACEN (National Academy of Customs, Excise, and Narcotics)
Mumbai, Maharashtra, India

Shailaja Sandeep Jaywant
MSc (OT) Assistant Professor
Dept of Occupational Therapy
Lokmanya Tilak Municipal Medical College and General Hospital
Mumbai, Maharashtra, India

Shubhangi Parker
DPM, MD, PGDHR, MSc, PhD
Professor and Head
Department of Psychiatry
Chief, Bombay Drug De-Addiction Center
Convener, MCI Nodal Centre
Ex DEAN In-charge
GS Medical College and KEM Hospital
Mumbai, Maharashtra, India

Unnati Nikhil Pandit
MPTh (CVR), PhD
Prof-Director, Dept of Physiotherapy
Padmashree Dr DY Patil university, Nerul, Navi Mumbai, Maharashtra, India

Preface

Philosophy of Physiotherapy: In last 50 years Physiotherapy profession has grown very fast to be recognized as an independent health profession. Unlike other health professions it deals with a ***Person with Pathology*** rather than dealing with Pathology of a person. The role of this profession came into limelight when WHO recognized that focusing on mortality alone is not adequate but the morbidity associated with pathology/injury is equally important from point of view of ***Quality of Life (QOL).*** Thus, when WHO classification got upgraded from ***'Medical' model*** [based on ***Mortality (ICD 10)***] to ***'Social' model*** [based on ***Morbidity:*** International Classification of Impairment, Disability and Handicaps (ICIDH)], it was established that 'If a ***doctor adds Years*** to the patient's ***life,*** the ***Physiotherapist adds Life*** to those ***years'.*** Thus, Physiotherapy has ***'Holistic' approach*** to care for a person in terms of his ***mind, body as well as spirit.***

Globally, in health care, the accepted and the most cost effective norm is ***Prevention is better than cure***. Therefore, in medical education, it has been observed that practically all the health related educational programs include a core subject on ***Community Health*** emphasizing the aspects of ***Primary Prevention and Health Promotion of Populations*** [for instance, Preventive and Social (Community) medicine, Preventive and Community Dentistry, Community Nursing to name a few]. Conventional medicine, at its postgraduate level, further adds one more specialty subject, namely, 'Physical Medicine and Rehabilitation' that unlike population health, deals with prevention of morbidity in established nonreversible disability or chronic health issues at ***individual*** level. This area of specialization involves the use of health care services for those individuals with ***established nonreversible and chronic disability*** at his/her home environment.

Physiotherapy profession emerged out of nursing profession for the same purpose to rehabilitate injured soldiers of First World War. The first Physiotherapy school was established in Washington DC after the outbreak of the war. This profession has grown by leaps and bounds to achieve the identity as an independent health profession but its scope in ***population*** related ***prevention*** remained dormant for a long time. In the recent past, the World Confederation for Physical Therapists (WCPT) has realized the importance of physiotherapy in preventive and community health, which has been emphasized in clinical practices as well as education, especially in the developed world. As opposed to this, in India, this area of specialization in Physiotherapy has not gained adequate recognition. It has been established through some research studies that this lack of recognition could be attributed to certain reasons like lack of awareness and motivation among students as well as Physiotherapists to pursue this specialization, lack of awareness among the communities about this profession and inadequate funding/incentives for program implementation. It comes as no surprise that ***Preventive and Community Physiotherapy*** is totally missing in the national health programs, despite proven benefits in the developed world, especially in the health care of mother and child, geriatric population, occupational health and lifestyle related non-communicable health issues like diabetes, hypertension, obesity, etc.

In the absence of the Central Council for Physiotherapy profession in India, the onus falls on the Physiotherapy educators to increase the awareness about this specialization and create a pool of skilled professionals who could promote this subject. Till the year 1996, the entry level Physiotherapy curriculum was highly diversified from 2 to 3 years diploma course to 3½ years degree course. Though the syllabus content still remains diversified to date, the Central Executive Committee (CEC-1996-98) of the Indian Association of Physiotherapists (IAP) recommended a 4½ years Bachelors degree (BPTh) program by adding two more core subjects, which are listed below and they are also elaborated in a chapter included in this book.

Functional Diagnosis

To fit within the philosophical domain of Physiotherapy, this paraclinical core subject was introduced to train the physiotherapist to 'diagnose' a given condition based on functional status of a person when WHO's classification of Health expanded from medical to social model. Concept of this subject is probably first of its kind in the international scenario of Physiotherapy and could help in first contact practice and establish Physiotherapy as an independent health profession.

Community Physiotherapy

This clinical core subject expanded the domain of prevention/health promotion in a wide range of ***healthy/vulnerable population*** (synchronous to Community medicine/Public health), 'Community based rehabilitation (CBR) of a ***disabled individual'*** (related to Physical Medicine and Rehabilitation). One more unique feature of this subject was that, the conventional term 'Community' was expanded by identifying various communities/subcommunities based on their ***'common risk factors'*** related to ***specific context*** such as—behavioral issues (sedentary lifestyle, stress, diet, substance abuse), age (pediatric and geriatric groups), industry (occupation related, including sports), gender (obstetrical and gynecological issues among women). Such expanded concept of 'community' broadened its domain from just ***outdoor locations*** to ***institutional population*** such as schools, mahila mandals, oldage homes, sports academies, etc.

Though IAP succeeded in establishing uniform duration of 4½ years for the Bachelors degree program in the country, it miserably failed in establishing uniform curriculum. Maharashtra University of Health Sciences (MUHS) was the first state health university to introduce both the subjects with correct concept in the year 1998. Few deemed universities of Maharashtra followed suit. However, in the last 19 years, the course on ***Functional Diagnosis*** has remained only in the Physiotherapy curriculum in the state of Maharashtra in spite of the fact that; in the year 2001, WHO identified the importance of documenting ***functional abilities in terms of capacity/performance*** and revised its classification from 'International Classification of Impairments, Activity limitations and Participation restrictions (ICIDH-II) to **'International Classification of Functioning, Disability and Health *(ICF)'*** and offered ***exclusive scope to physiotherapists to assess***/evaluate ***'functional abilities under prevailing contextual factors' and*** form ***'functional***

diagnosis'. It is high time that, this course gets its due recognition in the remaining parts of this country and surely proves to be a strong justification to demand for an independent Central Council for Physiotherapy professionals.

The course on ***'Physiotherapy in Community health'*** is still struggling to gain ground especially in certain part of the India. In certain universities across the country, it has been introduced with a modified nomenclature. For instance, a few universities in the state of Gujarat have named it as 'Rehabilitation/Community based Rehabilitation (CBR)', where the syllabus is limited to CBR of a disabled individual, when, in fact, the major component of this subject is designed to ***prevent disability***. The title 'Prevention Practice and Community Physiotherapy (PPCPT)' was therefore selected this textbook to highlight its scope directing towards an ***individual*** as well as ***specific population***. A chapter on 'Patient with Altered Consciousness' is included in this book which may appear offset to certain Physiotherapy professionals, but they should note that, manifestation of unconscious status is independent of its primary etiology (head injury, stroke, poisoning, etc). Moreover, in this status the patient is subjected to high-risk of developing bronchopneumonia which may not necessarily link with any primary respiratory etiology. Here the role of Physiotherapist in sustaining bronchial hygiene provides an evidence that domain of Physiotherapeutic preventive care is not limited to prevention of morbidity of a permanently disabled person, but has a much wider scope beginning right from ***saving patient's life.***

Formal education in Physiotherapy commenced way back in 1953 in this country. Still, to date, educators and students heavily refer to books published by foreign authors. India has produced some eminent Physiotherapists who have contributed tremendously for the growth of this profession via education and clinical practice. Despite this, very few senior physiotherapy educators in this country have disseminated their knowledge through textbooks/guides. Needless to say, there is a great paucity of textbooks available on the core subjects related to Physiotherapy in the Indian context.

As far as the role of Physiotherapy in prevention practice and community health is concerned, the case of India is unique, with huge cultural diversities and number of underserved communities. This poses a huge burden on the health care system, which struggles to treat the chronic health conditions that are escalating by the day. Given this distinctive scenario, the principles and solutions for these problems, as discussed by foreign authors in their books, might not be sufficient for planning cost effective community solutions to health problems in India. We (the editors) are therefore contemplating to publish this matchless book on prevention practice and community physiotherapy in an Indian context. One of the most important purposes of this publishing endeavor is to establish countrywide awareness about this neglected specialty.

In the global scenario today, attention is also focused on the non-communicable diseases (NCD) because of their highly adverse effect on the Quality of Life, nevertheless, effective preventive strategies can be applied in their management at all the four levels of 'Prevention, **i.e. Primordial, Primary, Secondary and Tertiary prevention** at the **population** as well as **individual** level. This ***theme of*** prevention is therefore incorporated in certain unique chapters of this book such as 'Developmental Health', 'Industrial Health', 'Health in Sports', 'Geriatric Care', 'Women's Health', 'Diabetic Footcare', 'Preventive Cardiology' and 'Hand Care' which cover all the four levels of prevention which will enable the students to understand selection of specific strategy at appropriate stage of the respective health issue.

The other exclusive feature of this book is that, many eminent Physiotherapy professionals, Occupational therapists and Medical experts in Public Health from all over the country and a Dietitian have contributed in this book. This was important since we aimed to create a holistic perspective about this specialization. Most of the contributors from Physiotherapy profession are holding PhD degree and/or are recognized PhD guides. Due to its national presence and diversity in approaches, this book caters to the needs of students from all over the country. In the recent past, many universities from abroad have tried to increase their collaborations with Physiotherapy departments across the country. This book could serve as a guide to anyone who wishes to understand the concepts of prevention practice and community physiotherapy, especially in an Indian context.

Yoga, 'the pride of Indian Philosophy and heritage' has established its recognition all over the world for sustaining/promoting physical, mental and spiritual health. However, the confusion persists all over between physical maneuvers of yogic practices and physical/breathing exercise. This book therefore includes two chapters on Yogic practices out of which, one chapter is exclusively devoted to elaborate on similarities as well as differences between the basic concepts and movement sciences related to Yogic practices (Asanas and Pranayama) and Exercise therapy (including breathing exercises).

Ideally, the only person who could have written a Foreword for this textbook, was none other than our beloved teacher Late Dr MG Mokashi—the main source of inspiration behind publishing this textbook. This is because, the concept of 'Preventive Community Physiotherapy' and 'Functional Diagnosis' is his brain child. He left for heavenly abode recently after putting up a fierce and prolonged fight against the deadly disease of cancer. Even during his rapidly collapsing health, he never stopped from encouraging us and guided as and when we felt the need during the proceedings of this publication. Unfortunately, he could not wait to witness the success of this endeavor; therefore we wish to dedicate this book to him as our tribute to this great man and the pioneer in introducing the concept of 'Functional Diagnosis' and 'Preventive Community Physiotherapy' in India.

We also wish to express our deep gratitude to have received his last creation—an article on 'Psychophilosophy of Yoga and its Remedial Value' which he wrote during his last days while bravely fighting with the excruciating pain of cancer.

We also express our deep gratitude to all the contributors, who graciously agreed to author this book just over a phone call. They are very busy a lot but have maintained high enthusiasm right from inception to completion.

We are positive that the success of this book will inspire many more Physiotherapy educators to join hands to disseminate knowledge through references and textbooks, which will not only help in the standardization of Physiotherapy education in India, but will also be acclaimed on an international level.

It has been published in two parts. The first one focuses on the basic understanding of the concept and applied sciences related to the same, while the other talks about clinical aspects of the subject. This book will also be available as an e-book'.

Bharati, Unnati and Pavithra (BHUPA)
Editorial Committee

Special Note

This publication intends to establish countrywide awareness about this novel clinical subject in Physical Therapy, hence includes National representation of multiple eminent authors which is first of its kind as far as Indian publication of any textbook on Physiotherapy is concerned. Therefore, this being a first trial, in order to obtain consent from the contributors to write a chapter in this book, the editorial committee did not impose any strict protocol on adhering to specific verbatim, style of writing and referencing but without compromising on the quality of content. Nevertheless, the authenticity and ownership of the content in the chapter shall be a complete responsibility of the respective contributor(s) and not the Editorial board.

Contents

PART I: INTRODUCTION

PART II: RESEARCH PERSPECTIVES AND PARADIGMS IN PHYSIOTHERAPY

PART III: BEHAVIORAL KEY COMPONENTS OF HEALTH AND WELLNESS

PART I

Introduction

1

Medical Perspective of Public Health

1.1 PUBLIC HEALTH IN INDIA

Prakash Doke

INTRODUCTION: DEFINITION AND CONCEPT

World Health Organization (WHO) has quite popularized the definition of health among medical and allied fraternity. But this ideal definition by many scientists is considered as individual based. As a community, we desire achievement of positive health by all members. Attempts towards improvement of health of all the members of the community by doctor consultation, compliance to advise given by a physician, etc. can only be theoretical way of achievement of this objective. For various obvious reasons such approach is never thought or practiced. It may require very long time and may not be feasible also. In history also there are not any countries or states which have exclusively resorted to this approach. On the other hand history is full of examples where contribution of other than medical system is acknowledged. In history although there were no precise measures of community health various countries at different times have witnessed huge differences in health of their citizens. Almost across the world such observations of disparity between health statuses of their constituent members have resulted socio-political and technical turmoil. The concept of public health has emerged in this manner.

Public health has been beautifully defined by Charles-Edward Amory Winslow as, 'the science and art of preventing disease, prolonging life and promoting health through the organized efforts and informed choices of society, organizations, public and private, communities and individuals.' The definition envisages a chain of continuum of objectives and assumes interlinking of prevention of diseases, prolonging life and promoting health. The best part of the definition is the advocated way of achievement. The only reason for such advocating is the realization of inevitability of executing joint efforts willingly for the achievement of the objective in true sense. The prolonging of life is not extension of life in critical care units in hospitals with life support systems. It expects increasing life expectancy. Public health is an applied science pooling disciplines like medicine, epidemiology, biostatistics, demography, social sciences together. Public health across the world is involved in some basic functions. The set basic functions include assessment of health status in the geographical area, developing guidelines for actions and assuring some provisions. The assessment includes periodical surveys, monitoring systems and linkages with subsystems and other systems. Assessment of risk factors forms integral part of health assessment in well-developed systems.

SOCIO-CULTURAL AND ECONOMIC INFLUENCE

The history of public health is full of examples illustrating the influence of socio-cultural factors on health. In London in sixteenth century there was tradition to publish Bills of Mortality on weekly basis mostly to know the deaths particularly due to plague. The first bill of mortality was probably published in 1532. This was not a regular feature. The difference between mortality among lower and higher socio-economic class was vividly explained after analysis of Bills in London. John Graunt's a small vendor of sewing articles became the first demographer after publishing his book 'Natural and Political Observations Made upon the Bills of Mortality (1662 Old Style or 1663 New Style)'. His attempt was towards creating a system of early warning for impending deaths due to plague. Sir Edwin Chadwick in 1842 published his report on, 'The Sanitary Condition of the Laboring Population'. This report generated local as well national movement which formed basis of and resulted in promulgation of the Public Health Act 1848 in United Kingdom. The Report clearly showed the correlation between the lack of sanitation and high morbidity, mortality and low life expectancy. Similar story happened in United States of America. Lemuel Shattuck an active person in civic affairs and turned into a book seller was appointed as Chair of Commission in Massachusetts. His Report of the Sanitary Commission of Massachusetts published in 1850 was a benchmark in public health. He described very lucidly the appalling status of sanitary conditions existing then. He also gave solid recommendations for improvements. Therefore he is called Architect of American Public Health. In last century, Thomas McKeown a British physician interested in history of medicine aggressively published his opinions from about 1955 to 1980. McKeown argued that the population growth of the United Kingdom post-1700 was due to economic conditions rather than improved medicine and public health.[1] This is popularly known as McKeown's thesis. Although vehemently opposed by medical fraternity, his contentions about role of socio-economic status in health and general improvement have been indirectly further expounded in another report. The Black report was a 1980 document published by the Department of Health and Social Security (now the Department of Health) in the United Kingdom. Sir Douglas Black was chairperson of the expert committee into health inequality. The report demonstrated that although overall health had improved since the introduction of the welfare state, there were widespread health inequalities, also found that the main cause of these inequalities was economic inequality. The report showed that the death rate for men in social class V was twice that for men in social class I and that gap between the two was increasing, not reducing as was anticipated.

In India the situation was more complex. Apart from socio-economic classes religion and casts also play major role. In NFHS 3 it was observed that among Jains 86.8% were from highest wealth quintile and only 1.6% were from lowest quintile. Whereas among scheduled tribes 5.2% were from highest wealth quintile and 49.96% were from lowest quintile.[2] Considering wealth quintile as proxy of socio-economic classes the class wise disparity in selected health indicators as given in Table 1.1.

The influencing factors may be internal or external. Study of the internal factors is almost exclusively domain of internal medicine. The external influencer can be grouped into physical and social environment. Evolution is a process of adoption to the physical environment. The influence is so powerful that in long run it modifies the genomic spectrum.

Table 1.1: Social disparity in health indicators, India

Wealth index	TFR	IMR	Institutional deliveries%	Anemia in women%
Lowest	3.89	64.8	12.7	64.3
Second	3.17	62.4	23.5	60.3
Middle	2.58	49.8	39.2	56.0
Fourth	2.24	46.2	57.9	52.2
Highest	1.78	27.4	83.7	46.1
Overall	2.68	41.5	38.7	56.2

TFR—Total fertility rate; IMR—Infant mortality rate

The broad term social includes cultural as well as the economical factors. Socio-economic factors are self-created by the community prescribing behaviors in day to day life. Their influences are equally strong to modify health status. The community is having different classes mostly as the product monetary consideration and religion including cast. Cultural factors are mostly generated from traditions in the religion and cast. But they are also influenced by geographic area where most common practices may percolate to other classes. The traditions affect the way of understanding and response to the problem. These factors affect understanding of signs and symptoms of the diseases and relating them some intuitive etiology. Accordingly the responses are based on such understanding. Thus they influence utilization of available health services. The influence on day to day life even may generate health problems. All the traditions are surely not harmful. Leisurely walking after dinner, washing hand and feet returning home and massage with oil to neonates, breastfeeding for one to year's are well acknowledged in modern medicine. Refraining eating papaya, eggs in pregnancy is very common practice which needs discouragement. Cultural practices also affect health seeking behavior. In all types of research the minimum age, sex and socio-economic status are the confoundable variables which are always considered.

Public health is solely function of economic system. There is always a competition among social sectors to grab largest pie in the financial allocation. In spite of recommendation of increasing health budget in national health policy, National Rural Health Mission (NHM) there is hardly any change. In Government budget social and community services are given code 'B' under revenue expenditure. As the investment in health sector does not generate any revenue, allocation to health is always comprised. About 1% GDP is allocated to public health sector. The overall health expenditure is about 4 to 5% of GDP and contribution of public sector is 20 to 25%.

Need for Public Health Response

The understanding and the redressal mechanisms for improvement in health status are really diverse. Moreover they may not be limited to health department. Apart from health system in the form resources, determinants of health include food supply, safe water supply and sanitation, air pollution. The obvious reflections are high morbidity and mortality due to gastroenteritis and subsequent dehydration due to consumption of contaminated water. Another set of vector borne disease like malaria and dengue are entirely due to mismanagement of stored/accumulated/stagnated collected water bodies. These problems are tackled through public health engineering. In 1972–73 Government of India initiated Accelerated Rural Water Supply Program (ARWSP) to improve the quantity and quality of drinking water supply. Later it was renamed National Drinking Water Mission (NDWM) in 1986. Lastly in 1991, it was again renamed after late Prime Minister of India as Rajiv Gandhi National Drinking Water Mission (RGNDWM). Almost all the states have water and sanitation departments. Safe water supply with widespread use of oral rehydration solution (ORS) has pushed the rank of diarrheal diseases to third or fourth position. Asthma and chronic obstructive pulmonary diseases (COPD) are emerging as leading cause of morbidity and mortality. These problems and solutions are beyond the scope of individualized curative medicine. The two main areas which need actions for overall betterment in health are behavioral communication and demand generation. Demand generation even compels government to device means and strategies for better behavioral communication. Persuasion from committed people directly or through courts sometimes has compelled government to enact health related Acts. Emerging chronic diseases and their complications directly affect productivity. The cost of treatment is very high and in most of the diseases the duration of treatment is long, may be lifelong. Many chronic diseases and their complications can be preventable through public health approach.

DEVELOPMENT OF HEALTH SYSTEM

Health sector planning is an integral part of social-economic development plan in all countries. In India the health sector planning has received inputs from various committees.

Bhore Committee

The first committee at the time of independence was named as, 'Health Survey and Development Committee'. The committee was appointed by Government under chairmanship of Sir Joseph Bhore in 1943. The report was submitted in January 1946. The report runs in to four volumes.[3]

Observations of the Committee

The health status of the community was poor and is reflected in following indicators are as follows:

- Crude death rate 22.4/1000
- IMR 162/1000 live births
- MMR 20/1000 live births
- Life expectancy 27 years

The committee also observed that many of the health problems were preventable. The committee opined that investment in prevention would give high returns, in the form of increased productivity and development. The committee stated that health and development are interdependent. An improvement in the related sectors other than health will certainly lead to improvement in health. The sectors recommended for indirect improvement in health were as follows—housing, communication, water supply, sanitation, improvement in nutrition, elimination of unemployment, improvement in agriculture, industrial production.

Recommendations

- Integration of and curative services at all administrative levels
- Major changes in medical curriculum including 3 months training in preventive and social medicine to prepare social physicians
- Development of health institutions
- Recommended area approach establishing basic health unit as close to the people as possible providing comprehensive services
- Long-term plan
  - First tier—75 bedded Primary Health Unit for 10,000–20,000 population, 6 medical officers, 6 public health nurses, 2 sanitary inspectors, 2 health assistants and other support staff
  - Second tier—550 bedded Regional Hospital Unit, to serve referral center for 30–40 PHUs
  - Third tier—2500 bedded District Health Unit to serve about 3 million population
  - Good communication system between PHU, RHU and DHU.
- Short-term plan
  - To be implemented in 5–10 years
  - Establishment of PHCs for a population of 40,000.

Primary Health Unit was expected to provide preventive, curative and rehabilitative services. The recommended staff for PHU was; 2 medical officers, 2 sanitary inspectors, 5 nurses, 4 midwives and some support staff. It is an important landmark in public health in India. The recommendations initiated concept of integrated development and also comprehensive medicine. Although not implemented, the present three tiers pattern of PHC, RH and DH is based on the recommendations.

Primary Health Care

The next landmark was covenant by many countries including India about Health for All. This theme was based on an international conference at Alma Atta in erstwhile Russia. The consensus was resorting to Primary Health Care approach for seeing objective of Health for All. A working group was formed by Planning Commission in 1980 appointing Secretary Health as chairman to set goals and objectives. The working group fairly evolved specific indices and targets to be achieved in the country by 2000 AD.

National Health Mission

Government of India after thorough assessment of health status in 2005 accepted 'mission mode' as redressal mechanism and launched National Rural Health Mission. In 12th plan it was subsumed in National Health Mission. All the national programs are brought under one umbrella. Substantial weightage is given to management. Funds are enhanced and deposited directly in the accounts of state level society. Adequate emphasis has been given to quality aspects by evolving Indian Public Health Standards for different types of health care institutions. Most importantly many systems like Accredited Social Health Activist (ASHA), Village Health Nutrition and Sanitation Committees, Rugna Kalyan Samittees etc. have been initiated. Bottom to top approach for planning incorporating some flexibility is established now. NHM gives special focus on reproductive and child health. Accordingly many new initiatives like Janani Suraksha Yojana (JSY), Janani Shishu Suraksha Karyakram (JSSK), Rashtriya Bal Suraksha Karyakram (RBSK) have been started.

Policies and Strategies

The constitution had given directive principles, health is a state subject. After 73rd and 74th amendment decentralization and power transfer to local self-governments has taken place remarkably. Government of India can give guidelines particularly about the implementation of national health programs. India responds to most of the international calls particularly from WHO and UNICEF while framing policies and strategies. In all the states the services are almost free and almost to all. Even if the charges are there, they are grossly subsidized. There is nominal fees for registration, investigations, etc. Generally patients needing services under national health programs including Reproductive and Child Health (RCH) services are not charged. Maximum weightage is given to primary health care services through public sector. First National Health Policy was evolved in 1983. Next National Health Policy was framed in 2002 and third policy is in draft stage. Government has sought comments from public on the draft health policy. Some goals were set in NHP 2002 and infrastructure development and increase in budget was envisaged.[4] In the same year National Policy on Indian Systems of Medicine and Homoeopathy (ISM&H) was also pronounced. Even before advent of NHM government always supported Non-Government Organizations (NGOs). All the policy documents mention involvement of NGOs. The most favorite areas for NGOs are family planning, leprosy and HIV/AIDS. Generally these policy documents clear guidelines of infrastructure development in rural areas. Hence in rural areas across the country there is uniformity in institutions.

Table 1.2: Norms for health care institutions in rural area

S. No.	Institution	Population norms	
		Plain area	Hilly/tribal/ difficult area
1	Sub center	5,000	3,000
2	Primary health center	30,000	20,000
3	Community health center	1,20,000	80,000

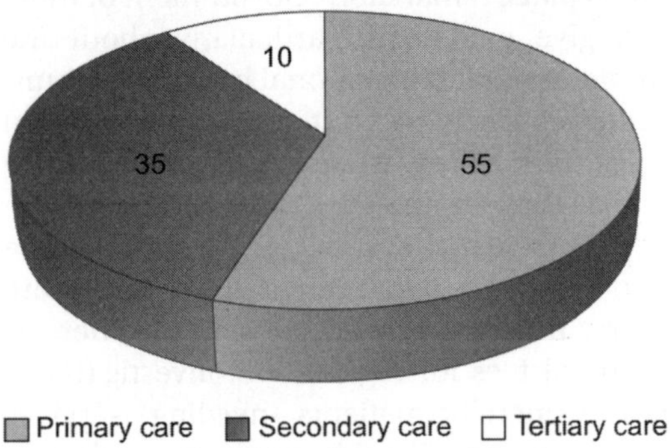

Fig. 1.1: Recommended budget allocation (%)

Urban area has been only considered seriously in 12th Plan. In 12th Plan concept of Universal Health Coverage has been extensively deliberated. It is recommended that states may start Universal Health Coverage first as project in limited geographical areas and then extend gradually. The recommended norms for establishing institutions are given in Table 1.2.

The budget for various levels of care recommended by NHP is shown in Figure 1.1. The policy also recommended that share of health department should be 8% of total budget. Most of the states lag far behind. It also recommends that central share in public health expenditure should be around 25%.

Private sector is strong in India and there no strict regulations for monitoring the performance or fees structure. Clinical Establishment Act 2010 has invoked only by nine states/union territories. Similarly National Pharmaceutical Pricing Authority time to times issues Drug Price Control Orders (DPCO) under Essential Commodities Act, 1955, announcing maximum price for selected essential and lifesaving medicines. However the resources with Food and Drug Administration limit the effective implementation of the orders.

The epidemiological transition has compelled government to divert attention towards non-communicable diseases and conditions. National Program for Prevention and Control of Cancer, Diabetes, Cardiovascular Diseases and Stroke (NPCDCS) in 2010–11.

The decisions to formulate policies, strategies are taken at highest level in Delhi or state capitals. The Central Council of Health and Family Welfare is the apex body consisting of Union Health Minister and Health Ministers from all the states with their secretaries. The council meets once in two years to formulate policies and strategies. Generally heterogeneous group consisting of people's representatives, administrators and senior technical experts evolve and shape the policies. The dissemination is executed in the form of resolutions, orders or gazettes from the Government. Generally vulnerable sections find some place in these guidelines.

Organization

India is a federation of 29 states and 7 territories. States are largely functioning independently usually following guidelines given by central government. There are multiple systems of medicine apart from modern medicine which is generally termed as Allopathy. The parallel systems under National Health Mission are grouped under AYUSH (Ayurveda, Yoga, Unani, Siddha, and Homeopathy). India has mix health system private and public.

Health and Family Welfare ministry has separate wings for Family Welfare, Health Services, National AIDS Control division and National Health Mission. There is separate department for AYUSH and Medical Research. Cabinet and State Ministers are

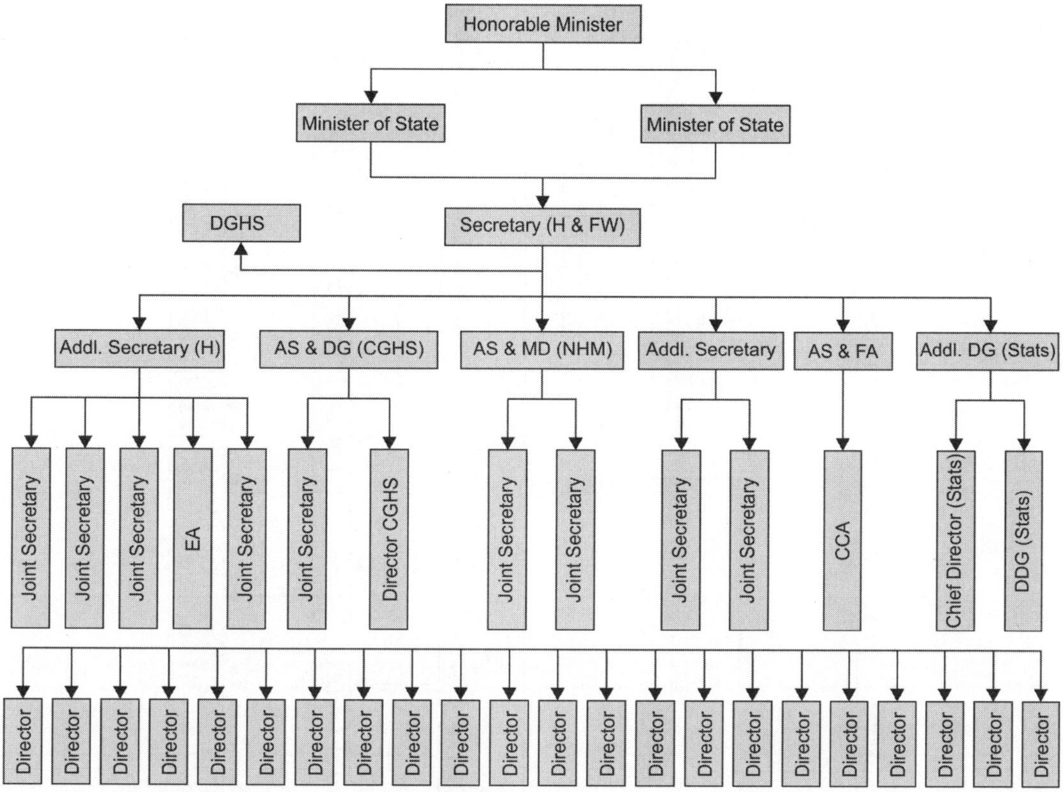

Fig. 1.2: Organogram of Health and Family Welfare Ministry, Government of India

DGHS—Directorate General of Health Services; CGHS—Central Government Health Scheme; H and FW—Health and Family Welfare; NHM—National Rural Health Mission; EA—Economic Advisor; CCA—Chief Controller of Accounts; DDG—Deputy Director General

Source: Adopted from website of Ministry of Health and Family Welfare, Government of India

elected representatives from some political parties. The secretary and his administrative colleagues are from Indian Administrative Services. Directorate General is the executive technical wing headed by senior technical person but not necessarily from Public Health. Food Drug Administration is theoretically under Directorate General of Health Services. The organogram of ministry is given in Figure 1.2. The organogram of Directorate General of Health Services pertaining to technical wing is given in Figures 1.3 and 1.4. The Directorate General of Health Services also supervises various national programs. Each program usually is headed by an officer of the rank of Deputy Directorate General of Health Services. Similar arrangement exists in state governments. In most of the states medical education and health services are different departments which may be headed by one minister or two different ministers. In some states the in-charge of is called as Director of Health Services and in some states Director General of Health Services. In states like Gujarat, Madhya Pradesh Director is replaced by Commissioner, an administrative officer.

As per the norms for health care institutions are spread over in all the states. The subcenter is the most peripheral public sector institution manned by one female and male health worker. The female health worker Auxiliary Nurse Midwife (ANM) is trained in midwifery to enable her to conduct

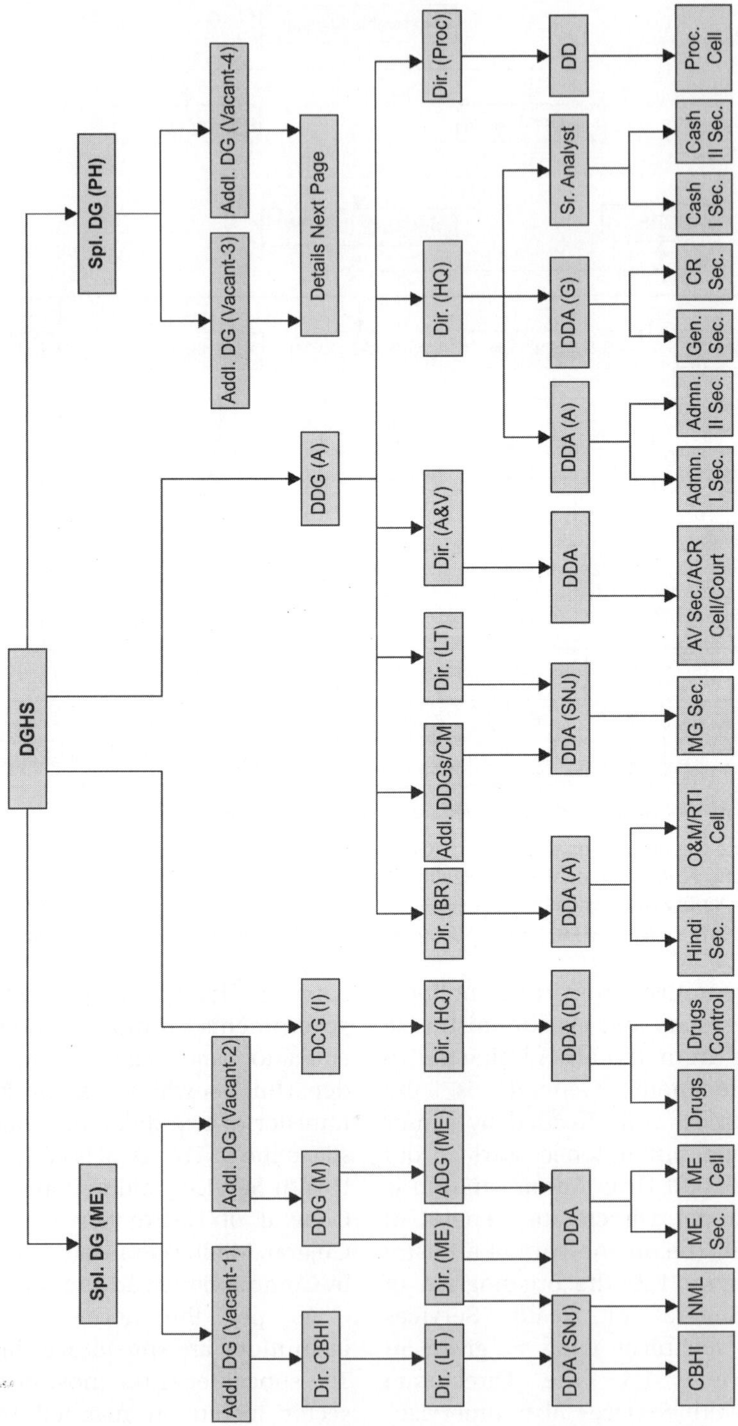

Fig. 1.3: Organization chart of Directorate General of Health Services (Technical Matters)

Source: Adopted from website of Ministry of Health and Family Welfare, Government of India

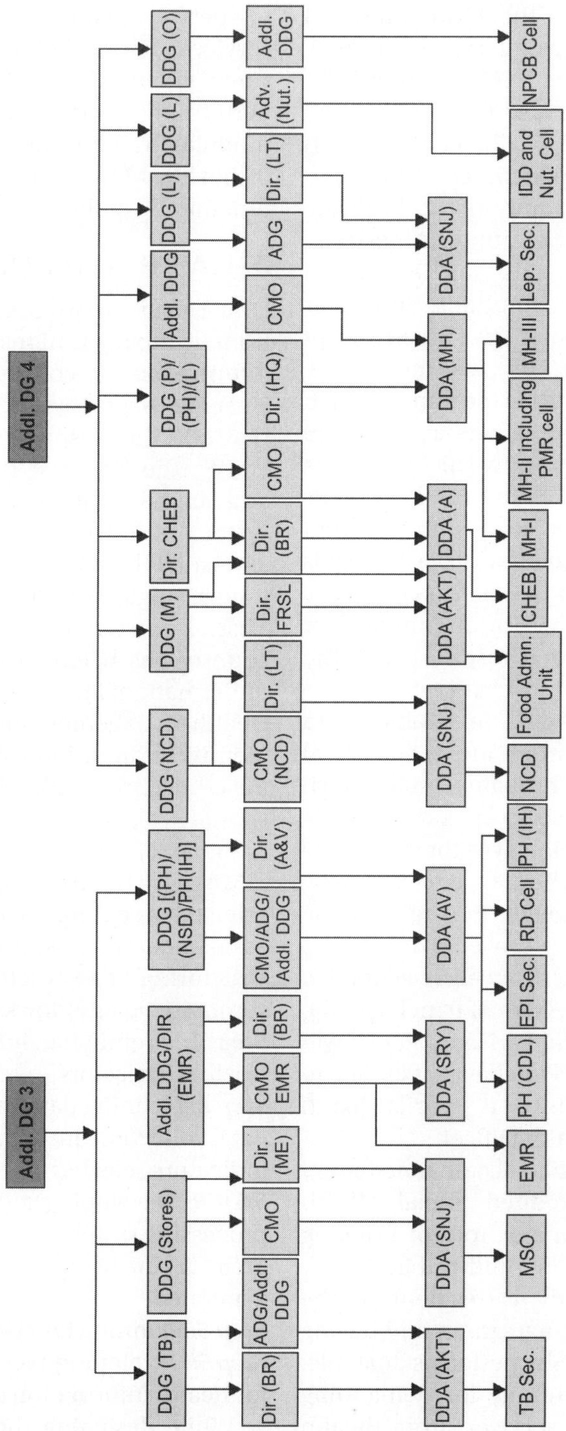

Fig. 1.4: Organization chart of Directorate General of Health Services (Technical Matters)

Source: Adopted from website of Ministry of Health and Family Welfare, Government of India

deliveries in subcenter. The ANM is the real backbone of public sector services. In many subcenters after advent of NHM second ANM on contractual basis is also functioning. The next level is primary health center which manned by about 15 personnel and headed by a medical officer. Some medical officers are from AYUSH background. Almost all primary health care needs can be satisfied in these two types of institutions. Subcenter and primary health center have area concept in their development; the institutions are responsible for the health of the population in the designated area. The secondary level care is partly given by Community Health Centers and District Hospitals. Some rural hospitals considering the work load and location have been upgraded to subdistrict hospitals where the number of specialists increases from three to five/eight. The minimum bed strength in district general hospital is 200. The civil surgeon is overall in-charge of curative and administrative field. In Maharashtra community health centers are called Rural Hospitals and are brought under civil surgeon. Specialists' services are available in these institutions. However there is acute shortage of specialists. Tertiary care is usually offered by medical colleges. In rural area the District Health Officer is overall in-charge. The Panchayat Raj System is well developed in rural area. Three tier system of Panchayat Raj exits in the form of Zilla Parishad, Panchayat Sammitte and Gram Panchayat. Parallel to this system in health, there is District Health Officer and Taluka Health Officer.

Although not a public sector functionary in each village Accredited Social Health Activists are playing major role of bridging gap between community and public health functionaries. The lady is resident of the village in reproductive age group and having schooling completed. She performs dual role. She is with the community for demanding regular and quality services from health personnel. She is with health personnel to peruse people to seek the available services. She is voluntary worker but gets some financial benefits based upon her performance. After selection ASHAs receive modular training for seven different aspect of health. More than nine lakhs ASHAs are functioning in the country.

HEALTH INFORMATION SYSTEM

Direct health information in details is available from health institutions. A large chunk of that information is collected through Health/Hospital Management Information System (HMIS). The hospitals also have their own HMIS. The National Programs were having and still have their own management health system and which still continue. Now as almost all the national programs are brought under single umbrella of National Health Mission since 2005 a unified HMIS across the country has been started. All the programs under national health mission are covered in Health Management Information System. The identification of indicators for monitoring is the crucial stage. Like objective the indicators should also be Specific, Measurable, Assignable, Realistic and Time-bound (SMART). Usually quantitative indictors are selected excepting exist interviews for quality assessment in hospitals. Steps involved in structuring or restructuring of HMIS can be summarized as follows:

Step 1: Identifying information needs and feasible indicators

Step 2: Defining data sources and developing data collection instruments for each of the indicators selected

Step 3: Developing a data transmission and processing system

Step 4: Ensuring use of the information generated

Step 5: Planning for HMIS resources

Step 6: Developing a set of organizational rules for health information system management.

While designing the HMIS some quality checks including validity are incorporated.

The NHM present HMIS has 30 validity rules while monthly data are being entered.[5] Any values of indicator X which cannot have value more than Y indicator is not accepted. For each indicator as validity measure outlier figures are also confirmed. HMIS monitors 255 indicators and many attributes from 17 major groups. Presently district wise information is available on the website of National Health Mission.[5] Most of the hospitals both from public and private sector also have their own HMIS. Hospital generally requires slightly different information like Bed Occupancy Rate, Bed Turnover Rate, Average Length of Stay, Mortality, Turn-Around Time for Investigations, Down Time for Critical Equipment's, mortality rates, stocks of material supplies, financial indicators, etc.

Civil Registration System[6]

Apart from HMIS health related data is also generated through non-institutional sources. Some of the systems are briefly described here. Statistics about birth and deaths is collected by Registrar General Government of India. Although registration of births and deaths is mandatory under Registration of Births and Deaths Act 1969, the actual registration is far from satisfactory. This continuous system of registration of births and deaths is called Civil Registration System. Latest level of birth registration in year 2013 is about 85.6%, and death registration about 70.9% (Office of the Registrar General). Over and above this most of the countries conduct National Level Health Surveys. Surveys with specific objectives like measuring incidence of tuberculosis are intermittently conducted. In India following surveys and systems collect health pertaining information regularly conducted.

Sample Registration System[6]

Although birth and death are vital events in the community the registration is not hundred percent. In many states it is even less than 75%. Therefore Office of Registrar General, India, in 1964–65 started a system of collecting information on births and deaths through samples on pilot basis. Encouraged by the results the Sample Registration System (SRS) was extended across the country in 1969–70. The system has two phases; in first phase a part time enumerator collects information about births and deaths in the sampled units. Then a full time supervisor independently and six monthly confirms the events. The discrepancy if any is verified. Since 2014 a total of 8,861 are covered under the scheme. The details are given in Table 1.3. The statistics generated through SRS is considered the most valid information about vital events in India hence it is extensively used in planning and research.

Table 1.3: Number of sample units under Sample Registration System

Residence	2014
Rural	4964
Urban	3897
Total	8861

National Family Health Survey[2]

In the absence reliable data about population health indicators, in most of the countries National Level surveys are conducted to generate the desired information. In India it named as National Family Health Survey (NFHS). It is a multi-round survey conducted across the country in a representative sample of households. For conduction of NFHS International Institute for Population Sciences (IIPS) is the nodal agency. NFHS receives financial support from international agencies. The first National Family Health Survey (NFHS-1) was conducted in 1992–93. The second was conducted in 1998–99 in 26 states of India. The third round was carried out in 2005–06 in 29 states. Fourth National Family Health Survey (NFHS-4) was recently carried out in 2014–15. The fourth round in addition to the 29 states included all six union territories for the first time. The most important feature is that it providing estimates of most indicators at the district level.

District Level Household Survey[7]

These surveys collect slightly different information then NFHS. The only difference was this system was giving district wise information. The first survey in this series was carried out in 1998–99. This was the only reliably valid data in public domain at district level. In addition the survey included assessment of public health institutions. In fact it is named as District Level Household and Facility Survey. The fourth round was conducted in 2012–13.

Annual Health Survey[6]

Annual Health Surveys have been started by Government of India 284 districts in nine states (eight Empowered Action Group and Assam). The single most reason for selection of these states was the extent of scope. These states have about 50% of India's population and have high birth and death rates. Reliable information for district level was not available. Total population covered is 1.82 crore constituting 36 lakhs households. The mean households covered per district are about 13 thousands. There are 20,694 sampling units; villages in rural areas and census enumeration blocks in urban areas.

Medically Certified Cause of Death (MCCD)[6]

The health care institutions are giving death certificate to relatives of deceased persons with mention of cause of death. Similarly even if the death occurs in home, the physician attending to the deceased fills the requisite form. A copy of the certificate is submitted to the Local Registrar of Birth and Deaths. This is in accordance with Registration of Birth and Death Act 1969. The statistics generated is of good quality as it is filled by a qualified doctor. But the compliance was not satisfactory. Only about 20% of reported deaths appear in the system. Hence from year 2014 submission of reports has been made mandatory to all health care institutions including from private sector. The sole purpose is generating statistics as per International Classification of Diseases, so that the data becomes comparable.

COMMUNITY ACTION

Some communitization mechanisms have been mentioned in National Health Mission. Community action has been built on two pillar concepts; people have right to health and health is significantly affected by social determinants. It is always envisaged that the people and communities will be active involved in the achievement of health. Community actions improve the access and quality of health services. The process passes through tackling social determinants of health. Nationally and internationally many women group are active particularly about Reproductive and Sexual Health and Rights. The pilot project of Community Based Monitoring which was launched in initial phase of NHM is well established now. This ambitious project was launched in 2007. This is a very large project implemented nine states (Assam, Chhattisgarh, Jharkhand, Karnataka, Madhya Pradesh, Maharashtra, Odisha, Rajasthan and Tamil Nadu). In each state three to five districts are selected. The project is implemented by state level non-NGOs with the help of field level NGOs. The CBM is built on NHM structures like Village Health Sanitation Nutrition Committees and Rogi Kalyan Samiti (RKS), and having one or few representatives from the concerned NGOs. The NGOs have frequent dialogues including *Jan Sunwai* with health care system. They monitor and prepare report card for functioning of Primary Health Center. Presently CBM is covering 25 states.

NGOs like Centre for Enquiry into Health and Allied Themes (CEHAT), Mahila

Sarvangeen Utkarsh Mandal (MASUM) and Dr Sabu George working in gender equality issues were worried by the declining child sex ratio in India and particularly in Maharashtra. They filed one Public Interest Litigation (PIL) in Supreme Court and thus were instrumental in finalizing the amendments in the Pre-Conception and Pre-Natal Diagnostic Techniques (PCPNDT) Act. Similarly responding to another PIL by Ramadan Ray in an order Supreme Court directed Government of India to frame insurance scheme for unfortunate fatalities during or after sterilization operations and improve quality of services by way of formulating guidelines about operating procedures and quality assurance committees.

HEALTH RESEARCH AND TECHNOLOGY

Health and medical field have not only very vast scope but also experience fast expansion. Indian Council of Medical Research (ICMR) is the apex body for conducting and encouraging health/medical research in India. It had its roots in the erstwhile Indian Research Fund Association (IRFA) established in 1911. After independence in 1949 it was renamed as ICMR. The Government of India envisages role of coordinating and funding medical research in the country. It is headed by Director General and many scientists of different cadres. The post of Director General ICMR has been upgraded to secretary health research. It has institutions working dedicated towards important aspects in health research. National Institute of Virology, National AIDS Research Institute, National Institute of Malaria Research, National Institute of Nutrition, etc. are cherished internationally. ICMR offers grants to research proposals from individuals as well as institutions. Under graduate as well postgraduate students are also given grants for small projects under Short Term Research Studentship program and thesis support scheme. The focus areas include use of biotechnology, genetics, etc. Recently Department of Health Research (DHR) has been established under ICMR exclusively to promote health care or services. Health system research has been identified as one the priority areas. It has many collaborative projects with international institutions conducting research. The thrust areas are listed here:

1. Communicable Diseases
2. Tribal Health
3. Reproductive and Child Health
4. Nutrition
5. Non-Communicable Diseases
6. Basic Medical Sciences
7. Traditional Medicine

Ethical Issues

The horrible stories of torture under the disguise of research after Second World War and then the Tuskegee syphilis experiment in USA were highly criticized across the globe. As humanly response various codes of conduct of medical research have been formulated. The first was Nuremberg Code consisting of ten points. The Belmont report is a classical document guiding ethical issues. The report lucidly deliberates on three principles—respect for persons, beneficence and justice. In India also ICMR has issued guidelines for conducting biomedical research. The basic principles remain the same. In Ethical guidelines for Biomedical Research on Human Participants published in 2006 following twelve principles have been described.[8]

1. Principles of essentiality
2. Principles of voluntariness, informed consent and community agreement
3. Principles of non-exploitation
4. Principles of privacy and confidentiality
5. Principles of precaution and risk minimization
6. Principles of professional competence
7. Principles of accountability and transparency

8. Principles of the maximization of the public interest and of distributive justice
9. Principles of institutional arrangements
10. Principles of public domain
11. Principles of totality of responsibility
12. Principles of compliance

ICMR as well as Central Drugs Standard Control Organization have given guidelines about ethics committee. Registration of all ethics committee is mandatory from 8th February 2013.[9] Similarly all clinical trials must be registered. This decision was necessary to avoid about 500 deaths each year due to clinical trials.[10]

IDENTIFICATION OF ISSUE

Past experiences and literature exploration adequately define and describe the health problems in the community. But the usual systems of collecting health data like HMIS may not provide in depth information. In such circumstances larger surveys are planned and conducted. Many projects resort to surveys to study the desired variables. The national level surveys are described in brief above. Although health indicators like IMR, MMR are declining there is wide statewise gap and many states have unacceptably high rates. Even within the states generally tribal areas, slum population, the indicators are unfavorable. Malnutrition among children and anemia among women particularly pregnant women is about 50% and there are no signs of any decline. Diseases like pneumonia and diarrhea continue to take their toll in child population. Non communicable diseases like coronary artery disease, cerebrovascular stroke, depression, cancer, chronic obstructive pulmonary disease/asthma, etc. are increasing rapidly. The cost of treatment is increasing and many families find it difficult to afford medical care particularly in private sector which is poorly regularized. The total fertility is still high in Empowered Action Group (EAG) states adding to total population. In the total population of India geriatric population is increasing and child sex ration is declining. There is acute shortage of trained manpower and other resources including required budgetary provision.

Modes of Survey

Survey is non-interventional method of collecting detailed information which in generally not easily available from a comparatively larger population. While conducting survey the selection of the individual subjects from the population is a critical issue and standard statistical methods and formulas are used for estimation of sample size. Most of the surveys are observational and sometimes analytical. Census which is carried out every ten years is probably largest face to face carried out survey. Paper and Pencil Interviews (PAPI) is speedily decreasing and Computer Assisted Personal Interviews (CAPI) or Tablet Assisted Personal Interviews are in vogue. These methods avoid use of paper, time-saving and easier for analysis. The way of interaction has changed and has been made easy but the art of preparing questionnaire still requires thorough homework. In the context of literacy and willingness to participate schedule is used more frequently than questionnaire which expects people to fill the proforma. Both schedule and questionnaire may be structured (in a sequence) or unstructured and the responses may be close ended (designed choices) or open ended.[11] For yield of standard scientific information the planning and implementation of the survey must rigorously follow the necessary steps. The survey instrument is usually tested for different types of validities. Whenever more than one person is involved inter-observer as intra-observer reliability needs to be minimized. Apart from face to face interviews telephone and web interviews are also in vogue; each method has its advantages and disadvantages.[12]

Planning and Implementation

All the information generate through census, HMIS, all types of national level surveys, estimates from national and international agencies is assessed and made use directly or indirectly in national level planning. In India Five Year Planning has been accepted as the major system to bring change. Presently 12th plan is in operation. Plan document deliberate existing situation, review last plan's performance and decide national level goals and objectives. In January 2015 Planning Commission was dissolved and National Institute for Transformation of India (NITI) Aayog was established. Prime Minister is Chairman of NITY Aayog. Apart from elected representatives subject experts are members of NITY Aayog. Health sector along with education is grouped under social sector. The states have Planning Boards which work with close liaison with planning department. The chairperson is Chief Minister and Executive Chairperson is political appointment. The state boards were formed in 1972 and reconstituted in 1995. District Planning District Planning Committees (DPC) constituted as per article 243 ZD of 74th Amendment of the Constitution. The District Planning Committee consolidates the plans prepared by the Panchayats and the Municipalities in the district and prepares a draft development plan for the district as a whole. The total number of members is proportionate to population but 4/5 are elected members. The planning as well implementation under NHM has been shifted to District Level Society.

Education and Training

Medical and allied sciences education is governed by constitutional bodies. For medical education there is Medical Council of India. Central Council for Indian Medicine governs systems like Ayurveda, Unani, Sidha and Sowa Rigpa. Homeopathy has a separate council. For dental education Dental Council of India takes the leading role. Similarly nursing education is governed by Indian Nursing Council. There is no separate council for physiotherapy and occupational therapy and professional associations develop guidelines and generally they are accepted. These are autonomous bodies. The members mostly elected persons and few are nominated. The President is elected among members. The foremost objective is to maintain consistently acceptable quality of medical education for postgraduate as well as undergraduate. It includes curriculum, manpower, infrastructure and the existence is confirmed by inspections; then only recognition is awarded to institution and qualification. The regulations are stringent but lately the role of MCI has become controversial due to alleged malpractices by the body. Similar objectives and systems have laid down for other councils.

Postgraduation in Public Health or Community Medicine is available in most of the medical colleges. Education in Public Health has percolated from doctors to non-doctors particularly from other systems of medicine and biological sciences. One of the reasons is students are more attracted to clinical specialties and later superspecialties. The earnings from these branches far exceed than public health in private sector. Some states including Maharashtra, Tamil Nadu, etc. have public health cadre; in these states public health specialties are preferred for senior administrative post. There are many institutions imparting education in public health like All India Institute of Health and Hygiene, Kolkata, National Institute of Health and Family Welfare (NIHFW), Delhi, etc. Public Health Foundation of India, Indian Institute of Health Management and Research, Jaipur, Tata Institute of Social Sciences, Shree Chitra Tirunal Institute of Medical Sciences, etc. offer public health qualifications which are not under the purview of MCI. All these institutions are also carrying out short-term trainings. NIHFW is the apex institute in public sector for conducting tailor-made training courses for government of officers. On similar lines most of the states have State Health and Family Welfare Training Centers. At regional levels they are named as Health and Family Welfare Training Centers (HFWTC). HFWTC mostly train medical officers, senior paramedicals and also conduct basic training courses for male multi-purpose workers. In most of the states there are District Training Centers and District Training Teams which conduct routine training for male and female health workers.

REFERENCES

1. Colgrove J. The McKeown Thesis: A Historical Controversy and Its Enduring Influence. Am J Public Health. 2002;92(5):725-9.
2. International Institute of Population Sciences (IIPS) and Macro International. National Family Health Survey (NFHS -3), 2005-06: India: Volume I. 2007 Mumbai IIPS.
3. Report of the health survey and development committee. Published by the Manager of Publications, Delhi, 1945.
4. Ministry of Health and Family Welfare, Government of India. National Health Policy, 2002.
5. Ministry of Health and Family Welfare, Government of India. Health Management Information System. Available at; https://nrhm-mis.nic.in/SitePages/Home.aspx. Accessed on 16 April 2016.
6. Office of the Registrar General Government and Census Commissioner, India. Available at: http://censusindia.gov.in/. Accessed on 16 April 2016.
7. International Institute of Population Sciences. District Level Household Surveys.
8. Indian Council of Medical Research. Ethical guidelines for Biomedical Research on Human Participants. 2006.
9. Ministry of Health and Family Welfare (Department of Health), Notification. GSR 72(E). 8th February 2013.
10. Aarti Dhar. Registration of Ethics Committee to approve clinical trails made mandatory now. The Hindu. New Delhi February 21, 2013.
11. Epidemiology and Management for Health. Sathe PV and Doke PP. Fourth Edition. 2014. Vora Medical Publishers, Mumbai.
12. Phellas NC, Bloch A and Seale C. Structured Methods: Interviews, Questionnaires and Observation. In; researching society and culture. 3rd edition. Editor; Seale C. 2012 Sage Publications Ltd., London ECIY ISP.

1.2 MAGNITUDE, PREVENTION AND CONTROL OF NON-COMMUNICABLE DISEASES IN INDIA

Damodar Bachani

GLOBAL SCENARIO

Globally, 14.2 million people die prematurely every year from non-communicable diseases (NCDs) between 30 and 69 years of age. About 86% of these premature deaths from NCDs occur in developing countries. Deaths due to communicable diseases, maternal, perinatal conditions and nutritional deficiencies accounted for 27.2% of all deaths in 2008 (Table 1.1). It is projected that in the year 2030, this proportion would shrink to just 13.8%. NCDs on the other hand would rise from 63.2 to 76.1% in the same year. While deaths due to cancer, heart diseases and stroke will increase, deaths due to communicable diseases, perinatal conditions and injuries will reduce during the next 15 years.

NCD BURDEN IN INDIA

India is also going through a time bomb of chronic non-communicable diseases epidemic at present, with over 60% of the deaths in the country already attributable to non-communicable diseases, particularly the four biggest killers, namely cardiovascular diseases, diabetes, cancer and chronic obstructive lung diseases. The picture is worsening fast as evident in the Figure 1.1.

While the nation's priorities in terms of other longstanding health problems such as maternal and child health as well as various communicable diseases, have shown significant decline over the last two decades, there still seems to be a long way to go and the government has been consistently focusing on the challenges posing them. However, it also realizes that India is running against time in combating large epidemics of various chronic illnesses in the coming years due to an increasing lifespan besides rapid changes in lifestyle and the physical environment owing to economic progress and urbanization.

A WHO report has suggested that India is projected to spend $237 billion (1.5% of the GDP) as a result of heart disease, stroke and diabetes from 2005 to 2015. A World Economic Forum report (2014) reported that India is expected to lose $4.58 trillion before 2030 from expenses in the care for NCDs and mental health conditions. Of this, $2.17 trillion is expected to be consumed by cardiovascular diseases alone.

Table 1.1: Causes of death in the year 2008 and 2030

	2008		2030	
Cause of death	Projected deaths (million)	%	Projected deaths (million)	%
Total	58.766	100	67.790	100
Communicable diseases, maternal, perinatal conditions and nutritional deficiencies	15.980	27.2	9.370	13.8
Non-communicable conditions	37.124	63.2	51.619	76.1
Injuries	5.663	9.6	6.801	10.0

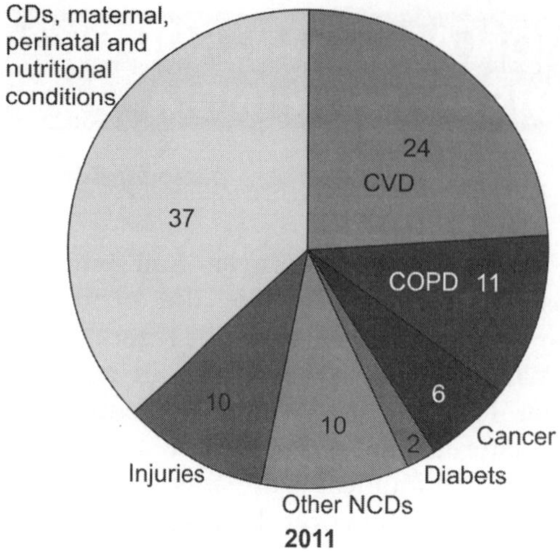

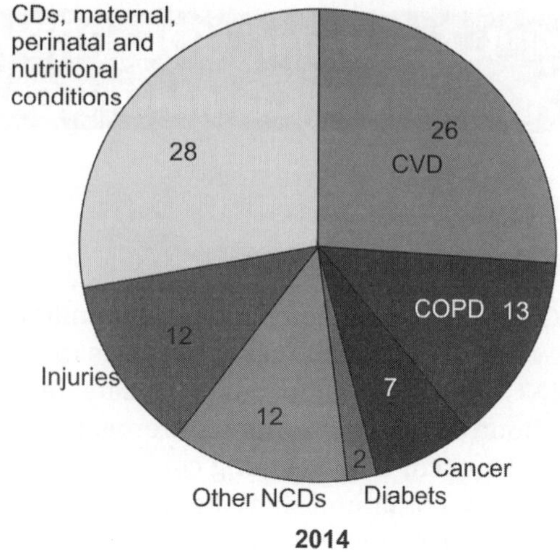

Fig. 1.1: Proportional mortality in India (% of all deaths, all ages, both sexes)

Source: WHO NCD Country profiles

REASONS FOR RISE IN NCDS (TABLE 1.2)

Increase in life expectancy and unhealthy lifestyle behavior are two main reasons for this epidemiological transition. Tobacco use, both smoking and smokeless forms, unhealthy diet rich in salt, sugar and saturated/trans-fats, physical inactivity and alcohol use are key risk factors associated with this trend. Increasing levels of air pollution and mental stress have also been attributable to this trend.

RESPONSE TO THREAT OF NCDS IN INDIA

National response to NCD epidemic has been praiseworthy in recent times, though far from adequate, given the magnitude of the burden and the challenges in its control. A National Programme for Prevention and Control of Cancer, Diabetes, Cardiovascular Diseases and Stroke was launched by the Ministry of Health and Family Welfare in 100 select districts in 21 states in 2010–11 and being expanded to all the districts in a phased manner. Key strategies of the program include health promotion for healthy lifestyles to reduce exposure to risk factors, early diagnosis through periodic/opportunistic screening of population and better diagnostic facilities, infrastructure development for management of NCDs, capacity building of human resources in public health facilities, facilitating rapid referral in medical emergencies (e.g. heart attack and stroke) to

Table 1.2: Prevalence of risk factors (India)

Risk factors	Prevalence
Proportion of insufficiently active population (15+ age group)	14%
Per capita alcohol consumption in liters of pure alcohol (2010)	4.3%
Proportion of population (>25 years) with raised blood pressure (140/90 mm Hg)	33%
Proportion of population (above the age of 20 years) who were overweight	11%
Proportion of population (>25 years) with raised blood glucose	10%
Proportion of population (> 25 years) with raised total cholesterol	27%

Table 1.3: Goals to prevent and control NCDs by the year 2025

Indicator	Year 2025
Relative reduction in premature mortality from NCDs	25%
Obesity and diabetes prevalence	Halt the rise
Relative reduction in prevalence of insufficient physical activity	10%
Relative reduction in the prevalence of raised blood pressure	25%
Relative reduction in mean intake of salt/sodium intake	30%
Relative reduction in alcohol use	10%
Relative reduction in prevalence of current tobacco use	30%
Eligible people receive drug therapy and counseling to prevent heart attacks and strokes	50%
Availability of essential NCD medicines and basic technologies to treat major NCDs public/ private facilities	80%
Relative reduction in household use of solid fuel	50%

reduce mortality and providing treatment to persons with NCDs including rehabilitation and palliative care. The government is also planning to introduce population-based interventions wherever applicable through multi-sectoral approach.

Long Term Targets

The Ministry of Health and Family Welfare has also prepared a monitoring framework to prevent and control NCDs and their risk factors by the year 2025 with some goals as shown in Table 1.3.

The Way Forward

To achieve these targets, it would be necessary to introduce healthy public policies, involve whole of Government, rope in Government, NGO and Private health sector and have massive campaign to make people realize to imbibe healthy lifestyle consisting of healthy and balanced diet, being physically active and abstain from use of alcohol and tobacco. Population-based intervention would require subsidies for healthy option, raising taxes on unhealthy food, tobacco and alcohol, controlling air pollution, providing clean energy in rural areas and bringing up children and adolescents in healthy lifestyles. Government should also realize that investment on health promotion and prevention and capacity building to manage NCDs will be cost-effective in the long run by means of averting premature deaths and disability in the productive age group and reducing out-of-pocket expenditure on these chronic diseases.

USEFUL WEBSITES

- World Health Organization: www.who.int/mediacentre/factsheets/fs310/en/index1.html
- World Health Organization: www.who.int/nmh/publications/ncd-profiles-2014
- Harvard Initiative for Global Health 2013. The Economic Impact of Non-communicable Diseases in China and India: Estimates, Projections and Comparisons. http://www.hsph.harvard.edu/pgda/WorkingPapers/2013/PGDA_WP_107.pdf
- World Health Organization: www.who.int/gho/publications/world_health_statistics/2012

2

Community Based Rehabilitation (CBR) of Differently Abled Persons: A Physiotherapeutic Perspective

Neeta Jayprakash Vyas, Megha Sandeep Sheth

DEFINITION OF DISABILITY

Community based rehabilitation (CBR) has been introduced in the previous chapter.

Disability is the inability of an individual to carry out activities required to be performed daily. The person with disability may be able to perform his activities of daily living but with difficulty. Disability can be defined as a physical or mental condition that limits a person's movements, senses or activities. It is a disadvantage or handicap, especially one imposed or recognized by the law.

According to WHO (World Health Organization), disability is any restriction or lack (resulting from any impairment) of ability to perform an activity in the manner or within the range considered normal for a human being.[1] ILO (International Labor Organization) defines a disabled person as an individual whose prospects of securing retaining and advancing in suitable employment are substantially reduced as a result of duly recognized physical or mental impairments.[2]

Disability is the consequence of an impairment that may be physical, cognitive, mental, sensory, emotional, developmental, or some combination of these. A disability may be present from birth, or occur during a person's lifetime.

Types of Disability[3]

- ***Visual disability:*** The blind are those who suffer from either of the following conditions:
    - Total absence of sight.
    - Visual acuity not exceeding 6/60 or 20/200 (on Snellen chart) in the better eye with corrective lenses.
    - Limitation of the field of vision subtending an angle of degree 20 or worse.
- ***Speech and hearing disability:*** This includes loss or difficulty in hearing and speech.
- ***Locomotor disability:*** It is a person's inability to execute distinctive activities associated with moving either himself or an object, from place to place and such inability resulting from affliction of either bones, joints, muscles or nerves.

  Locomotor disability can be categorized as, mild-less than 40%, moderate- 40% and above, severe-75% and above or profound or total which is 100% disability.
- ***Intellectual disability (Mental retardation):*** It is a condition of arrested or incomplete development of mind of a person which is specially characterized by subnormality of intelligence. It ranges from mental retardation to cognitive deficits like specific learning disabilities. A different category would also include pervasive developmental disorders including autistic spectrum disorders.

ICF AND RELEVANCE OF DISABILITY WITH ICF[4,5]

ICF is the International Classification of Functioning, Disability and Health. ICF belongs to the 'family' of international classifications developed by WHO for application to various aspects of health. The aim of ICF classification is to provide a unified and standard language and framework for the description of health and health related states.

Functioning is an umbrella term encompassing all body functions, activities and participation. Disability is an umbrella term for impairments, activity limitations or participation restrictions and not used as a name of a component. An *impairment* is a problem in body function or structure; an *activity limitation* is a difficulty encountered by an individual in executing a task or action; while a *participation restriction* is a problem experienced by an individual in involvement in life situations.[5] Thus, disability is a complex phenomenon, reflecting an interaction between features of a person's body and features of the society in which he or she lives.

Injury to the femoral nerve is a structural impairment, which leads to reduced muscle power of quadriceps muscle which is a problem in body function. So femoral nerve injury and quadriceps weakness are impairments. Because of that weakness, difficulty encountered in walking, squatting or getting up from squat position are activity limitations. Inability to attend office on the second floor in the absence of a lift because of weak quadriceps is a problem encountered in a life situation becomes a participation restriction. This then leads to inability of the person to fulfil his social responsibilities to financially support his family and makes him disabled.

WHO recognizes that words in the classification can be stigmatizing and labeling and hence the word 'handicap' was dropped early in the process. ICF uses the term disability to denote a multidimensional phenomenon resulting from the interaction between people and their physical and social environment.

The components of functioning and disability in ICF can be expressed in two ways. They can indicate non-problematic aspects of health and health related states termed under the umbrella term of 'functioning' or they can be expressed as problems such as impairments, activity limitation or participation restriction summarized under the umbrella term 'disability.' The components of functioning and disability are interpreted by means of four separate but related constructs. Body structure and function can be interpreted by changes in the anatomy and physiology. For the activities and participation two constructs are available—capacity and performance. A person's functioning and disability is conceived as a dynamic interaction between health conditions and contextual factors (personal and environmental). One may have

- Impairments without activity limitations
- Performance problems and capacity limitations without visible impairments
- Performance problems without impairments or capacity limitations
- Capacity limitations without assistance and no performance problems in current environment.

STRATEGIES OF MANAGEMENT OF DISABILITIES[6]

CBR Guidelines by WHO

Management of disabilities includes prevention and rehabilitation.

Disability prevention aims at measures to reduce occurring of impairments, limiting or reversing disability caused by impairment, and preventing its transition into participation restriction.

Rehabilitation includes measures aimed at reducing the impact of disabling conditions and at enabling the person with disability to achieve social integration, by training a person to adapt to the environment and then intervening at environment and society level to facilitate social integration. It can use the primary health care approach with appropriate supervision and referral. Primary health care provides promotive, preventive, curative and rehabilitative services.

Community based rehabilitation involves measures taken at the community level to use and build on the resources of the community, including the persons with disability, their families and the community as a whole who would be part of the rehabilitation team.

Government Policies and Support

Disability rights are provided for persons with disability as they face persistent barriers to enjoyment of basic human rights like education, employment, access to buildings, transportation and participation in public life. It is the state's responsibility to promote welfare of people and rehabilitation and that social, economic and political justice should be delivered. It is a matter of right and not charity for the persons with disability. The objective of social welfare is to secure for each human being economic necessities, decent standard of health and living conditions and equal opportunities with fellow citizens.

However the limitations of the state are limited financial resources, education and medical facilities, availability of trained personnel, efficient sympathetic administrative machinery and public cooperation.

Through the years at the national level, employment exchanges, job reservations, national institutes and district rehabilitation centers have been established. Various Acts like the Lepers Act (1898), Mental Health Act (1987), Workman's Compensation Act (1923), The Indian Factories Act (1948), Employees State Insurance Act (1948), Rehabilitation Council of India Act (1992), The Persons With Disability (PWD) Act (1995) and the National Trust Act (1999) have been passed by the government for benefit of the persons with disability.

Persons with Disabilities Act (1995–96) was passed to fix responsibilities of Central and State Government according to their resources, to provide services, create facilities, give support to PWD, enable them to have equal opportunities in participating as productive citizens of the country to the fullest extent of their abilities.

Assistive Technologies

Assistive technology is a generic name for devices and modifications for a person or in the community that help overcome disabilities. They can range from a simple cane or wheelchair to fully automated wheel chairs and computer aided devices. Other examples are washroom modifications in public places like malls, ramps in malls, voice/speech detections in computers.

Management of Disabilities at the Workplace

Precautions needs to be taken for safety of workers during their work with machinery, lifting devices and weights, protection of eyes, precaution against fumes, etc. Ergonomic advice for prevention of disabilities should be followed, e.g. advice regarding chair and table height for people working on computers. Occupational disease notification should be done. Specifications for age and hours of work also are regularized to prevent disabilities.

On the other side, job reservations for people with disabilities will improve inclusive rehabilitation. Job modifications can be advised according to the disabilities so they may continue the earning responsibility to the family.

Members of the Rehabilitation Team[7]

A single individual is most of the times incapable of managing disabilities. A rehabilitation team would be better equipped to complete this task. The team comprises of medical persons and sociovocational members. All members have their own roles.

Table 2.1: Members in a rehabilitation team

Medical members	Paramedical members	Sociovocational members
Physiatrists	Physiotherapists	Patient
General surgeon	Occupational therapist	Social worker
Physician	Prosthetist/ Orthotist	Vocational counselor
Neurologist/ neurosurgeon	Nurse	Family members
Psychiatrist	Biomedical engineer	Community workers
Gynecologist/ obstetrician	Vocational therapist	Employment agency workers
Oncologist	Speech therapist	Nongovernment organizations
Pediatrician	Movement therapist	Special educators
	Horticulture therapist	Funding agencies
	Music and dance therapist	

Table 2.1 shows the possible members in a rehabilitation team.

Medical members in the team would be according to the condition. Their main role is in diagnosis, prescribing medicines or performing surgeries where indicated.

A **farmer (patient)** living in a remote village, presenting with a non healing ulcer needs to be diagnosed as having a peripheral vascular disease. This is done by a **cardiothoracic surgeon**. If he needs to undergo an amputation for the same, a **general surgeon** comes into the picture. A **physician** will also have to look into the preoperative fitness of the farmer. There may be other medical specialties required in the team as well.

A **physiotherapist** is concerned with identifying and maximizing quality of life and movement potential within the spheres of promotion, prevention, treatment/intervention, habilitation and rehabilitation. This encompasses physical, psychological, emotional and social well-being.[8] Following a thorough assessment; impairments, activity limitations and participation restrictions are concluded. Exercises and instructions may be prescribed accordingly. These can be taught to **family members** who would encourage the patient to repeat the exercise program through the day and continue after discharge. Ambulation with a walker or crutches needs to be taught as well.

An **occupational therapist** restores, reinforces, and enhances function or performance and decreases disability.[9] He/she would work in coordination with the vocational counselor to help the patient regain required activities. They would provide training of management skills for independence at home and at work, care and use of aids and adaptive equipment and adaptations taking into account personal, social and cultural characteristics.

An **orthopedic surgeon** would grade the level of disability and issue a permanent physical impairment certificate. Government would provide aids and facilities according to the level of disability.

A **prosthetist** would take limb measures when appropriate and prepare the prosthesis. He would be responsible for the design, fabrication and fitting of the artificial limb. He would communicate with surgeons, physiotherapists and engineers to decide best aid. Patient and family members would be advised about its care.

In case patient is bedridden for a prolonged time, a **rehabilitation nurse**, plays a role in maintenance of health and self care activities. This would include transfers, sanitation, personal hygiene, medications and care of adaptive equipment.

A **social worker** interacts with the patient and family helping them to get adjusted to the presenting situation. They assess the patients living situation, lifestyle, resources and impact of the impairment (loss of limb). They would suggest modifications and alternatives. He would provide references for **vocational therapists, placement officers, NGOs and funding agencies** according to the patient's abilities, attitudes and hobbies. He would also make the patient aware about the benefits provided to a person with disability.

The **community** may also join in for financial aids or work options. A social worker would also play a role in educating the community about the condition, causes and treatment options.

For psychological issues following the amputation, a **psychiatrist or psychologist** may be suggested.

The patient may not be able to go back to farming which involves field work, and so a **vocational counselor** would identify the right vocation or skill of the patient and further train the patient for a new money earning option.

For the **specially abled children** following members also play a role in the team.

Special educators are required who understand the abilities and limitations of the child and teach each child accordingly. A **music therapist** uses instruments or vocal performances either by the person with disability for rehabilitation, or helps them to appreciate music by attending shows. Dancing to music helps improve coordination and also proves to be relaxing for the child. **Dance therapy** or creative movement therapy improves gross and fine motor control, relaxes the body and improves group activity.

SUMMARY

Disability is an umbrella term for impairments, activity limitations or participation restrictions. CBR of differently abled persons can be done following CBR guidelines by WHO, government policies and support, using assistive technologies and with the help of a rehabilitation team.

REFERENCES

1. International Classification of Impairments, Disabilities and Handicaps (ICIDH), World Health Organization, Geneva, 1980.
2. Vocational Rehabilitation and Employment (Disabled Persons) Convention, 1983 (No. 159), http://www.llo.org.
3. Office of the Chief Commissioner for Persons with Disabilities Disability Guidelines, http://pbhealth.gov.in.
4. ICF, International Classification of Functioning, Disability and Health, World Health Organization, Geneva, 2001.
5. Disabilities. World Health Organization, Geneva.
6. Disability Prevention and Rehabilitation. Report of the WHO expert committee on Disability Prevention and Rehabilitation. World health Organization Technical Report Series 668, WHO Geneva 1981.
7. S Sunder. Textbook of Rehabilitation, 3rd edition, Jaypee Brothers Publishers.
8. World Confederation of Physical Therapy, position statement, http://www.wcpt.org/
9. World Federation of Occupational Therapy, www.wfot.org.

3

Concepts of Prevention Practice, Functional Diagnosis and Community Physiotherapy

Bharati Vijay Bellare

Abstract: This chapter conceptualizes three inter-linking domains of Physiotherapeutic health care related to prevention, i.e. Basics of prevention practice in physiotherapy, functional diagnosis and community physiotherapy. With brief review on determinants of health, and with various examples and case studies, this chapter elaborates as how to these three concepts can be put into clinical practice of physiotherapy under a specialty subject 'Prevention practice and community physiotherapy (PPCPT)'.

Keywords: Health, Prevention, Community, Physiotherapy, ICF, Contextual factors, Functional diagnosis

INTRODUCTION

Role of Physiotherapy in community based rehabilitation (CBR) of a physically ***handicapped*** person is well established ever since the inception of this profession but its role in ***'preventing'*** the persons from becoming ***handicapped*** was not highlighted till recent years. Earlier, Physiotherapists used to follow a medical model for the evaluation and assessment that was based on clinical diagnosis derived by the medico and accordingly, the intervention was offered. However, in last 50 years this profession has grown very fast globally and has attained recognition as an independent health profession that deals with a ***Person with Pathology*** rather than dealing with pathology of a person and follows ***social model*** with ***Holistic approach*** in terms of person(s)'s ***mind, body as well as spirit***. Thus, the concept of '***Functional diagnosis*** is based on this principle which is ***independent*** of clinical diagnosis'. This chapter discusses basic concepts of prevention practice, functional diagnosis and community physiotherapy from point of view of **Indian Physiotherapy perspective**; therefore, certain ***standard definitions are modified wherever necessary***.

Determinants of Health

In the year 1948 the World Health Organization (WHO) proposed **definition of 'Health'** as ***'physical, mental, and social well-being, and not merely the absence of disease and infirmity'***[1] whereas, Public Health Agency of Canada has elaborated the factors that determine health.[2]

Reader should note that the sequence given in the Table 3.1 does not specify any priority of determinants; in fact all of them interlink to determine the health status.

- ***Wealth status:*** Higher economical status enables selection of healthy and active lifestyle that also includes desirable higher education and employment, power and luxuries. Nevertheless, misuse of wealth can cause negative health effect such as obesity and its related disorders due to consumption unhealthy (fast) food associated with sedentary lifestyle by misusing cellphone/computer technology

Table 3.1: Determinants of health from point of view of physiotherapy perspective in India

1. Wealth status
2. Social support from family, friends and community
3. Literacy and education
4. Environment (physical/occupation related)
5. Lifestyle behavior related to health
6. Influence of genetic components
7. Healthy development of a child
8. Cultural influence on behavior and attitude
9. Gender
10. Government policies-labor law

and falling easy prey to substance abuse instead of adopting active lifestyle by participating in sports. Similarly, misuse of 'power' of wealth can lead to indulging into socially/ethically unacceptable activities. Whereas, poverty can strongly influence health behavior and show certain typical 'culture of poverty'(see details later in this chapter).

- ***Social support:*** Family bondage by healthy interpersonal relationship, support from friends and social community can always help a person in need and boost up his morale to face any adverse situation confidently.
- ***Literacy and education:*** It enables selection of healthy lifestyle by differentiating between what is 'good and bad'. Aging effect on brain can be delayed by building needful neural network by acquiring higher education and sustaining long-term desirable careers.[3]
- ***Lifestyle and health behaviors:*** Health status is influenced by the balance in lifestyle (sedentary vs active), nutrition and diet (balanced vs fast food), eating habits (regular vs irregular), substance abuse (smoking, alcohol consumption, drugs), sleep, rest and leisure activities.
- ***Environmental health:*** It is determined by two components as follows:
  1. ***Physical environment:*** It depends upon factors surrounding indoor and outdoor area. There are certain factors beyond control such as climatic situation, water supply (depending upon rainfall), etc. but there are large number of factors within control; such as, maintaining cleanliness and good hygiene, improving greenery, controlling pollution of air and sound, avoiding congestion, and preventing contamination of water and food, etc. Conducive physical component of *work environment* needs free space for movement, temperature control in place where extreme temperatures are likely, provision of safety gadgets like helmets, etc. Such controllable factors can prevent diseases, injuries and create health-supporting environment.
  2. ***Psychosocial environment:*** It needs to be conducive at home as well as at work place. At home the interpersonal relation should be warm, full of caring and sharing. Unlike nuclear family system adopted in the developing countries; in India a joint family system exists even today. Though the differences of opinion are likely due to generation gap, the younger and working generation (specially women) should always realize about the responsibility (physical/moral) shared by the senior members of the family in domestic activities, child care, etc. At the same time, senior members should also realize about the change in thinking process prioritizing practical approach in behavior and attitude by the younger generation, hence they should not impose rigid traditional rules on their matured children. Thus,

cordial relationship built between generations living together can provide very healthy and cheerful psychological environment. Whereas, at the work place, psychologically conducive environment includes adequate work without feeling of exploitation, healthy competition among co-workers, fair and cordial relation between the employer and employee, etc. According to WHO, the key for fair employment is descent work, adequate safety measures at work place and minimum wages that are fair to the type of work allotment.[4]

- ***Cultural influence on health behavior and attitude:*** The cultural impact on beliefs, attitude, directives for decision making, expression of emotions, type of diet and self-image, etc. reflects greatly on health behavior and attitude towards availing health care facilities.[5] In spite of global civilization, even today certain communities in our country believe in the traditional faith healers like 'babas'/village priests, who claim to treat any illness with magic and witch craft because according to them, it is an ill effect of 'curse' of the departed souls or 'evil desire of existing spirits'. Any culture that is influenced with such belief can force a person to refuse modern medical treatment though offered free of cost.
  - Poverty can cause strong influence on health behavior, e.g. laborers working on daily wages are generally deprived of any benefits such as paid sick leave or free medical care, etc. Such situation forces them to ignore future and think only about current situation; leaving no option but to continue with work even if rest is mandatory for healing. This situation is totally in contrast to the cultural environment of developed countries and corporate industry in our country, where absenteeism due to aches and pain forms a major concern in spite of providing all the health facilities and sick leave benefits (see Case Study 1).
  - Nevertheless, poverty can also force a person to take some nonacceptable and drastic decisions when the 'thought of future' is prioritized (see Case Study 2).
  - ***Culture shock:*** While planning any intervention or ergonomic advice etc. Physiotherapist must take into account the ***socioeconomical and cultural dimensions***. This is because many health professionals hailing from better economical background but not exposed to poverty related issues are most likely to get highly frustrating experience while managing poverty stricken patients with standard protocol of intervention acquired during professional education (see Case Study 3).

Note: Both Case Studies 2 and 3 are real life events which were narrated to the author when she visited tribal health center in north-east Maharashtra in the year 2014.

- ***Early childhood development:*** Type of upbringing is known to establish specific physical and mental behavior during adulthood. Healthy nutrition, good physical and social development (by using healthy cultural concept of caring and sharing including polite behavior with elders and cordial relation with peer group, etc.), by grooming the child to sustain balance between studies and leisure activities, balanced healthy food and tasty but junk food, etc. is very much needed. Emotional development (impulse control) is also essential in addition to motivating the child to participate in sports and cultural events. Positive effect of healthy development builds resiliency but inadequate or negative impact increases vulnerability.

Case Study 1

Mathadi work (load of 50-100 kg carried on head) is a secured employment but its remuneration is based on daily wages. Unpublished postgraduate study supervised by the author in the year 2014 showed more than 80% prevalence of fair to severe musculoskeletal aches and pain among Mathadi workers; low back pain being most prevalent. Further, in spite of this fact, their rate of absenteeism was found to be 0%. Free basic medical services were offered to them by their employer but they hardly availed them.

The following 'Focus group discussion' (FGD) with 15 Mathadi workers conducted by the author represents typical health behavior that forces a person to ignore future and to focus only on 'today'.

Q1. From which source do you get the strength to continue working in spite of prevailing aches and pain?

Ans. How can we afford to pamper pain? We live under hand to mouth status and work on daily wages. Fear of failure to provide two meals to our family is the biggest force that enables us to ignore pain even if it is severe and we continue to work till the pain supersedes our tolerance. We are always aware that the moment we stop working it is THE END for our family.

Q2. Why do not you avail the free medical facility provided to you?

Ans. We work on daily wages and there is no provision of sick leave or time relaxation to avail the facility; more over, one day absenteeism would deprive us from the income of that day.

Q3. Do you offer regular prayers to get strength to withstand this stress?

Ans. God does not come down to bear the load which we carry every day.

Q4. Do you smoke or consume alcohol to relieve physical stress?

Ans. One need not have to be a Mathadi worker to smoke or consume alcohol.

Q5. We are informed that one overseas company wanted to donate advanced equipment to your organization to reduce the work stress.

Ans. We unanimously protest against such technology that substitutes human efforts and deprives a person from employment.

Q6. Your work is often accident prone, are you aware of protective gadgets and will you use them if provided?

Ans. We will surely use them provided they do not limit our work speed and efficiency.

Case Study 2

A 6-month-old baby suffering from severe bronchopneumonia was brought by her mother to a community hospital situated within tribal location. Looking at baby's critical condition, the doctor advised mother to admit the baby immediately and to stay with her in the hospital. However, mother refused and went away with her sick baby. Next day the same baby was brought again to the hospital in a gasping status by her 8 years old sister and by the time the doctor (who had already attended her on the earlier day) could start some emergency intervention, the baby expired. Doctor got extremely furious and asked the elder sister to go home and bring some senior members of the family immediately to pick up the dead baby. Mother arrived after few hours with an absolutely blank expression. Doctor threw tantrums and accused the mother for being so irresponsible. Mother remained silent till the doctor finally stopped talking. She then replied. 'Doctor, I am a mother of 4 children and this baby was born three months after her father died due to snake bite. I am the only person left to feed my children. When I work for ten hours, I can manage to prepare a single meal for them. I was aware that this baby was not going to survive even if I had stayed with her in the hospital losing my wages for that day. Therefore I felt, it would be wise to at least take care of my elder healthy kids, two of whom will be able to help me in earning after couple of years. May I ask you doctor, what would you do if you were in my situation?'

- ***Gender*** refers to the collection of rules and regulations empowered by the society to differentiate between two genders in terms of dominance in relationships, behaviors, attitudes, values, decision-making powers etc.[6] Male dominance prevails in this country. ***Self neglect***, dependency on male partner or senior member of the in-laws for all the decisions (including seeking medical help for self); least priority to access anything that is beneficial to self are the common social issues encountered by Indian women specially hailing from lower income groups and communities who

Case Study 3

Low back pain is highly prevalent among tribal community of North Maharashtra, during the season when they work for 8-10 hours for sowing paddy saplings in ankle deep wet mud. They work on basis of daily wages and their work involves continuous bending position. A Physiotherapist hailing from an upper middle class family of urban set up volunteered to offer services at same tribal health center mentioned in Case Study 2. She had hardly put up six months of service but started contemplating to leave because of poor job satisfaction. She was unsuccessful in rendering standard modes on intervention for aches and pain which she learned during professional education, e.g. while treating low back pain, if she advised the farmers to destress their back by stretching it after every 10-15 minutes while at work, they refused to comply because it would adversely affect their speed of bound task. Further, whenever she used to advise them to do at least some back exercises at home; they would make a mockery of such advice with a comment that there is no need of such treatment since they were already 'Over-exercising'.

are extremely rigid about their cultural beliefs.

- ***Government policies:*** In most of the countries globally, the central government takes responsibility of health care hence it becomes mandatory for each citizen, even in good health to undergo certain health checkup periodically as stipulated by the government. Unfortunately in our country this rule is not mandatory. Though government focuses on the 'health for all' policy and attempts to reach the grass root level, there are lot of lacunae. Various National Health Policies are implemented in the country but Physiotherapy is totally missing in spite of its proven benefits, e.g. Antenatal and Postnatal Physiotherapy is not included in our National Health Program for Maternal Health.

Any imbalance within the factors determining health can alter physical and mental states and result into dynamic processes of 'disease and disabilities'. Prevention is always considered to be better than cure and its practice can be applicable at the level of an individual or certain population or community.

As per Mosby's medical dictionary (8th edn 2009), ***the definition of 'Disease prevention' is*** 'Activities designed to protect an individual or community from actual or potential health threats and their harmful consequences'.

Team approach: Working mode of health care system always recommends a team approach in which various disciplines work together for a ***COMMON GOAL***. In the management of health care there are three modes of team work as follows:

1. ***Multidisciplinary: Individual*** management by each discipline but communication with others by referral system as seen in large tertiary hospitals.
2. ***Interdisciplinary:*** Each case is reviewed jointly by various health disciplines and management goals are set together. This is a most preferred model of team work which is not feasible at large tertiary hospitals but generally observed at health care centers rendering services to specific health conditions such as rehabilitation center for physically handicapped persons, cancer hospital, etc.
3. ***Transdisciplinary:*** One discipline takes over the tasks of another when the latter is not available as seen at the Primary/Community health centers, or mode used during disaster management.

CONCEPT OF PREVENTION PRACTICE

Prevention strategies: Impact of illness/disease can be interrupted at ***FIVE LEVELS during*** its process of development—i. Primordial, ii. Primary, iii. Secondary,

iv. Tertiary and v. Quaternary. The first two levels deal with a healthy status, the third level deals with an asymptomatic/preclinical/vulnerable status; whereas the last two levels deal with established manifested status after affection of disease/injury. ***Physiotherapy has a major role to play in 2nd, 3rd and 4th level prevention***.

Primordial Prevention

It is used ***before the emergence*** of risk/hazardous factors in the environmental, economic, social, behavioral or cultural pattern of living which are known to increase the risk of disease[7] or injury.

Intervention: It deals with individual or mass education and motivation to avoid/prevent emergence of potential risk factors. This mode is mainly incorporated within National policies and rules, e.g. rule to prevent accidental injuries; law ***against*** breaking traffic rules; (non-compliance of wearing seat belts or helmets while driving four or two wheelers respectively); law against activities that are likely to disturb ecological balance (cutting trees); law against developmental health issues (school bags weighing more than stipulated weight), etc. every citizen of this country has to take the responsibility to follow primordial prevention; the health professional have an extra responsibility to educate the masses in this regards.

Primary Prevention

It is used when ***potential risk factors are already emerged but persons are not yet affected***. The objective of this strategy in Physiotherapy is to identify the ***extent of known*** potential risk factors first and then to use preventive modes to eliminate them and also to provide protection against their exposure (by building resistance against them) exactly like immunization against epidemics.

Intervention: Aims at ***Health promotion***, a process that includes, ***education*** to create awareness about the potential risk factors and to ***motivate*** an individual or population to adopt healthy behaviors by creating ***necessary modifications in the lifestyle*** and ***to build healthy social and physical environments*** to support these behaviors.[8]

Lifestyle modification is a ***self-implemented*** process that not only needs ***determination, patience and perseverance*** to achieve positive changes in the behavioral pattern and ability to sustain the change till it becomes a natural part of life (risk of relapse is likely before as well as after achieving full success), e.g. contemplation on weight loss or giving up alcohol consumption/smoking. Other examples include maintaining balance between diet, physical activity and rest; use of mask while working in area with anticipated air pollution, adopting ergonomically safe lifting mechanism, work hardening before participation in sports or high impact occupational activity, etc (Flowchart 3.1).

Healthy physical environment: Special care to be taken to sustain indoor and outdoor space clutter free, clean and free from stagnant water; hygiene to be maintained at public places like gardens, sports grounds, theaters, public toilets and to establish smoke free environment by creating smoking zones, prevention from spitting after consuming paan/tobacco, etc.

Secondary Prevention

It is used when the subject is already affected but yet in an ***asymptomatic (pre-clinical)*** stage. Hence the main aim is to ***prevent*** asymptomatic status from ***turning symptomatic***.

Intervention: The main objective is to identify ***extent*** of exposure of ***known contextually*** (see details later) ***associated*** risk factors and immediate intervention before the person becomes symptomatic, e.g. early intervention in high-risk neonates, care of childhood obesity, addressing compromised mobility

Flowchart 3.1: Stages of self-implemented lifestyle modification

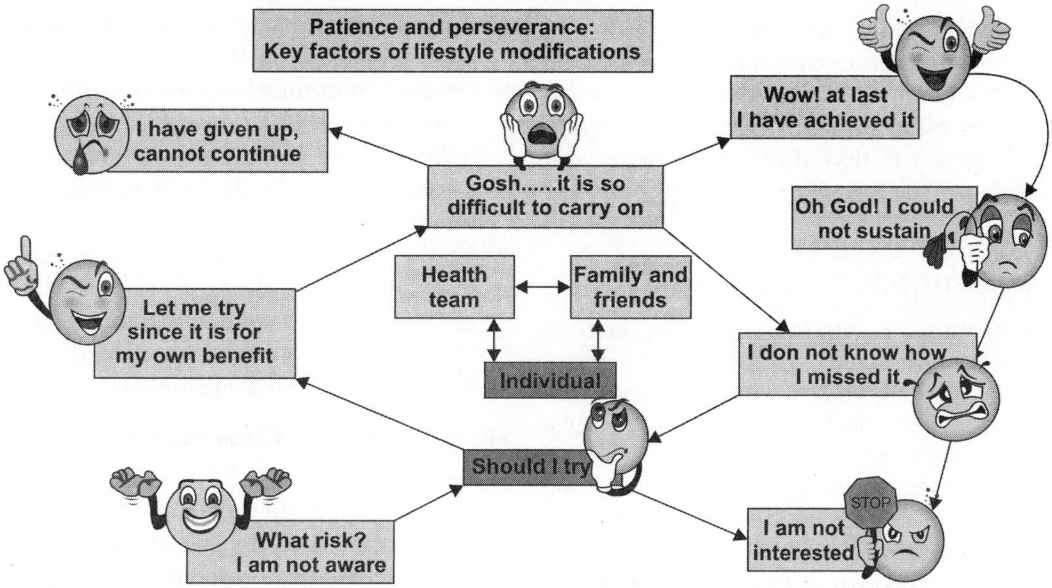

during height spurt (due to mismatch in the growth on bones and surrounding soft tissue) among children regularly involved in sports, etc.

Tertiary Prevention

It is used when person is ***symptomatic*** after the exposure to risk factors. Application of this strategy includes wide range from a critical to slowly progressive or non-reversible steady disabling status, which if neglected can lead to death, due to cause which may not directly link with primary pathology. Examples are as follows:

- ***Critical tertiary prevention:*** This strategy is applied to critically ill ***individual***. When an unconscious patient is admitted to the intensive care unit (ICU), irrespective of his cause of unconsciousness (cerebrovascular accident, head injury, diabetic, coma or poisoning, etc.), promoting bronchial hygiene to prevent life-threatening bronchopneumonia forms the major preventive strategy.
- ***Early disaster management*** applies to affected ***population***, when ***transdisciplinary team*** approach may be undertaken to prevent/minimize disability irrespective of type of calamity, i.e. floods, earthquakes or manmade calamities like bomb blast, train accident.
- ***Acute tertiary prevention*** of an ***individual*** is a part and parcel of ***restorative care*** for a specific pathology (e.g. domain of other clinical physiotherapy specialties such as musculoskeletal, neurological or cardiopulmonary physiotherapy) in which, in addition to remedial intervention, care is taken to ***prevent morbidity*** (hypomobility, muscle weakness, etc.) specially when the recovery period is long.
- ***Long-term tertiary prevention:*** It applies to an ***individual*** suffering from slowly progressive or nonreversible steady disability. The main aim here is to limit/delay the development of ***MORBIDITY*** following impact of ongoing pathology or risk of secondary complication in steady crippling health issue (e.g. paraplegia). Since this strategy is to be applied on long-term bases, it is rendered via ***Community based rehabilitation (CBR)***.

Quaternary Prevention

Methods to minimize or avoid results of unnecessary or excessive interventions in the health system.[9] This aspect largely applies to ***medical management*** (side effect of long-term administration of any drug) hence ***not within the scope of Physiotherapy.***

CONCEPTUALIZATION OF FUNCTIONAL DIAGNOSIS

Philosophy of physiotherapy: In last 50 years, Physiotherapy profession has grown very fast globally and has attained recognition as an independent health profession. Unlike other health professions, it deals with a ***Person with Pathology*** rather than dealing with Pathology of a person, thus follows ***Holistic approach*** to health care and links closely with ***Quality of life.***

'Wellness' is not just an absence of disease or infirmity but it describes a positive state of well-being in terms of physical, mental, socio-emotional, and spiritual dimensions enabling enjoyable life.[10]

Quality of life (QOL) is a broad multi-dimensional concept that usually includes perception of both ***positive*** and ***negative*** aspects of life.[11] It is defined as individual perception about high levels of well-being ***(wellness)*** and satisfactory physical, mental and spiritual ***functioning*** in which ***wellness*** and ***functioning*** form a ***perceptual*** and ***motor*** component respectively. The component 'Functioning' brought Physiotherapy profession into limelight because ***Physical functioning*** deals with **'Movement'**.

Health-related quality of life (HRQOL): This concept and its determinants have evolved since the 1980s to encompass those aspects of overall quality of life that can be clearly shown to affect health—either ***physical or mental.***[12-15]

- On the individual level, HRQOL includes physical and mental health perceptions (e.g. energy level, mood) and their correlates—including health risks and conditions, functional status, social support, and socioeconomic status.
- On the community level, HRQOL includes community-level resources, conditions, policies, and practices that influence a population's health perceptions and functional status.
- On the basis of a synthesis of the scientific literature and advice from its public health partners, HRQOL is defined as 'an individual's or group's perceived physical and mental health overtime.'[12]

History of WHO's Classification of Health

The first International Classification of Disease formulated by WHO (***ICD-10***) is based on Medical model focusing on ***'Mortality'.*** The first revision was made in the year **1980** when it was taken into account that, survival with disability causes ***morbidity*** which adversely affects ***quality of life (QOL).*** Therefore, this classification was modified from ***medical*** to ***social*** model as ***International Classification of Impairment, Disability and Handicaps (ICIDH)*** which became a turning point for Physiotherapy profession to attain its recognition by justifying that—'If a ***doctor adds Years*** to the patient's ***life***, the ***Physiotherapist adds Life*** to those ***years'.***

The next revision was done in the year **1993** when the term **ICIDH** was modified to **ICIDH-II.** In this revision the terminology of second and third domains, i.e. 'Disability and Handicaps' was modified to ***'activity limitations'*** and ***'participation restriction'*** respectively and the definition was reformed as ***'International Classification of human functioning at the level of body, the whole person and the person within the complete Psychosocial and physical environmental context'.*** The domains were description as follows:

- ***Impairment*** (based on systemic medical model). It involved specific anatomical structure(s), i.e. organs, limbs or their parts and physiological/psychological functions, e.g. pain/weakness/incoordination/hypomobility/depression, open wound.
- ***Activity limitations:*** They included difficulties in performing task or activities related to daily activities including occupational work, e.g. difficulty in walking, traveling, domestic activities, etc.
- ***Participation restriction:*** It included difficulties in dealing with various life situations, e.g. loss of job, problem in socialization due to vitiligo.

During this revision it was also taken into account that, activity limitations and participation restrictions may not necessarily associate together with impairment every time, e.g. a young girl with vitiligo patches on face may not have any activity limitations, but she has great participation restriction in socialization during community events.

Therefore it was necessary to take into account the positive (facilitator) or negative (Barrier) influence of **'Contextual factors'**, which were based on the determinants of health discussed earlier in this chapter and this concept is not changed till to date even after the next revision done in the year 2001.

Flowchart 3.2 elaborates as to how ICIDH-II links with ***contextual factors*** via functional outcome of impairment.

Flowchart 3.2: Showing link between ICIDH-II and contextual factors via functional outcome

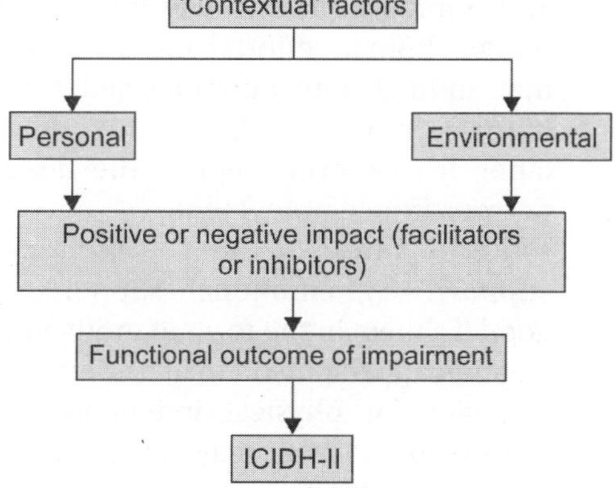

'Contextual factors' determining 'barriers or facilitators':

- ***Internal contextual factors:*** They include personal and co-morbid factors:
  - ***Personal factors:*** They include Gender/education/social background/personality/coping ability with unchangeable surrounding (e.g. change of environment when a girl goes to stay at her in-laws' residence after marriage).
  - ***Co-morbid factors:*** They include age/non-reversible health issue like diabetes, genetic factors, permanent locomotor disability (e.g. paraplegia).
  - ***Past and current experiences:*** Certain unforgettable incidences can create deep rooted positive or negative impact on the human mind.
- ***Environmental/External contextual factors:***
  - ***Natural and human made environment*** at home/workplace-indoor/outdoor surroundings, e.g. in case of a paraplegic subject, conventional provision of a wheelchair and tricycle for physical independence during indoor and outdoor ambulation respectively, would not serve the purpose if the subject lives in a 10' × 10' slum development and its access to main road is a long stretch of muddy, uneven terrain.
  - ***Geographical:*** Examples are various locations such as hilly/forest area or extreme climatic conditions can create barriers during ambulation and work respectively.
  - ***Sociocultural:*** Examples are Puerperal woman may refuse to attend postnatal follow up clinic within 40 days even if it is necessary because of sociocultural taboo imposed on outdoor activity during this period.

- ***Products and technology:*** Advanced technology makes work easier, faster and improves productivity but it may reduce human efforts and a person may indulge into adopting sedentary lifestyle; moreover, by cutting down labor, it may even deprive the needy persons from employment.
- ***Physical/financial and emotional support:*** e.g emotional supports is good if shown in the form of motivating a handicapped person to learn self-care activities for physical independence, but overpampering may cause exactly opposite reaction.
- ***Attitude:*** It is very much influenced by ***cultural impact*** on custom, ideology, values/norms and religious beliefs, etc. e.g. attitude of self-neglect among Indian rural women creates a strong barrier while availing health care facilities for themselves.
- ***Service system:*** Policies (public-private-voluntary) regarding provision of facilities/services for health care at community—regional, State and National level are always facilitatory.

The establishment of ICIDH-II enabled conceptualization of ***functional diagnosis which is independent of clinical diagnosis.*** Following three cases are the examples (see Case Studies 4–6) based on three age matched women having ***same clinical diagnosis*** and same impairment (off and on pain and swelling in knee) but their ***functional diagnosis is totally different*** in terms of variable activity limitations and participation restrictions (black boxes) because of influence by variable contextual factors. Thus the concept of functional diagnosis directs appropriate planning of ***individual need based intervention even though clinical diagnosis is same.***

Next and latest revision of ICIDH-II was done in the year **2001** which is sustained till to date. It takes into account a mismatch between 'capacity' and 'performance' of a ***'Functional'*** outcome. Therefore it is modified as ***'International Classification of Functioning, Disabilities and Health'*** which is abbreviated as ***ICF***, in which ***'capacity'*** determines as to how well a ***person can do*** in a ***standard/controlled environment***; whereas, ***'Performance'*** determines as to how a person ***actually does in the routine environment*** (Case Study 7).

Since ICF has emphasized on 'Functioning', the concept of ***'FUNCTIONAL DIAGNOSIS'*** is highlighted, hence demands patient assessment under three domains—i. Impairment

Case Study 4

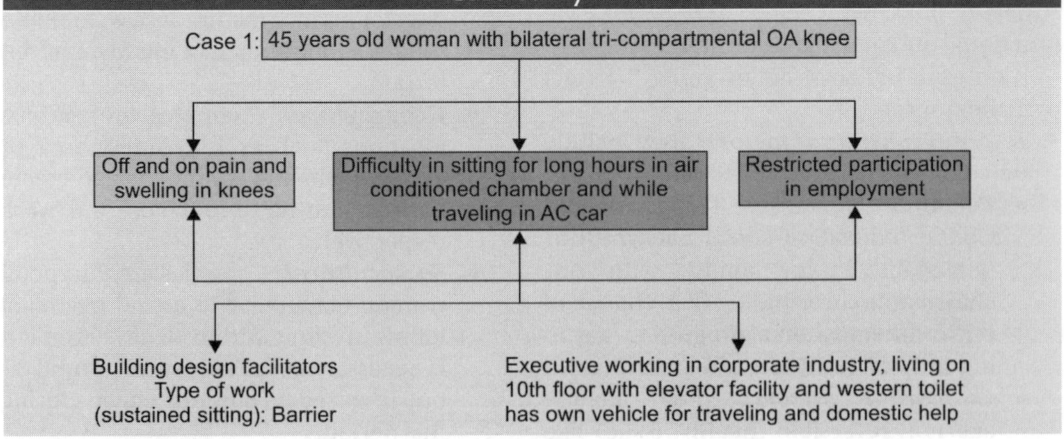

Case Study 5

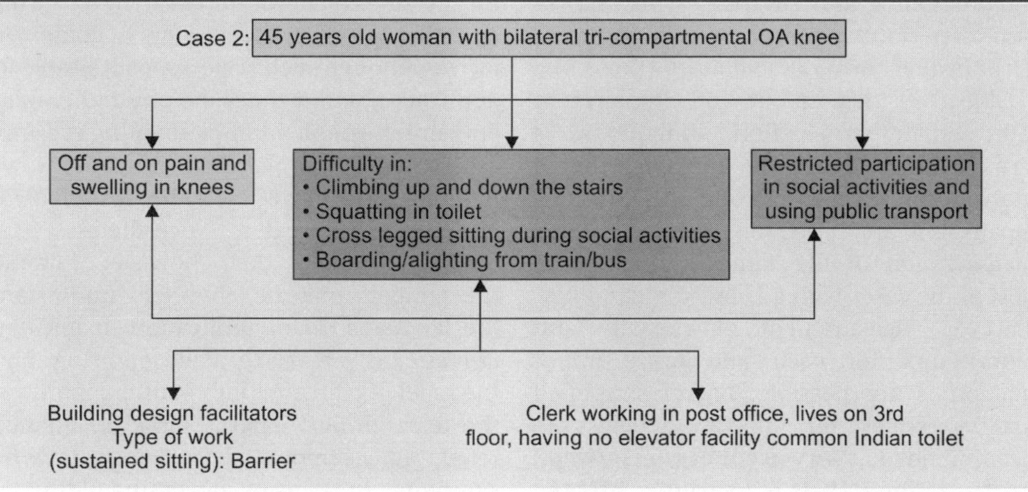

Case Study 6

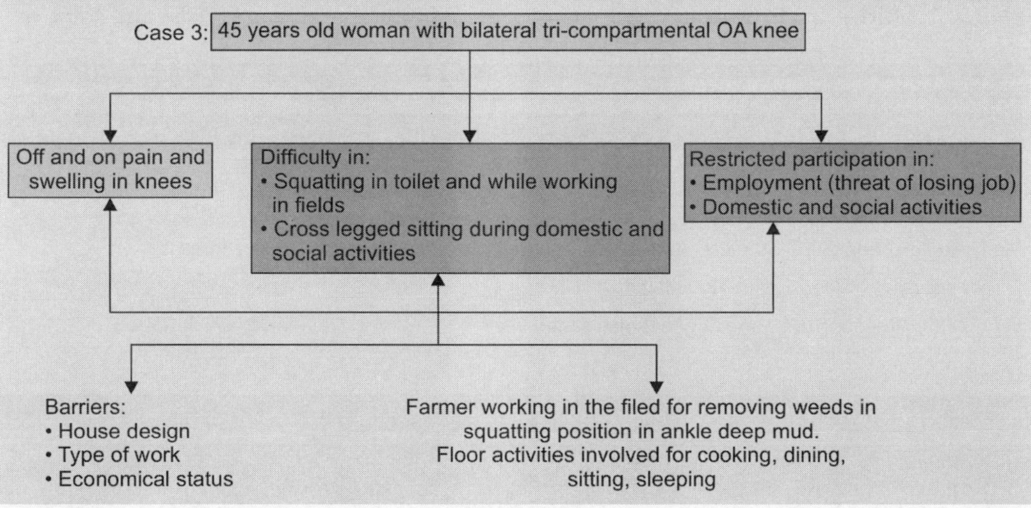

Case Study 7

Prabhat is a brilliant student but he scored only 45% marks (Performance) in the last examination (*controlled* environment). Having both the parents working and nobody to guide him at home after school hours, he was distracted towards a cellphone and watched movies, or played videogames on it constantly, neglecting his studies (barriers in the routine environment). However, as per the counselor's advice, Prabhat's parents took away his cellphone with a promise to return it after exams. His mother also took leave from work during his preparatory leave before the examination and motivated/coached Prabhat (facilitator in the routine environment). As a result Prabhat scored 85% marked (capacity) in the recent examination (standard/controlled environment).

(as per medical model) (Box 3.1); ii. Status of 'Functioning and Disability' (Box 3.2) in terms of performance and capacity; iii. Status of 'contextual barriers/facilitators' (Box 3.3).

Objective assessment of impairment and activity/participation limitations is very essential to analyze the outcome of intervention. Since objective modes to assess impairment are based on medical model, quantification of the same is possible in most of the cases with advanced technology. However, measurement of capacity and performance for each and every minor function is not possible. Lot of simplified qualifiers/scales for specific activity are recommended at **www.wcpt.org/sites/wcpt.org/files/files/GH-ICF_overview_FINAL_for_WHO.pdf**

Five point generic scale from 0–4 (0:Nil, 1:Mild; 2:Moderate; 3:Severe; 4:Complete/very severe) is recommended for the assessment of impairment and while quantifying barriers/facilitators of contextual factors. Though such scale appears simple for application, many times the physiotherapists encounter trouble in implementing it during assessment of impairment if patients are illiterate and have cognitive problem in understanding scales. Nevertheless, it is always observed that, however illiterate the patients may be, they can understand the language for quantification in terms of ***currency*** as ***'paisa'***, e.g. while reporting about the relief of pain after intervention; many use the term 25/50/75 paisa 'farak' to quantify relief. Many senior citizens also quantify the symptoms in terms of 'aanaa'-the old Indian currency coins which were discarded more than 50 years ago, e.g. char aana (25%), aath aana (50%), barah aana (75%) and solah aana

Box 3.1: Assessment of impairment

Qualifiers for Impairment [I]	Scale	Frequency of affection [F]
Nil affection	0	Never
Minimal affection/25%/25 paisa [Chaar ana]	1	Very Rarely
Moderate affection [50%]-50 paise [Aath ana]	2	Sometimes
Severe affection [75%]-75 paise [Baarah ana]	3	Frequently
Very severe affection:100%-one Rupee [Solah aana]	4	Always/Continuous

Box 3.2: Assessment of status of functioning and disability

Functional grade	Qualifiers of activity and participation limitation performance vs capacity	Disability grade [D]
IV	No problem in routine function-can do more [100% performance = CAPACITY]	0
III	Can just complete routine function but no more [25% performance affection]	I
II	Function completed with help [50% performance affection]	II
I	Incomplete function in spite of help [75% affection]	III
0	Nil performance [100% or complete affection performance]	IV

Box 3.3: Assessment of status of contextual barriers and facilitators

Contextual factors	Facilitators (0–4)	Barriers(0–4)
Environmental: Home/workplace		
Water/electricity/lighting/pollution		
Sanitation/Gen Hygiene		
Housing design-stairs/elevators, Indian/ western toilet		
Indoor space for movement		
Terrain (outside housing)		
Working environment		
Accessibility for medical aids		
Policies/Facilities		
Care giver's support		
Internal/Co-morbid factors		
Age/education/sex/Metabolic		
Financial support		
Social support		
Type of occupation		
Any other		

(100%) farak/relief. Therefore, equivalent terms of qualifiers are recommended in Box 3.1 to quantify impairment (I). Whereas, in Box 3.2, the scale 0–4 shows reciprocal relation between 'disability' and 'functional ability'. The highest scale (4) of Functional ability is recommended to be taken into account as 'Capacity' of the concerned function if 'standard environment' is not available.

CONCEPTUALIZATION OF COMMUNITY PHYSIOTHERAPY (CPT)

The concept of new clinical specialty ***'Prevention Practice and Community Physiotherapy' (PPCPT)*** relates to the health care that clubs two independent allopathic specialties, i.e. ***Community medicine*** and ***Physical medicine and rehabilitation,*** who deal with ***population*** and ***individual person*** respectively. Thus, this specialty has a wide span of prevention practice from 'womb to tomb' which spreads from ***Primary to long-term tertiary*** prevention. In this specialty subject the term 'community' is used in two different contexts as follows:

- ***Community based rehabilitation (CBR):*** This part which is based on the specialty 'Physical medicine and rehabilitation' deals with ***long-term tertiary prevention of an individual with nonreversible disability***. This section forms a ***small*** but already well established component of PPCPT where the term 'Community' relates to ***'outdoor/extra-institutional' location,*** similar to the connotation used in 'Community Medicine' CBR is elaborated separately in the next chapter of this book; therefore, the reader may refer to the same for details in this aspect.
- ***Community Physiotherapy (CPT):*** This is a ***novel*** but ***a MAJOR*** component of

PPCPT that deals with ***group/population*** with regards to ***primary, secondary and early tertiary prevention similar to specialty subject 'Community medicine'***. However, here the term 'community' does not restrict to outdoor location(s) alone but also ***includes intra-institutional*** population. This is because the term ***'COMMUNITY'*** referred here relates to ***specific 'Contextual factor'*** and represents under its umbrella; the various **sub-communities**/population, ***each*** *having* ***COMMON RISK ISSUES***. The Flowchart 3.3 identifies ***four major contextual factors*** (black boxes) and their respective major communities (grey boxes). To understand this concept, one can consider the socio-cultural concept of specific religion (contextual factor) and the communities/subcommunities covered under it (e.g. Hindu religion has four 'vernas/communities' out of which, according to the culture of Maharashtra state-a 'brahmin' ***community*** has various subcommunities such as Kokanastha, Deshastha, Karade, Saraswat, etc).

Community physiotherapy thus includes a wide span referring right from small groups of various subcommunities belonging to a single location/institution (e.g. occupation related communities like surgeons, physiotherapists, nurses, labor staff, etc. working in the same hospital) up to a large group of one subcommunity belonging to multiple locations (e.g. adolescent students within the age group of 12–15 years from various schools of Mumbai), etc.

Flowchart 3.3: Communities related to specific contextual factors

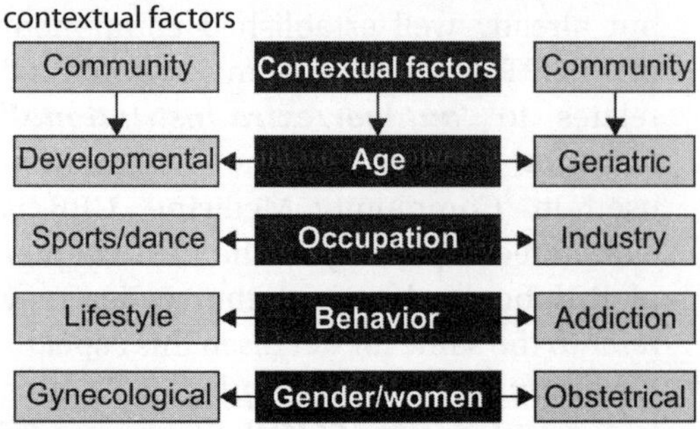

With reference to the Flowchart 3.3, certain examples are given here to simplify communities and their subcommunities covered under a specific contextual factor:

- ***Age related:***
  - ***Community:*** Pediatric/developmental: Subcommunities: neonates/children going to play school/students from primary schools/students during maturity/children belong to tribal areas.
  - ***Community:*** Geriatric: Subcommunities: Young old/Middle old/Old-old/Elderly from rural area/Institutionalized elderly.
- ***Occupation related:*** This contextual factor is strongly influenced by biomechanical impact. The communities 'sports' and 'dance' relate mainly to 'occupational activity' even though both are basically ***recreational*** activities.
  - ***Community:*** Industry: Subcommunities based on specific occupational activity: Executives/clerks/computer operators/security persons/transporters/labor staff
  - ***Community:*** Sports: Subcommunities based on specific type of sports: sprinters/marathon runners/swimmers/hockey players/gymnasts/wrestlers
  - ***Community:*** Dance: Subcommunity based on specific style of dance: Bharat natyam/Kathak/Salsa/Lokanatya (Tamasha) etc.
- ***Behavioral:***
  - ***Community:*** Lifestyle related: Subcommunities: Sedentary/Physically active/mentally stressed
  - ***Community:*** Addictions: Subcommunities: smokers/alcoholics/consumers of narcotics and drugs.
- ***Women's health related:***
  - ***Community:*** Gynecological: Subcommunity: Young women with PCOD/Climacteric/menopausal women

- *Community:* Obstetrical: Subcommunity: antenatal/puerperal/postnatal (after 6–8 weeks postpartum).
- ***Other co-morbid factors:*** This contextual factor is not shown in the Flowchart 3.3. since 'Age' which is one of the co-morbid factors is already included. However, as an option, 'Other co-morbid issues' can be included **as Fifth contextual factor** in which two major communities can be included such as:
  1. ***Community:*** Diabetic population, since its prevalence is tremendous in our country. Its subcommunities can be—i. Juvenile diabetics, ii: non-insulin dependent diabetics, and iii: Insulin dependent diabetics
  2. ***Community:*** Physically handicapped: This community should mainly include ***Paraplegics*** as its main subcommunity because it exists in large population globally and forms various national/international groups related to sports activities. Similarly, institutions offering exclusive care to this subcommunity (Paraplegic homes) also exist.

Major Difference Between PPCPT and Other Clinical Specialties in Physiotherapy

The major component of PPCPT is 'Community Physiotherapy'(CPT) which refers to ***'Population'*** right from its ***healthy*** and ***asymptomatic*** status; whereas, other Physiotherapy specialties deal with ***restorative*** care of an ***individual*** with ***established health issue***. Further, the risk factors to be dealt in CPT relate to ***various Contextual factors*** (age, gender, occupation and lifestyle, etc.) rather than any ***pathology of specific system*** (musculoskeletal, neurological, cardiopulmonary, etc).

However, the **'CBR'** component of this clinical specialty ***OVERLAPS*** with ***all*** the other clinical specialties of Physiotherapy.

Strategies of Management in Community Physiotherapy

Conduct of survey (reader can refer to the model of formats given at the end of the chapter).

Conduct of survey is essential to assess the extent of exposure of a known health risk issue within a specific subcommunity at specific (intra/extra-institutional) location(s). It is to be conducted in a following sequence:

- ***Goal[s] selection:*** e.g. To assess the prevalence of hypomobility following mismatch between growth of bones and soft tissue during height spurt among adolescent students (subcommunity) belonging to XXXX school(s) [location(s)].
- ***Type of survey:***
  - Population survey which needs some communication with population.
  - Environmental survey needs observational strategies.
  - ***Population survey:***
    - ***Selection of Location(s):*** To access the target population (e.g. Mahila Mandal, old age home, primary/secondary school, etc.)
    - ***Selection of mode:*** i. To select the mode of survey based on the cultural dimensions, level of literacy and feasibility (e.g. if door to door survey is planned). ii To prepare a specific tool for collecting data (e.g. validated questionnaire).
    - ***Approach to community:*** If the location for survey is situated within any institution then informed consent from the chief administrator is necessary (permission is required from the Principal of the school for the study of prevalence of childhood obesity, among students of that school). Whereas, for any outdoor/field survey, it is necessary to communicate with the local

leaders, politicians who have an ability to motivate the community and obtain the necessary consent and background information needed as per the objectives (e.g. cultural dimensions about health behavior of a religious community for the objective of formulating interventional services in obstetrical care).

- ***Environmental survey*** to be conducted if need, e.g. indoor and outdoor environment of school to assess in terms of facilities for physically handicapped students. Detailed format needs to be prepared for specific observation related to respective risk factors.

Conduct of survey and data analyses to determine outcome (models of formats for conducting survey are given at the end of the chapter).

Education: Communication with respective leaders/administrators/motivators, etc. regarding the outcome of survey (extent of exposure, statistics of population falling under various stages of exposure).

To create awareness about the consequences if risk factors are neglected.

Intervention program development: Intervention planning regarding patient education, training of target group or care givers should be done in consultation/collaboration with respective community leaders which enables better acceptance and compliance.

Conduct of intervention:

- Patient education including motivation for necessary lifestyle modification. Initial training with further home program if need be, ergonomic advise, special instructions on 'Dos and Don'ts'.
- Education and Training of Health workers and care givers/motivators from family.

Evaluation → Pretest evaluation → post-test/intervention evaluation → data analysis for assessing outcome measure.

Follow-up survey to assess impact of intervention

To interact and facilitate the Community Group in each of the above: The readers are recommended to refer to SF 36[16] and prepare the evaluation format for assessing constructs of activity limitations and participation restriction as per their own discretion.

SUMMARY

This chapter gives comprehensive outlook for prevention practice, Concepts of Functional Diagnosis and Community Physiotherapy, interlinking all under the umbrella of a new clinical specialty in Physiotherapy-'Prevention Practice and Community Physiotherapy'. The formats provided at the end are just the models hence reader is advised to prepare own need based assessment sheets as and when required.

REFERENCES

1. Constitution of the World Health Organization. In: World Health Organization: Basic documents. 45th edn. Geneva: World Health Organization; 2005.
2. Public Health Agency of Canada. What determines health? Available at: http://www.phac-aspc.gc.ca/ph sp/determinants/determinants-eng.php. Accessed October, 2010.
3. McDowell I, Xi G, Lindsay J, et al. Mapping the connections between education and dementia in the elderly. J Clin Exp Neuropsychol. 2007;29:127-41.
4. World Health Organization. Closing the gap in a generation: health equity through action on the social determinants of health. 2009; Available at:http://www.who.int/social_determinants/thecommission/finalreport/en/index.html. Accessed January, 2010.
5. Helman C. Culture, Health and Illness, 5th edn. New York: Oxford University Press; 2007.
6. Health Canada. Health Canada's gender based analysis policy. 2000; Available at: http://www.hc-sc.gc.ca/hl-vs/pubs/women-femmes/sgbapolicy-politique-ags-eng.php. Accessed July 28, 2011.
7. Porta M. Dictionary of Epidemiology. New York: Oxford University Press; 2008.
8. Green L. National Policy on the Promotion of Health. Int J Health Educ. 1979;22:161-8.
9. Gofrit ON, Shemer J, Leibovici D, et al. Quaternary prevention: a new look at an old challenge. Isr Med Assoc J. 2000;2(7):498-500.
10. Last JM. A dictionary of public health. New York: Oxford University Press; 2007.
11. The WHOQOL Group. The World Health Organization Quality of Life Assessment (WHOQOL). Development and psychometric properties. Soc Sci Med. 1998;46:1569-85.
12. Centers for Disease Control and Prevention. Measuring healthy days: Population assessment of health-related quality of life. Centers for Disease Control and Prevention, Atlanta, Georgia, 2000.
13. Gandek B, Sinclair SJ, Kosinski M, et al. Psychometric evaluation of the SF-36 health survey in Medicare managed care. Health Care Financ Rev. 2004;25(4):5-25.
14. McHorney CA. Health status assessment methods for adults: past accomplishments and future directions. Annual Rev Public Health. 1999;20:309-35.
15. Selim AJ, Rogers W, Fleishman JA, et al. Updated U.S. population standard for the Veterans RAND 12-item Health Survey (VR-12). Qual Life Res. 2009;18(1):43-52.
16. https://en.wikipedia.org/wiki/SF-36

INDUSTRIAL SURVEY

[Mark √ where ever relevant]: Urban/Urban-rural [slums]/Rural/Tribal

Location/address: ______________________________

1. **ACCESS ROAD broad enough for**–truck/tempo/car/2 wheeler/two persons/one person

   A. **Terrain:** Concrete/tar/tiled/wet mud/dry mud/sand/pot holes

2. **Surrounding:** Sea/lake/jungle/garden-park-farm/barren land/main road/railway track/Airport/railway station-yard/dockyard/warehouse/shed for poultry–cattle/structure under construction/housing colony-residential area/scattered/school/community hall/cinema theater/market/mall/huge dumps/open drain–nullah/putrefying garbage in open bins–scattered/dirty water collection/Other______________

3. **Housing[factory]: Material** manufactured ______________________________

   [A] Byproducts causing potential health hazards: No/Yes ______________________________

   [B] Construction: Planned concrete/barrack/temporary tin shed/open shed/open unsheltered area

   [C] Flooring: Cemented/tiled/mud/wooden/uneven natural terrain; Risk of fall due to slippery cluttered terrain–too many obstacles while crossing

   [D] Lighting: Adequate/Not adequate

   [E] Ventilation: Central AC, Cooler, Fans; Ventilation: Adequate/Not adequate

   [F] Toilets: [a] Provided/Not provided; [b] If provided: i] adequate–not adequate, ii] Western-Indian, iii] Clean–dirty

   [G] Drinking water: a] Electronic Filters—Hygienic–not hygienic; b]-Clean water cans containing edible water/non-edible water containers/No supply

4. **Prevailing pollution:** Yes-Noise/air: dust-strong odor of chemicals-paints-drugs–asbestos/vibrations/Other ____________/Not perceived, **Refuse:** Stored in closed—Open bin/cluttered, **a] Disposal of waste**–satisfactory/unsatisfactory: Piled up dumps–open drainage–contaminated water collection

5. **RISK AT WORK:**

   [A] Direct contact: Sharp tools/crushing machinery/paints–chemicals–poisonous items: No/Yes; If yes then protective devices provided/not provided

   [B] Fall from height due to suspended seat: No/Yes; If Yes then protective harness provided/not provided

   [C] Fall from height due to climbing on narrow-ramp-steps without railing: No/Yes

   [D] Fall of heavy objects on head: No/Yes; If yes then helmet provided/not provided

   [E] Injury to eyes: No/Yes; If yes then protective glasses provided/not provided

   [F] Musculoskeletal injury while maneuvering heavy objects: No/Yes; If yes then protective gadgets provided/not provided

   [G] Other ________ Protective device provided/not provided

6. **WORK ERGONOMICS: Job profile:** Executive level I-II/Table [computer] work/Technical/Security/Transport/Skilled work/heavy labor/Farming/Cottage industry/Collecting jungle products/Other ______

[A] Job description ____

____

____

____

[B] Risk of fatigue due to

- **Sustained posture:** No/Yes: Seating ergonomics satisfactory/Not

  Satisfactory–Describe ____

  ____

- **Repetitive stress**: No/Yes: working ergonomics satisfactory/Not Satisfactory–Describe____________

  ____

- **Overuse:** No/Yes: Working ergonomics satisfactory/Not Satisfactory–Describe __________________

  ____

[C] Restricted freedom of movement due to crowding: No/Yes, **D] Desirable mechanization:** provided/not provided, **E] Breaks during duty:** Not provided/provided, Adequate/not adequate

[F] Leisure activities during breaks: provided/not provided

[7] EMERGENCY SERVICES: **A] Medical:** Yes/No, **B] Fire:** Yes/No, **C] Risqué operation** Facility-No/Yes, **D] Electricity failure:** Yes/No

[8] GENERAL CLENLINESS and HYGIENE: Good/satisfactory/unsatisfactory/poor

Domestic pests _ Rats–Rodents/lizzards/cockroaches/houseflies/mosquitoes

[9] WILD/STRAY ANIMAL THREATS: No/Yes–dogs/snakes/scorpions/other ___________

[10] Any specific observation:____

____

____

____

FAMILY SURVEY

[Mark √ where ever relevant]: Urban/Urban-rural/Rural/Tribal

Location/address: ____

1. **ACCESS ROAD--broad enough for**–truck/tempo/car/2 wheeler/two persons/one person

   [A] Terrain: Concrete/tar/tiled/wet mud/dry mud/sand/pot holes

2. **SURROUNDING:** Sea/lake/jungle/garden-park-farm/barren land/main road/railway tract/airport/railway station-yard/dockyard/warehouse/Shed for poultry–cattle/structure under construction/Industry: with-without chimney/scattered huge dumps/Cinema-community hall/market/mall/open drain–Nullah/putrefying garbage in open bins–scattered/dirty water collection/other ______________________

3. **HOUSING**: Bungalow/Well planned Colony/Overcrowded buildings–slums/single building–shanti/Well planned Cottage/Chawl–Barrack/other______________

   [A] Floor-Elevation level-ground/1st, 2nd, 3rd, 4th, >4th ____-/Elevator provided-Not provided–Total no. of steps to climb_____/Railing provided–Not provided

   [B] Level of main door—a] same/raised/below the level of outer access; b] If raised:-Steps–No/Yes–no. of steps _______/average height of step_____'/-Ramp—cement–wooden--/width ______ angle: steep/average/Railing provided—Yes/No

   [C] Height of main and other doors: Adequately high/low height

   [D] No. of rooms _________/Kitchen-independent/not independent

   [E] Space in each room-adequate for maneuvering aids: Tricycle–Yes/No, Wheel chair: Yes/No, Walker–Yes/No

   [F] Status of House: a] Floor: Tiled/cement/mud, **b] Walls:** Cement/only bricks/mud/cow dung/asbestos/tin/bamboo/wood, i] Status: well Painted–no leakage/plaster fallen/water leakage evident-slight-moderate–heavy, **c] Roof:** Cement/tin/asbestos/tree leaves/bamboo–wood, i] Status-Well covered/water leakage evident–slight-moderate–heavy; **d] Ventilation:** Good/satisfactory/unsatisfactory-windows per room ______________; **e] Light**–Natural adequate-not adequate/Electrical: adequate/not adequate-nil/other means

   [G] Kitchen: Separate–Yes/No; **a] Floor:** Tiled/cement/mud/cow dung, **b] Cooking Type:** On floor/platform, **c] Overhead storage:** Yes/No, **d] Smoke vent:** adequate/not adequate, **e] Drinking Water** supply: Inside/outside [distance____]/nil/Non-edible supply outside, **f] Fuel** for cooking: Gas/kerosene/wood–dried cow dung/charcoal

   [H] Bathroom: Washing—Inside/Outside-distance ___________ **a] Size** adequate for wheel chair-Yes/No, **b] Water supply:** Inside-continuous-intermittent/outside, **c] Drainage:** adequate/not adequate

   [I] Toilet a] Inside-Western–Indian/Outside–Indian [distance _________] i] Size adequate for wheelchair: Yes/No [ii] Water supply-inside: Yes/No; **b] Outside**-in/open: Distance _______ i] Access suitable for wheelchair/Crutch walking, **c] Sewage:** Closed drains/open drainage

[J] Refuse Stored: in Closed-Open bin/Cluttered **i] Disposal**–daily/alternate day/> 2 days

[K] Furniture: Cot [Yes/No]/Chair [Yes/No]/Stool [Yes/No]/Only floor activity

[L] Any means of recreation: TV/VCR/Radio/Nil

[M] Domestic pets: inside/outside the house: No/Yes–Type ________

[N] Domestic pests: Rats–Rodents/lizzards/cockroaches/houseflies/mosquitoes/snakes/Any other ___________

Observed ______________________ Reported_______________

[O] General Cleanliness and Hygiene in the house: Good/satisfactory/unsatisfactory/poor

[P] Hygiene of Patient: Good/satisfactory/unsatisfactory/very poor

[Q] Any specific observation: ____

____

MGM SCHOOL OF PHYSIOTHERAPY
KAMOTHE-NAVI MUMBAI

Name of the student: ____________________ Class: ___________ Date: ____________

SCHOOL SURVEY

[Mark √ where ever relevant]: Urban/Urban-rural/Rural/Tribal

Location/address: ____

1. **ACCESS ROAD--broad enough for–**School bus/tempo/car/2 wheeler/1-2 persons

   [a] Terrain: Concrete/Tar/Tiled/wet Mud/dry mud/sand/pot holes

2. **SURROUNDING-**Sea/lake/jungle/garden-park-farm/barren land/playground/main road/railway track/airport/railway station-yard/dockyard/Warehouse/Shed for poultry–Cattle/Structure under construction/Industry: No-Yes: __________ with-without chimney/cinema-Community hall/market/mall/scattered huge dumps/open drainage–nullah/putrefying garbage: in open bins–scattered/dirty water collection/Pests: rodents-mosquitoes–lizards/Animal threats: stray dogs–cats–monkeys–snakes–other______

3. **SCHOOL STRUCTURE: A] Type:** Concrete multi-storied building/Barrack//Shanti/Open If multi-storied: i] Total floors _______ ii] Elevator for students: provided/Not provided, iii] Railing at steps/ramp at main entrance: Yes/No, iv] Railing at steps for higher floors: Yes/No

   [B] Level of Entrance door and corridor —a] same/raised/below the level

   [C] No. of classrooms _______ Adequate/Not adequate ________________________________

   [D] Adequate size of door to maneuver a] Wheel chair: Yes/No; b] walker-crutches: Yes/No

   [E] Adequate Space in each class room: a] For no. of students: Yes/No; b] For moving with aids: i] Wheel chair: Yes/No; b: walker-crutches: Yes/No

   [F] Status of Corrior and Classrooms: a] Floor—tiled/cement/mud, **b] Walls**–cement/only bricks/mud/cow dung/asbestos/tin/bamboo/wood. Status: well painted–no leakage/plaster fallen/water leakage evident-slight-moderate–heavy, **c] Roof:** cement/tin/asbestos/tree leaves/bamboo wood. Status-well covered/water leakage evident-slight-moderate–heavy

   [d] Ventilation–Good/satisfactory/unsatisfactory----windows per classroom ________________

   [e] Light–Natural adequate/not adequate/Electrical: adequate/not adequate-nil/other means

   [f] Domestic Pests: No/Yes: Mosquitoes/houseflies/lizards/cockroaches/insects/bugs

4. **ERGONOMICS: A] Class ergonomics: a] seating for students:** satisfactory/not satisfactory

   ____

   [b] Furniture for teacher/administration: satisfactory/not satisfactory ____________________

   ____

   [c] Audio-visual aids: Adequate/Not adequate ________________________________

   ____

[B] Storage space for library/books/notebooks: Adequate/Not adequate____________________

____

5. **SEPARATE SPACE for: a] lunch break**–Yes/No, **b] Physical training:** Yes–adequate-not adequate/No; **c] For Indoor/Outdoor games**–Adequate/not adequate/nil
6. **DRINKING WATER: a]** Electronic Filters-i]-Hygienic/not hygienic, b] Clean watercans containing edible water/Non-edible water containers/No water supply
7. **TOILETS: A] Indoor:** Not provided/provided–a]-Adequate/Not adequate ________________ b] Clean–Yes/No, c] Continuous water supply-Yes/No, d] Space adequate to maneuver; i]-wheel chair:Yes-No/ walker–crutches–Yes/No, e] Western toilet provided–Yes/No
8. **REFUSE:** Stored in Closed-Open bin/cluttered **i] Disposal**–daily/alternate day/> 2 days
9. **SAFETY DEVICES:** a] Grilled windows with safety gate-Yes/No, b] Grilled corridors with safety gates–Yes/No, c] Security at main gate—Adequate/not adequate
10. **EMERGENCY SERVICES:** a] Medical: Yes/No, b] Fire: Yes/No, c] Electricity failure: Yes/No
11. **GENERAL CLENLINESS AND Hygiene:** Good/satisfactory/unsatisfactory/poor
12. **ANY OTHER**____

____

____

4

Physiotherapy in Primary Health Care: A Review on Global Perspective

Lata Shroff Parmar

HISTORY

'European colonial period' was the period from the 16th century to the mid twentieth century, during which time several European and some American powers established colonies in Asia and Africa. Historians distinguished different types of colonization after 1960's and studied the impact of colonization, which was wide and varied from advances to enslavement to exploitation. The Indian independence movement began probably much before 1857 until 15 August 1947, when India got independence from the British Rule.

In 1945 diplomats of various countries met to form 'United Nations', one of agenda was setting up a global health organization. Jawaharlal Nehru also was one of the members who gave his opinion in favor of starting World Health Organization (WHO).

On 7th April 1948, WHO's Constitution came into force a date now celebrated every year as World Health Day. It was set up with the fundamental objective of 'the attainment by all peoples of the highest possible level of health.' This lofty goal was coupled with an equally ambitious opening statement that defined health as 'a state of complete physical, mental and social well-being and not merely the absence of disease or infirmity.'

This definition, according to Rodolfo Saracci (1997), director of research in epidemiology, ran in to most serious problems, which impaired its guiding role especially when the conflict between health needs and resources became of paramount concern, nationally and internationally. In fact, a state of complete physical, mental, and social wellbeing corresponded much more closely to happiness than to health. These two words designated distinct life experiences.

Alejandro R Jadad and Laura O'Grady (2008) concluded that, 'any attempt to define health is futile; that health, like beauty, is in the eye of the beholder; and that a definition cannot capture its complexity. Further, he said 'We might need to accept that all we can do is to frame the concept of health through the services that society can afford, and modulate our hopes and expectations with the limited resources available, and common sense'.

Marcos Cueto (2004) has presented a historical study of the role played by the World Health Organization and UNICEF in the emergence and diffusion of the concept of primary health care during the late 1970s and early 1980s. The author writes about number of people from within the public health and outside the public health who influenced the emergence of Primary Health Care (PHC).

The first International Conference on Primary Health Care (PHC), meeting in Alma-Ata, between 6th and 12th of September in the year 1978, expressed the need for urgent action by all governments, all health and development workers, and the world community to protect and promote the health of all the people of the world, which is the fundamental right of all. Alma-Ata Declaration was the landmark declaration expressing the need of PHC, since then all the member countries have accepted this approach.

The declaration reaffirmed the definition of 'Health' and also that it was a 'human right'. It highlighted the inequalities between the developed and developing countries and declared it as unacceptable. Participation of people as a group or individually was declared as a 'human right and duty'. The state would have a role in attainment of Health that will permit and lead people of the world to socially and economically productive life by year 2000. PHC has since then been adopted.

The Alma-Ata institutionalization of PHC has strong socio-political influences; it emphasizes need to address the underlying social, economical and political problems of poor health. PHC emphasizes close link between health and poorer sector of the community, strong participation of people affected is essential.

WHAT IS PRIMARY HEALTH CARE

Primary health care is about shifting the focus 'upstream' that is, providing care before individuals get sick or injured and seek urgent medical intervention. Primary health care, for most people, is the first point of contact for the prevention, diagnosis, treatment and ongoing management of many conditions that might otherwise make enjoying life a little difficult.

In other words, PHC is also defined as *'Socially appropriate, universally accessible, scientifically sound first level care provided by a suitably trained workforce supported by integrated referral systems and in a way that gives priority to those in most need, maximises community and individual self-reliance and participation and involves collaboration with other sectors.'*

Primary health care ensures continuity and coordination of care for patients across the lifespan from pediatrics to geriatrics, from prevention to acute care, and from rehabilitation to end-of-life care. Primary health care (PHC) refers to an approach to health care that includes all services that play a part in health, such as income, housing, education and environment.

Thus, internationally, there have been different interpretations of what primary health care is, often as a result of political intent, with a large number of varying programmes being developed in the name of primary health care. The hope of primary health care was that it would address the economic reality of health care with an increasing shift to primary disease prevention and health promotion, promoting self-reliance.

Principles of PHC

The 1978 Declaration of Alma-Ata proposed a set of principles for primary health care. PHC should:

1. 'Reflect and evolve from the economic conditions and socio-cultural and political characteristics of the country and its communities, and be based on the application of the relevant results of social, biomedical and health services research and public health experience.
2. Address the main health problems in the community, providing promotive, preventive, curative and rehabilitative services accordingly.
3. Involve, in addition to the health sector, all related sectors and aspects of national and community development, in particular agriculture, animal husbandry, food, industry, education, housing, public works.
4. Promote maximum community and individual self-reliance and participation in the planning, organization, operation and control of primary health care,

making fullest use of local, national and other available resources; and to this end develop through appropriate education the ability of communities to participate.
5. Be sustained by integrated, functional and mutually-supportive referral systems, leading to the progressive improvement of comprehensive health care for all, and giving priority to those most in need.
6. Rely, at local and referral levels, on health workers, including physicians, nurses, midwives, auxiliaries and community workers as applicable, as well as traditional practitioners as needed, suitably trained socially and technically to work as a health team and to respond to the expressed health needs of the community.

There is a set of 'core activities', which were normally defined nationally or locally. According to the 1978 Declaration of Alma-Ata proposed that these activities should include:

- Education concerning prevailing health problems and the methods of preventing and controlling them
- Promotion of food supply and proper nutrition
- An adequate supply of safe water and basic sanitation
- Maternal and child health care, including family planning
- Immunization against the major infectious diseases
- Prevention and control of locally endemic diseases
- Appropriate treatment of common diseases and injuries
- Basic laboratory services and provision of essential drugs
- Training of health guides, health workers and health assistants
- Referral services
  - Mental health
  - Physical handicaps
  - Health and social care of the elderly.

HEALTH PROFESSIONALS TEAM-ROLE OF PHYSIOTHERAPY

Primary care is an integral component of primary health care, but the two concepts must be distinguished from one another. The term 'primary care' includes the diagnosis, treatment and management of health problems with services delivered predominantly by physicians. Alternatively, primary *health* care 'incorporates primary care, but also recognizes and addresses the broader determinants of health including population health, sickness prevention, and health promotion with services provided by physicians and other providers often in group practice and multidisciplinary teams' (Health Canada, 2000). The role of physiotherapy at the primary care level, which has traditionally been based on the biomedical model, is well supported by the literature. Also, physiotherapy, or physical therapy, is a health care discipline well positioned to take on an increased role in primary health care.

Determinants of health extend well beyond the domain of traditional health services. Governments have recognized that they need to work with local communities and be responsive to their differing needs. This involves governmental and non-governmental organizations (NGOs) and the private sector all working together, to address such wider determinants, if we are to see real health gains and inequality reduction across society. The team providing is a team of health professionals inclusive of physicians, nurses, dentists, social workers, occupational therapists, physiotherapists and pharmacy among others. To be effective, it is integrated with secondary and tertiary health care, education, work place, child welfare and criminal justice systems. Between 2004–2006, the Canadian physiotherapy association was one of the 10 associations that participated in an initiative 'Enhancing Interdisciplinary Collaboration in PHC'.

Lina Rodrigues de Faria and Camila Aloísio Alves, the authors comparing Brazil to Canada, say that the questions concerning the composition of primary care teams and integration among its members are subjects of discussion and debate, and that these could be areas of implementation and barriers to primary care. According to the Brazilian Ministry of Health, the practice of physical therapy must be part of the multidisciplinary home care team.

The literature has highlighted the multiple possibilities of physical therapy in PHC. Physiotherapists have an important role to play in the movement towards primary health care. This has been recognized by the World Confederation for Physical Therapy (WCPT) which advocates the provision of primary health care that is mindful of:

- Local culture
- Socio-economic and political circumstances
- Provision of equitable access for all to effective services.

Physiotherapists are encouraged to work with the relevant agencies to promote and facilitate the development of primary health care identifying the core elements of:

- Promotion of good health
- Prevention of health problems
- Treatment/intervention
- Rehabilitation.

To meet these challenges, the need for the development of new skills and the dissemination of new experiences during training should be emphasized. Knowledge of primary care proposals and the principles of the health care system, both on the part of the students, as on the part of teachers, should be encouraged in the classroom, but few curricula include courses focused on the actions of comprehensive health care. More attention is to be given to patients' perceptions about the impacts of their disease, the suffering, and the experiences of the patients and their 'ways of life.'

According to Lesley K Holdsworth and Valerie S Webster 2014, General Practitioner open access to physiotherapy was introduced as national policy in 1981 (DHSS, 1981). The benefits attributed to open access have included a reduction in: patient waiting time, the costs associated with drug prescribing, tertiary referral rates, patient non-attendance and costs to patients. Fewer physiotherapy contacts, patient preference and convenience have also been associated with open access. Accordingly, Lesley K Holdsworth and Valerie S Webster (2014) state that 'direct access to physiotherapy is an example of innovative primary care service provision that is feasible, acceptable to both users and providers and has major implications for general practitioner workload. Its efficacy however, should be evaluated in a range of settings before being universally introduced.'

Several authors have reported 'Physical therapists increasingly provide direct access services to patients especially with musculoskeletal conditions, and growing evidence supports the cost-effectiveness of this mode of healthcare delivery.' However, against these advantages is the potential disadvantage of an increase in total cost owing to a larger number of patients being treated because of improved access to, and awareness of, physical therapies. More importantly, there is doubt about the overall health benefit of some forms of physical therapy. In the future, it is important to evaluate the consequences of direct access, both on quality aspects and on cost-effectiveness.

In 2007, PHC resource guide was commissioned by Alberta physiotherapy association and Canadian physiotherapy association. This was to help the physiotherapists to integrate their services into emerging service models. Within a primary health care context, a physiotherapist's role is varied and continues to evolve. It includes diagnosis and treatment of acute and chronic conditions within the scope of practice, management of patients with chronic disease, education in disease self-management, case management, and participation in health promotion and injury prevention initiatives. Emerging roles include provision of education to and consultation with other health care professionals, and involvement in research and policy development.

The Saskatchewan Ministry of Health's Health Care System Framework indicates:

'A strong primary health care system provides access to high quality care delivered by a team of health professionals that meets the needs of patients and their families of all ages, in any health care setting.' Physiotherapists deliver effective *and* efficient care and can support high quality PHC through a variety of roles.

Examples include:

- Physiotherapy delivered in primary care settings such as community health centers, emergency departments and family physician offices;
- Physiotherapy as a resource for primary care physicians and/or nurse practitioners;
- Physiotherapists as first contact health care providers; and
- Advanced practice physiotherapist roles.

Early intervention promotes a child's growth and development and supports the family during the critical early years. Early intervention services are not a cure for disabilities or risk conditions; however, services provided during the first three years of life can have significant effects on the cognitive and social development of young children with disabilities.

Services may include: medical services, for diagnostic or evaluative purposes only, assistive technology devices/services, family training, counseling and home visits, audiology services, nutrition counseling, nursing, physical therapy, occupational therapy, respite, psychological services, social work services, speech-language pathology, others as needed.

Rehabilitation personnel, including physical and occupational therapists and mid-level rehabilitation workers, have been identified as being well placed to facilitate the prevention of tertiary disability, whereas physicians and nurses are perhaps more familiar with primary and secondary prevention (World Health Organization 1995a). However, physical therapists have a valuable contribution to make across all levels of prevention.

WCPT policy PHC Sept 2011 Physical therapist entry level education and continuing professional development opportunities need to adequately prepare and equip physical therapists to practice in a variety of settings for both urban and rural communities. These opportunities also need to ensure that physical therapists' roles as facilitators and educators of other health personnel are recognized. WCPT encourages its member organizations and physical therapists to work with governments, NGOs and disabled persons organizations (DPOs) to facilitate the development of primary health care and promote the contribution of physical therapists.

Physiotherapists impact quality of life and the cost effectiveness of care by:

- Providing early assessment and intervention
- Improving exercise tolerance and helping maintain or restore optimal function
- Assisting in the prevention and treatment of pain
- Promoting fitness, health and wellness
- Improving client satisfaction in care, including education and guidance on maintenance or improvement in overall function.

Early assessment and treatment by physiotherapists result in:

- Reduced volume of referrals to specialists
- Reduced wait times

- Increased likelihood that patients will achieve their treatment goals
- Reduced absenteeism from work (for musculoskeletal injuries)
- Better outcomes for the patient
- Cost-effective care and efficient use of health human resources.

It is worth noting, however, that the issues concerning the composition of health care teams are still an obstacle in the recognition of the role of physical therapy in primary care.

With Regards to India

Delivering primary health care in India is a challenging issue, especially to a large population. The problems could be multiple viz. delay in seeking help, non-compliance with the treatment, culture and religion influences, psycho-social factors, etc. The Indian health care system can be broadly categorized into government and private sector. The government provides all levels of health care, i.e. Primary Health Centers, Community Health centers, District hospitals, regional medical institutes to provide dedicated tertiary care level, Information, education technology (IEC) using the mass media, folk media and other communication to reach out to the community. There is also promotion of public-private partnership. All kind of health systems modern and alternative systems are promoted. Rehabilitation units are being encouraged to encourage domiciliary services.

According to Mane Abhay and Khandekar Sanjay 'ASHA' (Accredited Social Health Activists) becomes an inevitable component in providing primary health care to the village level by creating awareness on health and its social determinants. They have mobilized the community towards local health planning that increased utilization of primary health care and thus placed the health in the hands of the people. Finally, recognizing ASHAs and giving them a greater role in activism and advocacy would provide them with greater recognition in their communities. They play a potential role in providing primary health care at the village level. More than 6 years after the launch of the NRHM, the ASHA has emerged as a significant factor in improving the health situation especially among women and children. Further improving and strengthening of the program can bring India's targets closer to MDG.

In 2011, the 'operational guidelines 'national program for health care of elderly' (NPHCE), by the ministry of health and family welfare, with elderly persons above age of 60 approx exceeding to 12% of the total population, 8–10% expected to be bedridden, India has released this policy. The main objective of this is to provide easy access to preventive, promotive, curative and rehabilitative services for the elderly. The NPHCE envisages dedicated services for elderly at all levels of health care delivery system, along with provision of long-term and short-term training of health care professionals to address the health care of the elderly.

Amy Goddard, June 3, 2014 writes *'As experienced physical therapists (PTs), we know that PTs are grossly underutilized in managing especially musculoskeletal (MSK) patients. Physical therapy is typically introduced late in an episode after more than four physicians are involved in the management of the patient. Yet, clinical and health policy research shows a 'physical therapy first' approach is most efficient and cost effective. This primary care role must be obtained so we can better influence value in a changing health care environment, which is searching for alternatives to pharma and surgery.'*

Dr Pawan Kumar Directorate of Health Services, Govt of NCT of Delhi in conference presented a paper and stated 'Physiotherapists are committed to deliver the quality health care'. In recent era it is well recognized that rehabilitation services need to be integrated to primary health care system. Across the world, physiotherapists are valuable members of multidisciplinary teams, making an important contribution to health care through their health promotion, prevention, screening, as well as triage, assessment and treatment activities and are able to improve the health status of individuals across the lifespan.

At present physiotherapy services are mainly confined to tertiary health care level only whereas it has huge scope and potential in primary care also. Under umbrella of National Rural Health Mission (NRHM) all national health programs are being implemented through public health care delivery system in India like National Programme for Health Care of Elderly (NPHCE) and National Programme for control of Diabetes, Cancer, Stroke and Hypertension (NPCDCS) etc. Keeping in consideration, all programs and population size of rural India, there is huge potential and opportunities for delivering physiotherapy services under primary health care system which can be achieved by integrating the physiotherapy services at all levels of health care delivery system.'

Today in India 'direct access' to Physiotherapist is not uncommon; the awareness about Physiotherapy is fast growing, 'Physiotherapy camps' are successfully conducted all over the country and the feedback from these camps invariably is not only of increased demand but also of increased frequency. This involves governmental and non-governmental organizations (NGOs) and the private sector all working together. The philosophy of these Physiotherapy camps is to maximize the individual's potential functional ability by educational, preventive, promotive and physical means and thereby improve their quality of life. In addition to the camps, there are support groups, a number of Institutes provide voluntary Physiotherapy services at the nearby PHC's and man community extension centers where in Physiotherapy/ Rehabilitative services are provided to the people of surrounding villages. The idea of the Health Universities/Institutes adopting villages would probably work wonders.

Thus, in India the role of Physiotherapist is visualized to be vital at all levels of the health care system, however necessary steps with regards to integrating this at the entry level and advanced training is the need of the hour.

Author acknowledges and is very grateful to the scholars/authors/editors/publishers of all those articles, journals and books from where the literature for this has been reviewed and discussed.

BIBLIOGRAPHY

1. Alejandro R Jadad, Laura O'Grady. Editorial 'How should health be defined'? BMJ. 2008;337:a2900
2. Alma-Ata 1978. Primary Health Care: Report of the International Conference on Primary Health Care Alma-Ata, USSR, 6-12 September 1978. Jointly sponsored by the World Health Organization and the United Nations Children's Fund. WHO GENEVA 1978.
3. Amy Goddard. PTs must play a primary care role in health care delivery…2014. Go Sports Therapy. http://www.gosportstherapy.com/2014/06/03/pts-must-play-primary-care-role-health-care-delivery/
4. Dr Pawan Kumar. Directorate of Health Services. Govt. of NCT of Delhi. Role of Physiotherapy in Primary Health Care: Opportunities and Challenge. Conference paper : 2nd International Conference and workshop on Physical Therapy AIIMS 2013 organized by AIIMS, New Delhi, At AIIMS, New Delhi. https://www.researchgate.net/.../262179007_Role_of_Physiotherapy_in_Primary_Health
5. Durant TL, Lord LJ, Domholdt E. Outpatient views on direct access to physical therapy in Indiana. Phys Ther. 1989;69(10):850-7.
6. https://en.wikipedia.org/wiki/Postcolonialism
7. John D Childs, Julie M Whitman, Phillip S Sizer, et al. A description of physical therapists' knowledge in managing musculoskeletal conditions. BMC Musculoskeletal Disorder. 2005;6:32.
8. Kevin C Patterson, Rachel A Patterson. Direct Access to Physical Therapy in Michigan is Overdue. EDITORIAL. MSRJ 2013 VOL: 03. Issue: Fall epub September 2013; www.msrj.org
9. Leemrijse CJ, Swinkels IC, Veenhof C. Direct access to physical therapy in the Netherlands: results from the first year in community-based physical therapy. Phys Ther. 2008;88(8):936-46.
10. Lesley K Holdsworth, Valerie Webster. Direct access to physiotherapy in primary care: Now? - And into the future? PHYSIOTHERAPY. June 2004 https://www.researchgate.net/publication/223884727
11. Lina Rodrigues de Faria, Camila Aloísio Alves. On caring: Preliminaries of a comparative study of Primary Health Care in Brazil/Canada. Saude soc. vol.24 no.1 São Paulo Jan./Mar. 2015 http://www.scielo.br/scielo.php?pid=S0104-12902015000100072andscript=sci_arttextandtlng=en
12. Mane Abhay B, Khandekar Sanjay V Strengthening Primary Health Care Through Asha Workers: A Novel Approach in India. Primary Health Care. http://dx.doi.org/10.4172/2167-1079.1000149
13. Marcos Cueto. The Origins of primary health care and selective primary health care. Am J Public Health. 2004;94(11):1864-74.
14. Maria Sandborgh - Screening, Targeting, Tailoring, and Implementation in Primary Health Care. An integrated physical therapy and behavioural medicine approach to persons with persistent musculoskeletal pain. 2008. http://www.diva-portal.org/smash/get/diva2:171907/FULLTEXT01.pdf
15. Martin Chadwick, Amanda Brown, et al. Engaging in Primary Health Care. New Zealand Society of Physiotherapists. Primary Healthcare Working Party Report.
16. Moni Fricke. Physiotherapy and Primary Health Care: Evolving Opportunities. Department of Physical Therapy, School of Medical Rehabilitation, University of Manitoba.Manitoba Branch of the Canadian Physiotherapy Association, 2005.
17. National Programme for Health Care of the Elderly NPHCE :: Ministry... http://mohfw.nic.in/showfile.php?lid=1403
18. Ojha HA, Snyder RS, Davenport TE. Direct Access Compared with Referred Physical Therapy Episodes of Care: A Systematic Review. Phys Ther. 2014;94:14-30.

19. Position Statement. Primary Health Care. The Canadian Physiotherapy Association position statements. https://www.physiotherapy.ca/getmedia/623371a0-4f99-4b25-bbc9-2c58db9a6072/Primary-Health-Care_en.pdf.aspx.
20. Primary Health Care and Physiotherapy, 2008. Australian Physiotherapy Position Statement. https://www.physiotherapy.asn.au/DocumentsFolder/Advocacy_Background_Papers_Primary_Health_Care.pdf
21. Primary Health Care. A Resource Guide for Physical Therapists, May 2007, College of Physical Therapists of Alberta, Alberta Physical Therapy Association, Canadian Physical Therapy Association. https://www.physiotherapyalberta.ca/files/primary_health_care_1.pdf
22. Robert G, Stevens A. Should general practitioners refer patients directly to physical therapists? Br J Gen Pract. 1997;47(418):314-8.
23. Rodolfo Saracci. The world health organization needs to reconsider its definition of health. BMJ. 1997;314:1409.
24. Roger P Worthington, Anupriya Gogne. Cultural aspects of primary healthcare in india: A case- based analysis. Worthington and Gogne Asia Pacific Family Medicine., 2011 10:8 http://www.apfmj.com/content/10/1/8
25. SV Subramanian, Daniel Kim, Ichiro Kawachi. Covariation in the socio-economic determinants of self rated health and happiness: a multivariate, multilevel analysis of individuals and communities in the USA. J Epidemiol Community Health. 2005;59:664-669.
26. The Primary Health Care Provider's Role in Early Intervention. California Early Start. http://www.dds.ca.gov/earlystart/docs/HealthCareProvidersRole08.pdf
27. Value of Physiotherapy to Primary Health Care in Saskatchewan. http://saskphysio.org/images/stories/pdfs/Value_of_PT_to_PHC_in_SK.pdf
28. World Confederation for Physical Therapy 2011. http://www.wcpt.org/policy/ps-primary-health-care
29. World Confederation for Physical Therapy. (2003) Primary Health Care and Community Based Rehabilitation: Implications for physical therapy based on a survey of WCPT's Member Organisations and a literature review. WCPT Briefing Paper 1. WCPT: London.

PART II

Research Perspectives and Paradigms in Physiotherapy

5

Public Health as Profession: An Indian Physiotherapist's Perspective

Nalin Kumar

Abstract: Improving equitable opportunities for safe and healthy survival for all and Improving quality of life of communities has been a long thrust of the majority of Public Health programs. A review of the public health programs indicate that a majority of the public health programs where driven by medical models of care where the focus was on improving health outcomes, morbidity and prevention of mortality. Now, for majority of the high and middle income countries there has been a higher growth in the Gross Domestic Product (GDP), there public health systems have strengthened over time and the equitable distribution of food has improved over time. Together with better health and nutritional status it has resulted in increase in the average life expectancy of an individual in India.

Physiotherapists are one of the key professionals who have expertize working on the diverse age spectrum of children, adults to the elderly population in our societies. Conventionally the model of care by physiotherapist was considered as a client based or a clinical discipline. Taking a step ahead, there is a vast scope on how the clinical skilled physiotherapists may contribute towards improving the community health. The current chapter is one of the key contributing on providing insights on the linkages of public health profession to physiotherapy. The author has the opinion that the physiotherapists would play a key role towards combating the growing epidemic of non-communicable diseases, occupational and human work related disorders, improving quality outcomes solutions for diseases of long-term origin and life-long diseases/disorders, disability and elderly population globally.
Keywords: Public health, Health promotion, Prevention, Global burden of disease, Quality of life, Health system, Center for Disease Control (CDC).

Learning Objective
- Introduction to public health
- Understand public health as a career option
- The linkage of physiotherapy with public health
- Understand the different perspectives related to public health physiotherapy

INTRODUCTION AND DEFINITION

There are numerous available career options after a 4½ years of a bachelors in physiotherapy. Many times the students find difficult in the selection of an appropriate subject for masters. Majorly students like to opt for a career in a clinical subject. This chapter has been written for the graduate and postgraduate physiotherapy students to help them understand more on public health and its relationship with physiotherapy.

People's health of any country involves the population needs of the country and the wise full utilization of the available resources. India has been one of the countries to have a plural system of health care, where the ancient form of care was more related to the cultural and religious practices. The modern form of care related to the modern medical science also known as the western medicine. However, the modern medical science is the widely known form of medical care in the country.

There are numerous definitions of the two specialities. The most accepted definitions of the two are mentioned in following Table.

Definition

Public Health[1]
'Public health is the science of protecting and improving the health of families and communities through promotion of healthy lifestyles, research for disease and injury prevention and detection and control of infectious diseases. Overall, public health is concerned with protecting the health or entire population.' **Center for Disease Control**
Physiotherapy[2]
'Physiotherapy is a health care profession dedicated to rehabilitation, prevention and education. Performing these roles, physiotherapists take the holistic approach to the individual. Physical agents and specialized techniques are used to help the individual attain maximum functional independence with minimum complications. Education of patients, families, and the public plays an important role in both the rehabilitation and prevention aspects of physiotherapy.' **University of Manitoba, School of Medical Rehabilitation**

Indeed the two professions (Physiotherapy and Public Health) are not much different and one contributing towards the other. In other sense we may agree that physiotherapy contributes towards improving the health of the communities and thus leading to an improvement in the public health.

The content of the chapter has been written in the context to provide a link of the two professions. Though the two professions are looked as two separate professions, but a larger understanding of the public health can help to improve the quality of care plan and the work of physiotherapist.

THE TEN ESSENTIAL SERVICES OF PUBLIC HEALTH[3]

The Center for Disease Control and Prevention (CDC) Atlanta has developed the frameworks for the essential services which are accepted globally. These principles are:

1. Monitor health status to identify the community health programs.
2. Diagnose and investigate health problems and health hazards in the community.
3. Evaluate effectiveness, accessibility, and quality of personal and population-based health services.
4. Inform, educate and empower people about health issues.
5. Mobilize community partnerships to identify and solve health problems.
6. Develop policies and plans that support individual and community health efforts.
7. Assure a competent public health and personal health care workforce.
8. Ensure laws and regulations that protect health and ensure safety.
9. Link people to needed personal health services and assure the provision of health care when otherwise unavailable.
10. Research for new insights and innovative solutions to health problems.

PUBLIC HEALTH AS A CAREER OPTION[4]

Considering choosing a career in public health may not be a choice of many physiotherapists as there is not much known about it. A major part of any public health professional goes on finding solution to the disease or condition by prevention.

Choosing a career in public health would require further exploration to the probe that what would give us satisfaction as a professional. Would we like to bring change just at the individual level or we also want to bring a change at the larger community level. Do we want our approaches to the treatment to be stronger in terms of research? An answer to some of these questions would help to reflect back our decisions for our life that we take.

Apart from integration public health strategies at the clinical level, the students may opt for a separate job opportunities in the field or public health with the government, NGOs, international agencies, UN, etc. Here is the list of few of the different available jobs in the sector of public health. However, this is not an extensive list, there would be more available job profile. The different job titles are:

- ***Public health specialist or consultant:*** The consultant or specialist is responsible for a specific project. He is selected for his expertize over the subject. Majorly some of the key areas or such selection of candidates are maternal and child health, tobacco control, public health nutrition, community mobilization, reproductive health, adolescent health, disaster management consultant, environmental and climatic health expert, gender expert, behavior change communication, etc.
- ***Public health manager:*** The public health manager is responsible to manage a large program/project. Depending on the projects he would be responsible for the overall projects performance. He has to take the lead in areas of project management, financial management, meeting the deliverables, documenting the project process and reporting to donor agency.
- ***Epidemiologist:*** The position of epidemiologist is usually involved in a program or research project. He would be responsible for the design of research, research conduction, monitoring of research, data analysis and reporting.
- ***Health specialist:*** The health specialist is responsible to manage a public health problem for a certain geographic context. Some of the examples of position are a health specialist for promotion of school health as an intervention.
- ***Researcher:*** The position of a researcher exists in different research project at organizations, universities and international agencies. Based on the desired methodology the position of a qualitative or a qualitative researcher is required. Sometimes even both the skills may be an asset. The researcher is responsible for the research design, conduction and final report preparation within the set protocol.
- ***Behavior change specialist:*** There is high demand for the behavior change specialist. He uses the knowledge base of research, sociology, health psychology to design an appropriate method for behavior change in respect to a local public health problem.
- ***Community mobilization specialist:*** Mobilization of the communities for a desired positive health outcome is a difficult task to achieve. The expert uses the base of science and links the facts of science in a demystified way so that even the person with least literacy skills may be included in the strategy. Usually, community mobilization experts are part of large public health programs.
- ***Health promotion expert:*** Health promotion specialist is one of the least focused area of the current job market in India. However, looking at the demographic need and the estimated increase in the non-communicable diseases the position is expected to be in high demand in coming years.
- ***Healthcare in IT:*** A specialization in the area of health care IT is one of the newer areas of expertize where the corporate working in IT sector recruit individuals with an understanding of health.
- ***Health economics, financing:*** Specialization in the area of health economics and health financing is a area which requires mathematical skills along with the health programs knowledge. This may be done as a post masters specialization.

- ***Health planning and policy:*** The masters in public health planning and policy may be done at master's level. Opportunities for work exist in the government health department, National Health Mission and all public health/development programs.
- ***Monitoring and evaluation officer:*** Every public health program requires careful planning and monitoring. The process of monitoring has to be systematically planned before the conception of the project and it continues periodically, to assess the projects trajectory to its specified objectives and goals.

The Benefits of Having a Career in Public Health

There may be numerous benefits of choosing this career, a few of the benefits of the career for physiotherapist in the area of public health are mentioned here.

Along with treatment the physiotherapy may also work on the prevention of disease. Thus decreasing the economical burden on the family.

- Health promotion could be a part of the individual health program or a community health program.
- A degree in public health would help in understanding the effective treatment method by research and not adopting anything that is driven by the market.
- It would help in improving the quality of the individual treatment protocol.
- It would help in improving the efficiency of the performance of the individual.
- It helps to broaden understanding from societal perspective.
- Improving behavior change at individual level and at community level.
- It gives dual advantage of jobs. One the individual is a physiotherapist so may always get the job of a physiotherapist. However, a public health degree would help him in increasing the portfolio in this new area.

The Different Courses Available in Public Health[5]

There are various courses available in public health. A short description of the course is mentioned below:

- MD in Community Medicine or Prevention and Social Medicine (PSM)—available to individuals with MBBS.
- Master in Public Health (MPH) or Diploma in Public Health (DPH) recognized by Medical Council of India (MCI)—these courses intake majorly individuals with MBBS and conducted under government institutions.
- MPH under Christian Medical College/JNU/BITS Pillani etc. They require masters in respective subjects (allied health science). Recently, AIIMS Jodhpur has begun MPH to candidates with a 4 years bachelor in Health science.
- MPH under Tata Institute of Social Sciences (TISS) and other private and government universities in India—require a completion of any graduation.
- Postgraduate Diploma in Public Health—those individuals who do not have a 2 years' time may opt for this or those who do not wish to upgrade to a doctoral program.

Suggestion: A career in public health preferably should be adopted after 2–3 years of work experience. As this would help in understanding the health system and the different academic subjects along with understanding once own interest to opt for a profession for life.

Note: Distance education masters in public health is not recognized by University Grants Commission, India.

Preventive Health Perspective

We all know that 'Prevention is always better than cure'. A career in public health provides the opportunity to understand how we could stop certain diseases or occurrences. As if

Table 5.1: Examples of primary, secondary and tertiary preventions targeting individual populations

Disease	Intervention	Primary	Secondary	Tertiary
Backache in nurses	Individual	Assess, identify and give strengthening exercises for nurse at risk	Treat those who report back pain and train on correctional rehabilitation and home care	Prevention of deformity and secondary complication
	Population	Screen all nurses for back pain and provide correctional exercises to the high-risk nurses	Preparing home exercises video for nurses with back pain persistent	Prevention of deformity and secondary complication
Fall in adults over 60 years of age	Individual	Assess, identify and provide balance training	Provide support to those who need ambulatory devices and balance training	Prevention of deformity and secondary complication
	Population	Community screening for those at high-risk	Provide support to those who need ambulatory devices and balance training	Prevention of deformity and secondary complication

appropriate timely prevention is done by disease screening and prevention of harmful behaviors or risk factors the disease may be stopped or delayed or deformities/disability may be prevented. There are three stages of prevention[6] (Table 5.1).

Primary Prevention

Primary prevention is concerned with preventing the onset of disease; it aims to reduce the *incidence* of disease. This involves strategies that are applied before there is any evidence of disease or injury.

Example 1: Include protection against the effects of a disease agent, as with vaccination. It can also include changes to behaviors such as cigarette smoking or diet. The strategy is to remove causative risk factors (risk reduction), which protects health and so overlaps with health promotion.

Example 2: Targeting all target clients who may be attending the weight training session for a core strengthening exercise. At this time the disease has not occurred and the training of the core muscles would help in the prevention of the disease.

Secondary Prevention

Secondary prevention occurs after the onset of the disease and it uses procedures to detect disease and treat preclinical pathological changes, and thus controlling the disease progression.

Example 1: A pap smear test is used to screen for cancer of the cervix, or a prostate-specific antigen (PSA) blood test for prostate cancer; other instances include teaching people about the early signs of disease that they should watch for, and what type of treatment to seek. This is the task of preventive medicine.

Example 2: A 34 years old female patient approaches a physiotherapy clinic after pain in neck and arms. There is a constant dullness in the pain for last 10 days. The physiotherapist diagnosis the condition and confirms the diagnosis. Here the efforts would be directed towards restoration of the lost functions and prevention of deterioration of the condition.

Tertiary Prevention

Once the disease has been developed and has been treated in its acute clinical phase, this stage is focused to soften the impact caused by the disease on the patients function, longevity, and quality of life. Tertiary prevention may require modifying a risk factor like assisting a neurological patient.

Flowchart 5.1: A classification of preventive strategy

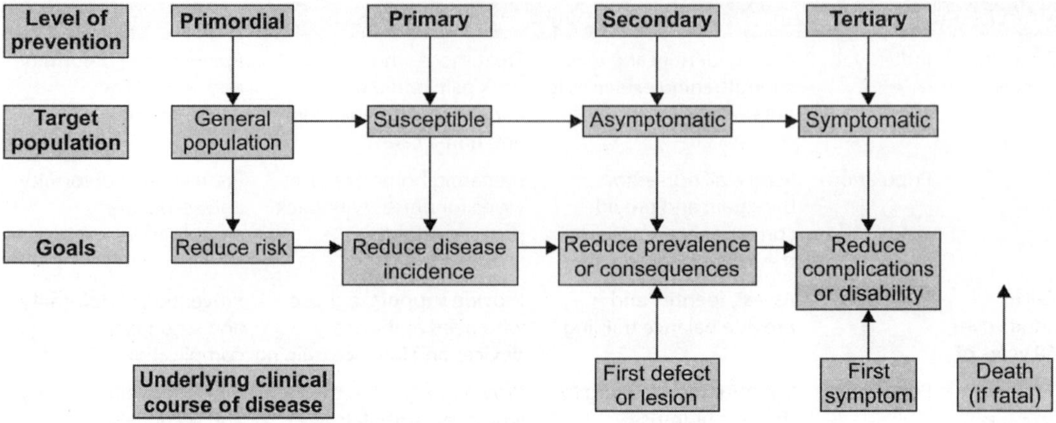

Source: https://www.med.uottawa.ca/sim/data/Prevention_e.htm

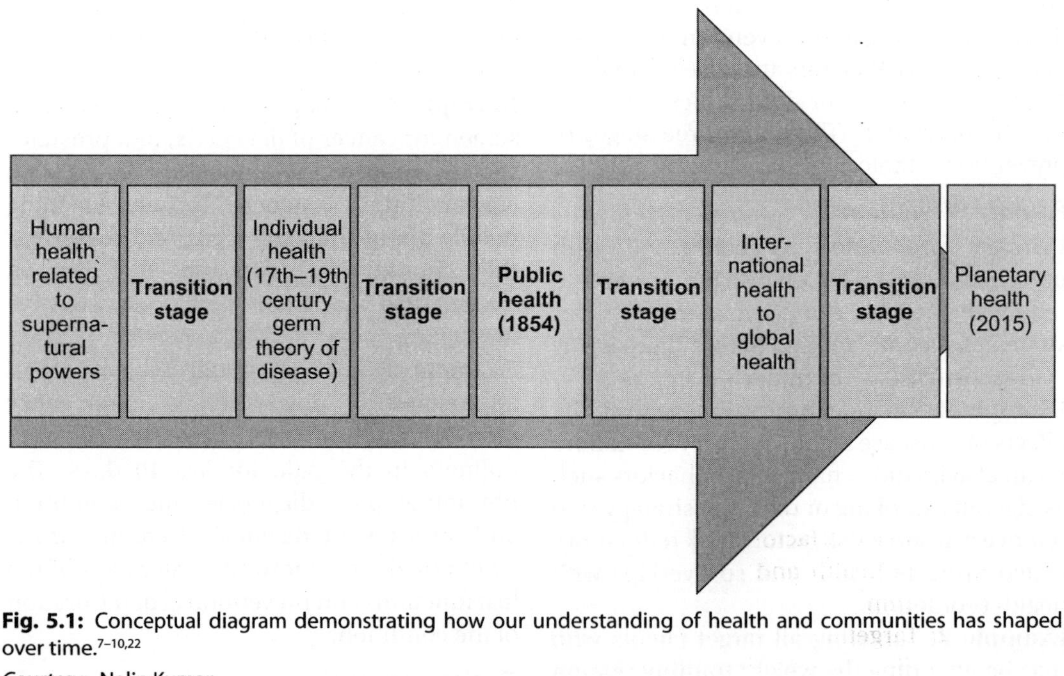

Fig. 5.1: Conceptual diagram demonstrating how our understanding of health and communities has shaped over time.[7–10,22]

Courtesy: Nalin Kumar

The strategies are focused on rehabilitation, assisting the patient to accommodate to his disability.

Example 1: There are environmental modifications and adaptations done for a child with cerebral palsy to accommodate his ability.

HUMAN HEALTH AND COMMUNITIES (CONNECTING THE PAST TO PRESENT)

There are empirical evidences which inform us about how the knowledge of health was available to the communities (Fig. 5.1). The evidences inform that the roots towards understanding the health of the communities were present in the past. The ancient civilizations of the Mesopotamia and the Harappan civilization they knew about how some of the determinants of the civic health were related to the health outcomes. Though, with time we have learned more and understood in a better way what seems to be integral in the public health planning and management. The recent development in public health is updated with high quality evidence it uses the integration of information from all the disciplines to solve the public health problems. The common tools used in public health are research, health policy, health planning, survey, monitoring and surveillance.

THE HISTORY OF PHYSIOTHERAPY IN INDIA[11]

Physiotherapy in India was provided as a certificate program during its initial years and form there it has grown to a degree program (4½ years) in Physiotherapy education. At that time polio was a huge epidemic and the profession had a huge contribution to the rehabilitation of the individuals affected by Polio.

There are three + 1 National Institutes in Physiotherapy and rehabilitation sciences. The national institutes are:

1. Swami Vivekananda, National Institute of Rehabilitation Training and Research (SVNIRTAR), Odisha-offers BPT, MPT
2. National Institute for Locomotor Disabilities (Divyangjan) (formally known as National Institute of Orthopaedic Handicapped), West Bengal-offers BPT, MPT
3. Pt Deendayal Upadhyaya Institute for the Physically Handicapped (formally known as Institute of Physically Handicapped), New Delhi-offers BPT
4. All India Institute of Physical Medicine and Rehabilitation (AIIPMR), Mumbai-offers Post BPT-Fellowship in Rehabilitation (Physiotherapy) and Master of Physiotherapy.

These institutes offered a Diploma (3½ years), to a BSc in physiotherapy and then upgraded to a BPT curriculum (4½ years). In the public sector there has been a large change also seen at that time where the medical colleges had been offering the BPT education. Certainly there were a huge number of physiotherapists which were trained by the private institutions. A lot of institutions have been setup in various states in India which have contributed by providing quality education to physiotherapist. But still in the low performing states which are poor in their health care delivery the physiotherapy colleges in the private or the government sectors is to name a few. This also shows the lack of will from the government or the private sector to invest in the area of people's well being.

There are majority of the institutions in private sector offering BPT/MPT/PhD program. From having a general set of skills now they had been specializing in the areas of musculoskeletal physiotherapy/manipulation therapy, neurological physiotherapy, pediatric physiotherapy, geriatric physiotherapy, cardiovascular physiotherapy, gynecological and obstetric physiotherapy, hand conditions physiotherapy, community-based rehabilitation, etc.

PERSPECTIVES TOWARDS PHYSIOTHERAPY

While understanding perspectives it is always important to know that with whose perspective we are referring too. I would further build upon the topic with examples and explaining the context around the perspective. A perspective building exercise is being considered as one of the highest level of evidence which requires more comprehensiveness, understanding of the topic, understanding of the problems, being unbiased and also to a great depth a lot of philosophical perspective too. Understanding, that I am not a subject expert and still, I am learning more about the subject, philosophy and about the science and society. The perspectives are not always the same, it also changes with time. Whatever, I am expressing as perspectives is just based on my learning's about the Indian social context and the relation of physiotherapy in the public health system over the years. I have known and learned from our senior professionals in the field. I express my apology, if at some point you may have any contradictory views. I have taken about 6 months to learn different subjects that would help me in bringing down the perspectives together along with my over 10 years of experience being a physiotherapist and having training in public health.

Perspective on Origin of Physiotherapy from East or West[23]

'All the independent health professions (Allopathic Medicine, Ayurveda, Homeopathy, Siddha and Naturopathy) have common strategy, i.e. to treat the **Pathology** and not the ***'Person'.*** Ours is the unique profession where we adopt a different strategy, i.e. we treat ***a person with pathology***, e.g. three persons with same pathology can have totally different intervention for functional independence. We have been using medical model for intervention so far hence could not establish ourselves as independent professionals. It is high time that we switch over from 'Medical' to ***'Social'*** model and conduct intervention based on the strategies that fit very well in the ICF model of WHO, i.e. in addition to the conduct of clinical examination, we must understand the 'contextual (internal and external/environmental) factors and by clubbing both we have to arrive at the ***'functional diagnosis'*** (Performance vs Capacity to function) and accordingly plan/execute intervention. Our ability to do 'Functional diagnosis' independently is the most powerful tool to establish ourselves as independent health professionals'.

Prof (Dr) Bharati Vijay Bellare, Mumbai

Although there exists many differences which divides the eastern and the western medicine. In the east the links between disease and human health was known, long before the origin of western medical science. In the east countries like China the diagnosis made in the Traditional Chinese Medicine (TCM) and acupuncture used meridians as one of the criteria to identify illness, along with the diagnosis of energy level (Yin and Yang). It was considered that any such imbalance in the energy level would lead to a disease. The treatment involved correcting the imbalance and the flow of energy by needling, moxibustion, cupping and by the use of Chinese herbal medicine.

In India there were several forms of medical care being given. The plural form of health care includes both the modern medical care and the Indian systems of care. The Indian system of health care are—Ayurveda, Siddha.[12] The concept on which the diagnosis in Ayurveda and Siddha was based on the science that the human body is made of three elemental substance the doshas (called the vata, pitta and kapha) and an imbalance in these elements may cause diseases. The diagnosis in this form of care was done by the pulse diagnosis, observation or stool, toilet, color, odor, etc. The treatment followed a prescription of change in life-style, diet pattern, herbal preparations and bahamas (powder). Siddha has the origin from Tamil Nadu and the training of Siddha is available in just Tamil Nadu as the literature of Siddha is in Tamil. The diagnosis of Siddha is based on Naadi (pulse diagnosis), Neerkuri (urine) and Neikuri (urine + oil).

The **germ theory of disease** was the main differentiation point between the east and the west. Now the western or the modern physician followed a scientific method of diagnosis by various scientific methods, tools and process. The treatment was followed by prescription of chemical drugs, hospitalization, surgery, radiation, etc. This is one of the most widely known form of care then any form of care from the east or any other part of the world.

Though there are many evidences available which informs about the origin of physiotherapy from the western medical science. Having the scientific base of physiotherapy as same as of the western medical science would always help it to be in an auto correction mode. However, there are numerous empirical evidence that exercises were as part of prescription much earlier than the western medical science. One of the earliest prescriptions of exercises was known by the Chinese physicians, where they prescribed 'Tai Chi' on their prescriptions.[20] In our own Indian Ayurveda, the physicians used to prescribe 'Yoga' as the form of exercises.[21] The exercise prescription by western physicians or modern medicine practitioners have been done only after the World War-II, when there were many casualties and exercises was known as a form of care and rehabilitation of the soldiers.

From an Equitable Health Perspective/ Primary Health Care

There are numerous evidences which inform that the people who are poor, the marginalized communities, the communities staying in distant areas, low resourced communities, aboriginals, the urban poor, women, disabled, people with long-term conditions, people with deformity and chronic conditions, cancer and HIV/AIDS have lower quality of life in comparison to their counterparts. The Alma-Ata Declaration[13] was the first time when distribution of equitable health services for the communities was perceived by the concept of primary health care. PHC were considered as the first contact point of the community for any of their health needs, which was available in their own communities. Since, then there have been various efforts done to make PHC more inclusive and available for the communities. From being an essential part of the health care system, were a majority of thrust was given on the primary health services, now in many countries physiotherapy is considered as a primary health care service.

Still in India the concept of PHC does not include physiotherapy services. People need to travel to a district hospital to receive physiotherapy services. Still equity in the distribution of the physiotherapy services has not been a concern for India which is the largest democracy in the world and has over 1.2 billion population (Census 2011). Not having such a provision leaves communities with restricted human functions and a decreased quality of life. There is economical loss related to this in the national Gross Domestic Product (GDP). It would be unwise to think of sustainable health care system, which does not look into the equity in the health care service provisions. There is a need to make efforts on how easily the communities may avail physiotherapy services in their own communities. This would ensure the adherence to the physiotherapy treatment and at the same time would help the communities to regain or return back to their usual life with less delay. Conditions were a long-term care is needed, may receive the treatment and rehabilitation services without compromising in the quality of services being offered to them.

Primary Health Care (PHC) is defined as: 'Primary health care is essential health care based on practical, scientifically sound and socially acceptable methods and technology made universally accessible to individuals and families in the community through their full participation and at a cost that the community and country can afford to maintain at every stage of their development in the spirit of self-reliance and self-determination. It forms an integral part both of the country's health system, of which it is the central function and main focus, and of the overall social and economic development of the community. It is the first level of contact of individuals, the family and community with the national health system bringing health care as close as possible to where people live and work, and constitutes the first element of a continuing health care process.'

(Declaration of Alma-Ata, International Conference on Primary Health Care, World Health Organization, Alma-Ata, USSR, 6–12 September 1978).

PHC is the essential health care clinic which is situated in the community, is easily accessible and acts the linkage to the community health needs. Though, the physiotherapy services are not being considered as part of the primary health care delivery system in India. Primary Health Care in Canada involves the public health care delivery system.

A physiotherapist supports individual and population wellness in their community by:*

- Promoting physical activity and overall health
- Preventing disease, injury, and disability
- Managing acute and chronic conditions, activity limitations, and participation restrictions
- Improving and maintaining optimal functional independence and physical performance
- Rehabilitating injury and the effects of disease or disability with therapeutic exercise programs and other interventions
- Educating and planning maintenance and support programs to prevent re-occurrence, reinjury or functional decline.

The following examples are some of the roles and activities of physiotherapists in primary health care:*

- Assessment, diagnosis, treatment including individualized exercise programs, self-management and education for patients with musculoskeletal complaints
- Assessment, diagnosis, treatment, education and management programs for incontinence and pelvic pain
- Assessment and treatment for those with neurological conditions such as stroke and Parkinsons
- System navigation assistance for those who need to access physiotherapy and other services in the community
- Mobility aids assessment and assistance in navigating funding options for devices
- Falls prevention programs including outreach programs in community
- Collaborative triaging for specialist care for musculoskeletal conditions
- Assessment and triaging for back pain including providing self-management program and education, referral to community-based treatment programs and identification of need for additional diagnostics, specialist referral
- Assessment, education, self-management programs and counseling for increased activity for those with obesity, pre-diabetes, diabetes, arthritis and other chronic diseases
- Facilitate linkages with community programs, assessment of appropriateness of programs for those with chronic conditions including pain management, providing counseling on safe participation for those with chronic conditions
- Pain management programs, counseling and education on self-management techniques for those with chronic pain issues
- Assessment, individualized self-management programs and treatment for those with mobility and pain issues related to cancer including those in palliative phase
- Support and education for caregivers for assistance of those with chronic diseases including prevention of injury programs for caregivers
- Return to work programs
- Individualized self-management and lung health programs which teach patients skills to manage their acute periods and

*By Ontario physiotherapist association[15]

counseling for those with chronic cardio-respiratory conditions such as asthma, chronic obstructive pulmonery disease (COPD) and deconditioning after illness

- Osteoporosis education and individualized self-management programs.

Health System Perspective of Physiotherapy

India has a plural form of health care where there is recognition of both the modern medicine and the traditional medical sciences. The recognized form of health care are:

1. Modern medical science (MBBS and BDS) and allied health sciences.
2. AYUSH (Ayurveda, Yoga, Unani, Siddha, Homeopathy)
3. ***Unrecognized form of care:*** Alternative medicines like bach flower therapy, acupressure, massage, acupuncture, electro homeopathy, magneto therapy, etc.

The Position of Physiotherapist in the Health Care System

Physiotherapist has been considered as an essential part of the health care delivery system. Now the role of physiotherapist is not just confined to the health system but they are also part of the educational system (Sarva Shiksha Abhiyan), their role also recognized by Ministry of Social Justice and Empowerment, Sports Ministry, Corporate Organization, various Civil Society Organizations, Agencies like the International and within various NGOs.

Within the health care system the physiotherapist are placed as the first point of contact under the national program for the health care of the elderly and the national program for the prevention and control of noncommunicable diseases (NCDs) under National Rural Health Mission (NRHM), at the Community Health Centers (CHCs). Although, their position within health system was conceived to be at the district hospital. The skills of physiotherapist are considered as an important skill and not they are part of the superspeciality hospital health care team. All the national institutes like the AIIMS, National Institute of Mental Health and Neuro Sciences (NIMHANS), Indian Spinal Injury Centers (ISICs) they all have the position of physiotherapists at the various department in the hospitals.

There are functional changes in our life as we develop more with time. With changes in human body either physiologically or pathologically, diseases, accidents or by ageing there is a change in our functional ability. Human functions are related to providing an individual with lot of confidence, pride and self-respect. Human functions are related to providing an individual with lot of confidence, pride and self-respect. We might not remember the very first day when we might have started using our hands to eat successfully as a developing child, but we surely notice the pride and dignity attached with this victory to feed self. Slowly with time the child learns more of the human functions and becomes as a self-conscious individual. By not providing the restoration of human functions, which might be possible we are taking away the pride and dignity of the individual. We are aware about the access barriers to the health care systems and the demographic and geographic location of the communities are quite dispersed. However, there also exist various other socioeconomic barriers to the access of the health facility which is far away from the communities. The location of CHCs or district hospitals is quite far off, which restricts the individuals towards access of the health care facility by a physiotherapist.

It is important for India to invest in making the increase in the health care expenditure as part of GDP. There is a need for increasing the proportionate distribution of the budget to the preventive and promotive health care. Physiotherapy as a health care profession has a major role in the disease prevention and health promotion. Integration of physiotherapy as part of the health care services would be an important step towards this. A primary health care center acts as a unit of care for about 30,000 populations for plain areas. By making physiotherapy services available at the PHC, the communities may easily adopt the service. Thus resulting in improved function, better quality of life and restoration of dignity to the individuals.

Health Promotion

One of the main targets of this chapter is to inform students about the curiosity to understand more on the aspects of the health promotion as a concept. The concept of health promotion advocates about the well-being of the individual in whatever stage he is in. This concept would need further exploration and I believe for many of the common diseases of the modern world have very common determinates which may be shared determinants.

WHO defines Health Promotion[14] as: Health promotion is the process of enabling people to increase control over, and to improve, their health. It moves beyond a focus on individual behavior towards a wide range of social and environmental interventions.

The Ottawa Charter for Health Promotion

In 1987, the Ottawa Charter for Health Promotion was prepared in an international conference (Fig. 5.2). The resulting Ottawa Charter proposed action 'to achieve health for all' by the year 2000. It included the following strategies:

- ***Building healthy public policy:*** This puts health on the agenda for all policymakers, directing them to be aware of the health consequences of their decisions.
- ***Creating supportive environments:*** This recognized the importance of environment for health, and proposed a socioecological approach to health (e.g. encouraging a family to support their relative who is trying to lose weight).
- ***Strengthening community action:*** Health promotion requires community empowerment and involvement in setting priorities, planning and implementing strategies to achieve better health.
- ***Developing personal skills:*** Health promotion supports personal and social development through providing information and enhancing life skills.
- ***Reorienting health services:*** Health promotion argues for shifting health resources towards a more equal distribution between health care and preventing disease. Essentially, health services should be expanded to include the four strategies above in addition to conventional medical care. Responsibility for health promotion services should be shared among individuals, community groups, health professionals, health services and governments.

With time know the profession having its strong deep roots in concept that was part of the oldest form of medical care and also adopts the modern scientific base. The profession has now taken a new shape, the followers of this form of care are now trained to diagnose, treat and rehabilitate. There was not much back when the effect of exercises was known to these professionals, but with the epidemic of non-communicable diseases. Globally, all states are concerned about this epidemic. There are for indicators mentioned by the United Nations high-level commission to combat NCDs (2011).[17] They are:

- Lifestyle modification
- Low intake of salt and cholesterol
- Prevent harmful use of tobacco and alcohol
- Increase in the level of physical activity.

Now, the role of physiotherapist has become more integral by not just treating the ailment, but also to provide health counselling about lifestyle correction, dietary intake, prevention of tobacco and alcohol along

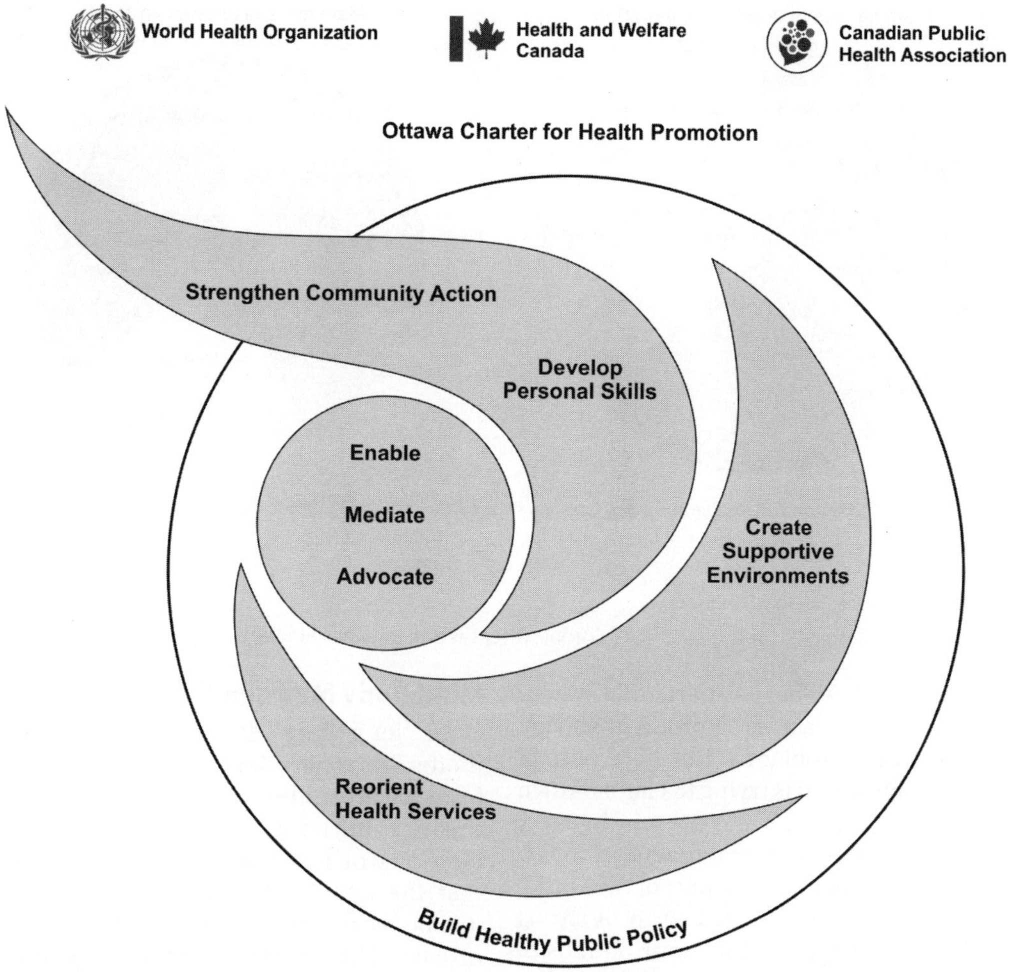

Fig. 5.2: The charter also identified seven prerequisites for adult health: peace; shelter; education; food; income; a stable ecosystem, and sustainable resources.

Source: http://www.med.uottawa.ca/sim/data/Health_Promotion_e.htm

with their own domain to increase physical activity.

Long back, there was not much known about the neuroplasticity, and it was known that as a person reaches his adulthood, not much could be done to train the individuals brain. It was perceived that the medical science could not do much in the adults with long-term conditions and were individuals have lost human functions. But with the information of how moderate physical activities, may contribute in the rewiring and relearning of the brain, has again strengthened the work what physiotherapist do in long-term conditions. The understanding of effectiveness of the treatment from a medical to a health care model has helped us again understand the different roles of other health care professionals and how we are contributing to the system. Even if we look at the systems theory and considering physiotherapy as a system of care. There are

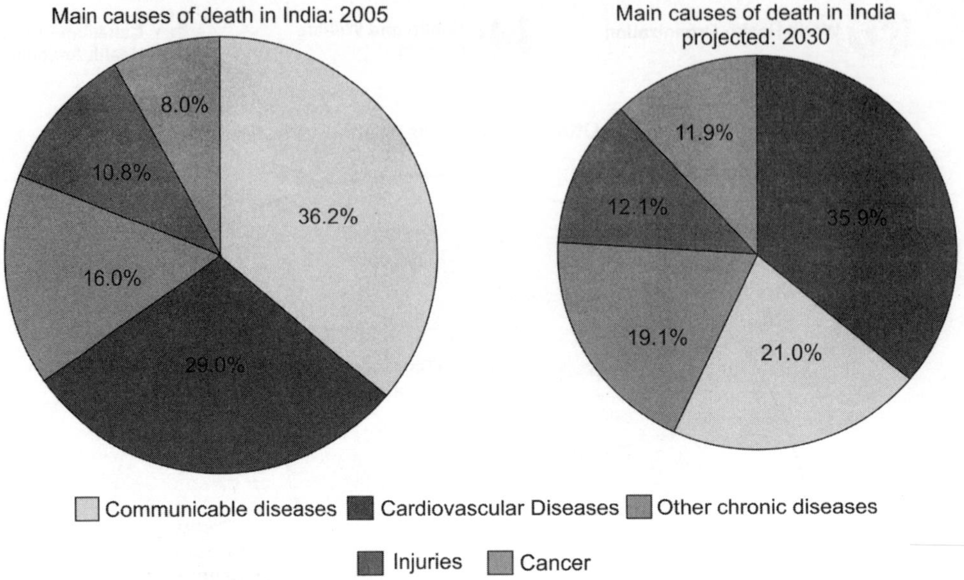

Fig. 5.3: Main causes of death in India

Source: Patel V, Chatterji S, Chisholm D, et al. Chronic diseases and injuries in India. Lancet. 2011;377:413-28.

not even evidences that any particular system has been able to act as a problem-solving to the existing problems. The best part of physiotherapy is as it is trying to claim its own form of system, though it is present in every system of health care being practiced today. No matter, whether it is any part of the world, or the practitioners with any form of strong belief on their systems. The contributions of the exercises towards human wellness are well advocated globally and there are large-scale movements to make exercises as part of daily routine.

One of the easiest concepts of health promotion is being adopted for NCDs by WHO is ABCDE.

A—Avoid alcohol

B—Be physically active

C—Cut consumption of salt and sugar

D—Do not consume tobacco and its products

E—Eat plenty of vegetables and fruits.

These concepts of health promotion may be appropriate in many of the diseases that we treat/rehabilitate.

Mind Body Medicine[16]

Until, long back the practitioners of the modern medicine did not focus on the mental form of care, rather it was more on the germ theory as the basis of care and treatment. The followers of mind body medicine advocate that the treatment of the disease may not just be based on the medical germ theory of disease. The treatment should also involve finding and treating the root cause. Many of the times the root cause apart from the germs are the psychosomatic illness, which are related to the patient's lifestyle or his mental status. The difference in the treatment of these physicians is they treat holistically—mind, body and soul. Here, there is an integration of the east and the west.

Societal Perspective

Many of the diseases, disorders and behaviors are based on the accepted social norm. As in many communities the social norm may be acting as a health benefit whereas for some other the social norms may also be misleading. These norms are decided by the community over the period of time as the community decides. Many of the positive social norms related to health are:

- It is considered important for the children to take care of their parents when they are aged. This is one of the accepted social norm with which there is a positive implications attached.
- In many families in India, for the first pregnancy the women visits to her parents place for the delivery. This is accepted as a social practice. With this practice it is being perceived that the women would get the best form of care at her parents place.
- The consumption of alcohol if being considered inappropriate in ISLAM, this is one of the accepted practices by the followers of Islam. Such a social norm prohibits the consumption of alcohol and decreases the health risk.

Social Norms with a Negative Health Implication

- In many communities the consumption of tobacco and alcohol is being considered as an acceptable social norm. There is always a risk attached if the social norms are approving behavior with health risks involved.
- In many communities visiting a Ojha, shrine or a traditional healer is being considered as an approved form of care. However, our role as health providers is not to break their belief but to make our clients of the scientific form of treatment for diseases and disorders. The both form of care may be continued. Unless the clients belief on other form of care is being dangerous, there should be efforts to work collaboratively on the both form of care.
- There are various health risks and taboos related to the menstruation. Various practices are often accepted by the community and then it becomes a social norm to practise it or not. This has a negative implication on the hygiene, poor health and overall wellbeing. Every individual has its own method to understand his/her health. Often it is based on cultural, societal factors and an individual/family and immediate environments plays a big role.

Life Span Perspective[18]

Major principles and techniques used in physiotherapy and public health are focused on the life span perspective. The scope of practice or intervention begins before the conception. While the public health principles in pregnancy are majorly directed towards making safe pregnancy and improving the quality of life of the mother undergoing pregnancy. In physiotherapy the efforts are directly towards the individual well-being and improving the quality of life of the mother by the antenatal exercises, advice on care during pregnancy. Slowly the two speciality focus on the different stages of life progressively from birth to the old age (Fig. 5.4). While the clinical physiotherapist focus on the care of individual clients, the public health professionals focus on the public health aspects of the issue.

Quality of Life Perspective[19]

Research on Quality of Life (QOL) provides patients and health care providers with vital information about the impact that disease and its treatment has on physical, functional, social and emotional well-being. QOL outcomes are also being recognized as important prognostic variables, which help to predict which patients are most likely to benefit from treatment. The physiotherapy treatment protocols are directed towards the outcome of benefiting the individual by improving his quality of life. In some conditions, diagnosis and treatment may reduce the impact of any particular disease without extending life expectancy or improving QOL. Older individuals with

Health Policy in Perspective: Physical Therapy as Partners in the National Health Agenda

Life stages	Infancy and childhood (birth–10 years)	Preadolescence and adolescence (11–17 years)	Young adult (18–44 years)	Middle-ged adult (45–60 years)	Older adult (61–74 years)	Senior and frail adult (75 years)
Health promotion	Motor development	Activity behaviors	Physical health with work and family	Active adult life	Independent living	
Prevention	Safe physical environment	Reduce unintentional injury	Health risk monitoring	Health risk management	Reduce unintentional injury for safe mobility in the home and community	

Life Course Consequences of Physical Inactivity or Poor Physical Health

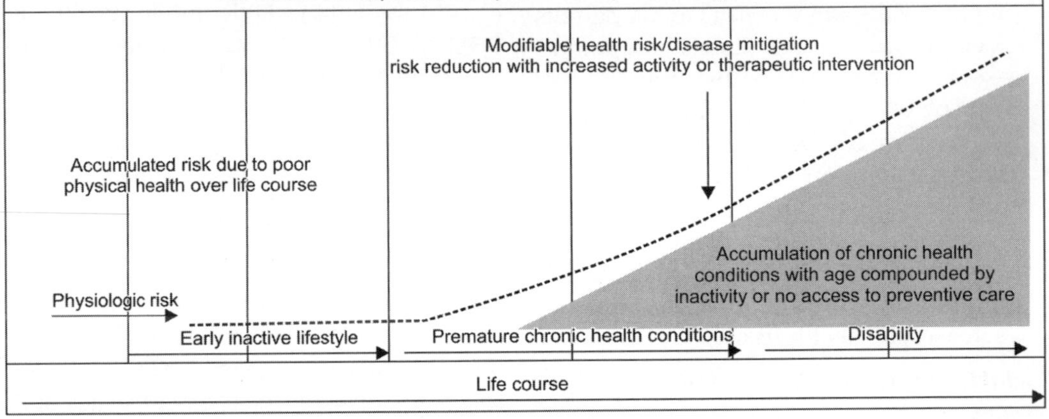

Fig. 5.4: Role of physical therapy in physical health promotion, disease mitigation, and injury prevention by life stage: age-related health risk by chronologic age

Source: Centers for Disease Control and Prevention. Life Stages and Specific Populations. Available at: http:/www.cdc.gov/Lifestages/. Accessed May 3, 2011.

multiple comorbidities may not benefit from treatments for a particular disease if competing health problems acts as a threaten to their life or reduce QOL.

There are different dimensions of assessing the QOL. WHOQOL-Bref dimensions are—Overall Quality of Life and General Health, Physical Health, Psychological, Social relationships, Environment.

8+1 Dimensions of Quality of Life[24]

This dimension towards the development has been decided for Europe and this would be a new dimension towards understanding the countries development. Based on academic research and several initiatives, the following 8+1 dimensions/domains have been defined as an overarching framework for the measurement of well-being. Ideally, they should be considered simultaneously, because of potential trade-offs between them:

- Material living conditions (income, consumption and material conditions)
- Productive or main activity
- Health
- Education
- Leisure and social interactions
- Economic and physical safety
- Governance and basic rights
- Natural and living environment

+1 Overall experience of life

The concept of QOL has been helpful in understanding the care in long-term

Table 5.2: Evidence supporting the role of physiotherapists in primary health care

Opportunity	Evidence
System effectiveness Research has shown that physiotherapy diagnosis and evidence-based treatments are effective and cost-efficient in treating a variety of physical health problems.	Strong evidence was found to support physiotherapy at the PHC level for the following conditions • Arthritis[26-29] • Coronary Heart Disease[30,31] • Chronic Lung Disease[31,34] • Incontinence[31,34] • Diabetes[31,34] • Osteoporosis[31,34] • Fall prevention[32] • Low back pain[31,34] • Total hip and knee replacements[32] • Urinary incontinence[31,32]
Cost effective methods of delivery	Cost-effective rehabilitation treatments include self-care education, group exercise, walking programs, strength training, hydrotherapy, splinting, adaptive equipment, postural training, and home adaptation[36]
Other conditions where with supporting evidence for physiotherapy	• PTs assume many roles within primary health teams that maintain an evidence based approach to health care delivery and collaborative interprofessional care.[37] • Imbedding PTs into a primary health care teams is ideal. Considerations for the most optimal health care delivery model for different communities and populations served is needed.[38]
Effectiveness of physiotherapy in primary health care settings	• Decreased wait times for surgery, increased return to work, fewer emergency room visits, fewer imaging studies and increased patient satisfaction[32] • Physiotherapist's monitoring of patient function through EMR in primary care can increase activity levels[33]
Physiotherapists in program design for obesity	Strategies to manage childhood obesity; target family and child. Physiotherapists have skills to design effective programs[34]
Reduced use of other health services	Stanford University which is renowned for their model for chronic disease management found rehab program resulted in reduced use of health services saving $780/patient[35]

Source: Physiotherapists in Primary Health Care. Ontario Physiotherapists Association, Canada. https://opa.on.ca

conditions and in concepts related to the end of life care or conditions in which there might not be a significant improvement. In 1997 the Institute of Medicine report on 'Approaching Death' identified six elements of quality end-of-life care:

- Overall quality of life
- Physical well-being and functioning
- Psychosocial well-being and functioning
- Spiritual well-being
- Patient perception of care
- Family well-being and perceptions.

Quality end-of-life care in the world is a large-scale problem that admits of no simple solutions. However there is a need to recognize quality end-of-life care as a global public health and health systems problem.

Cost-effectiveness Perspective[25]

For majority of the public health intervention to be effective, it requires there the minimum risks involved with its scalability, the intervention is simple and it gives effective solution and the intervention to be scalable. Based on the community needs many of the interventions are locally adapted to suit the audience.

Many of the evidences to support the cost-effectiveness of physiotherapy has been documented by the Ontario Physiotherapy Association. The details of the cost effectiveness are as follows:

'The department of physiotherapy (DPT) is one of the very few fully autonomous institutes in India. This means that physiotherapists can evaluate and address patient delivery on their own without any supervision by physicians. The DPT, Swami Vivekanand National Institute of Rehabilitation Training and Research (SVNIRTAR) is also one of the very few institutes that is engaged in an exclusive manual therapy practice. Persons with mechanical pain symptoms are assessed functionally. The ultimate goal of our department is to improve the functioning of the patients. This grossly contraindicated with the medical model of rehabilitation, where patients are treated for a diagnosis rather than functioning.'

Dr PP Mohanty PhD
Patitapaban Mohanty

CONCLUSION

Having known all this the question arises again. Is physiotherapy from east or west? We are the believers of the germ theory of disease and we also practice the traditional form of exercises as part of our treatment protocol. We are an evolving form of medical care and we accept newer forms of treatment with a scientific base, which are majorly non-chemical (pharmacological) or surgical.

'India has great potential here, given there are avenues for expanding the scope of practice of physical therapy, which has become more challenging in higher income countries.'

Elizabeth Dean, PhD, PT
Professor, Department of Physical Therapy,
Faculty of Medicine,
University of British Columbia, Canada

REFERENCES

1. CDC definition of Public Health. Available from: http://www.cdcfoundation.org/content/what-public-health.
2. Definition of Physiotherapy. University of Manitoba. Available from: http://www.umanitoba.ca/rehabsciences/pt/.
3. Ten Essential Principals of Public Health. Available from: http://www.cdc.gov/nphpsp/essentialservices.html.
4. Career in Public Health. Available from: http://www.explorehealthcareers.org/en/field/11/public_health.
5. Different courses in Public Health. Available from: http://www.nhsrcindia.org/index.php?option=com_content&view=article&id=289&Itemid=683.
6. Levels of Prevention. Available from: http://www.med.uottawa.ca/sim/data/Prevention_e.htm.
7. Belief-and-the-healing-arts-of-ancient-civilizations. Available from: http://www.wrf.org/ancient-medicine/belief-and-the-healing-arts-of-ancient-civilizations.php.
8. Germ Theory of Disease. Harvard University. Available from: http://ocp.hul.harvard.edu/contagion/germtheory.html.
9. Cholera. Available from: www.choleraandthethames.co.uk.

10. Theodore M Brown, Marcos Cueto, Elizabeth Fee. The World Health Organization and the Transition from 'International' to 'Global' Public Health, American Journal of Public Health. 2006;96(1): 62–72.
11. Shimpi A, Writer H, Shyam A, et al. Role of Physiotherapy in India—A Cross-sectional Survey to Study the Awareness and Perspective among Referring Doctors. Journal of Medical Thesis. 2014;2(2):11-15.
12. Ministry of AYUSH. Available from: www.indianmedicine.nic.in.
13. WHO called to return to the Declaration of Alma-Ata. Available from: http://www.who.int/social_determinants/tools/multimedia/alma_ata/en/index.html.
14. Health Promotion. World Health Organization. Available from: www.who.int/topics/health_promotion/en/
15. Ontario Physiotherapy Association. Available from: http://www.opa.on.ca.
16. Center for Mind Body Research. John Hopkins Center for Mind-Body Research. Available from. http://www.jhsph.edu/research/centers-and-institutes/johns-hopkins-center-for-mind-body-research/
17. United Nations High-level meeting on non-communicable diseases. Available from: http://www.un.org/en/ga/president/65/issues/ncdiseases.shtml.
18. Katherine J Sullivan, John G Wallace Jr, Margaret E O'Neil, et al. A Vision for Society: Physical Therapy as Partners in the National Health Agenda. 2011;91(11):1664-72.
19. Kaplan RM. Quality of life: an outcomes perspective. Arch Phys Med Rehabil. 2002;83(12 Suppl 2): S44-50.
20. Alice Jones, Margot A Skinner. Special Paper. The Current Status of Physical Therapy in China. Chinese Journal of Rehabilitation Medicine. 2013;28(6).
21. Denise Rankin-Box. The science of yoga-what research reveals. Elsevier, 2015.
22. United Nations Sustainable Development Goals. 2015. Avaliable from: http://www.un.org/sustainabledevelopment.
23. Physiotherapy/Physical Therapy. Available from: https://www.physio-pedia.com/Physiotherapy_/_Physical_Therapy.
24. Quality of life indicators - measuring quality of life. Euostat online publication. http://ec.europa.eu/eurostat/statistics-explained/index.php/Quality_of_life_ indicators_-_measuring_quality_of_life.
25. Physiotherapists in primary health care. Ontario physiotherapy Association.
26. Cott C, Devitt R, Wong R, et al. A Client-Centerd Health Service Model of Primary Health Care and Rehabilitation for Arthritis, 2005.
27. Fricke M. Manitoba Branch of the Canadian Physiotherapy Association and the College of Physiotherapist of Manitoba, Physiotherapy and Primary Health Care: Evolving Opportunities, 2005.
28. MacKay C, Devitt R, Soever L, et al. ACREU, An Exploration of Comprehensive Interdisciplinary Models for Arthritis, 2005.
29. Roddy E, Zhang W, Doherty M, et al. Evidence-based Recommendations for the Role of Exercise in the Management of Osteoarthritis of the Hip or Knee – The Move Consensus, Rheumatology,. 2005; 44(1): 67-73.
30. Restall G, Leclair L, Fricke Moni. Integration of Occupational Therapy and Physiotherapy Services in Primary Health Care in Winnipeg, School of Medical Rehabilitation, University of Manitoba, 2013.
31. Lacima RM, Pera M. Combined Fecal and Urinary Incontinence–An Update, Current Opinions in Obstetric Gynecology: 2003;15:405-10.
32. Richardson J, Letts L, Wishart L, et al. Rehabilitation in Primary Care: National and International Examples and Training Requirements, Ontario, Canada, 2006.

33. Richardson et al. BMC Family Practice 2013. http://www.biomedcentral.com/1471-2296/13/29.
34. Nick Kates. Provincial Lead, Quality Management Collaborative for Ontario's Family Health Team Accelerating Primary Care, 2008.
35. Stanford School of Medicine: Chronic Disease Self-Management Program. Information available at: http://patienteducation.stanford.edu/programs/cdsmp.html.
36. Cheryl Cott, Rachel Devitt, Rosalind Wong. ACREU: A Client-Centred Health Service Model of Primary Health Care and Rehabilitation for Arthritis, 2005;20.
37. Dufour SP, Lucy SD, Brown JB. Understanding Physiotherapists' Roles in Ontario Primary Health Care Teams. Physiotherapy Can. 2014;66(3):234-42.
38. Cott CA, Mandoda S, Landry MD. Models of integrating physiotherapists into family health teams in Ontario, Canada: challenges and opportunities. Physiotherapy Can. 2011;63(3):265-75.

6

Research Methodology in Community Physiotherapy

Pavithra Rajan

Keywords: Research, knowledge dissemination, statistics, pilot study

■ INTRODUCTION

Research is key to evidence-based practice in community health. The advances and the new methods of treatment in physiotherapy that have been adopted are only after it has been tested and approved through research. Hence, research plays a very important role in furthering of the profession of physiotherapy and creating a separate platform for recognition of this profession as an important entity in the field of allied and public health.

Certain concepts of research need to be revised before going ahead with the research design, statistics, drawing inferences and scientific writing for a hopeful publication in a good journal for knowledge dissemination. They are discussed as follows.

■ POPULATION

Population is defined as the entire community that is of interest. For example, if we wish to conduct a study on underprivileged urban slum school children, this forms the population of interest. Other examples would be postmenopausal women in India, HIV/AIDS children in Africa, school children in Maharashtra, etc. All the members in a population cannot be part of a research study because it is not feasible to contact each and every person for data purposes. Hence, we recruit a 'sample' of the population.

■ SAMPLE[1]

Sample is the representative portion of the population. For example, if we wish to study the incidence of urinary incontinence in all the post menopausal women in India, it is not feasible as we might not be able to reach each and every woman in the country. For the purposes of this study, we recruit some postmenopausal women and get the information about urinary incontinence. This forms the 'sample' that is representative of the population of interest. How many women do we recruit and from where and how, are questions that are answered in the following sections. We study the sample to get an idea about how the pattern is in the population.

■ PARAMETER[2]

A parameter describes the characteristic of a population. Sample is used to understand population parameters. For example, if a sample is correctly chosen, it can tell us many things about the population. In a study if we find that school children at urban slum areas in five cities in Maharashtra report backache, it can be concluded that urban slum school children in the state of Maharashtra have backache.

Please note that a population parameter is *always unknown.* It can only be known if we perform a complete study of the entire population. The concept of statistical inference is important for this reason.

STATISTIC

A statistic describes the characteristic of a sample. This is used to describe the population parameters. Certain limitations of this statistical inference need to be noted. Firstly, since sample is only a small part of the population, the numerical values of a sample are not expected to give true information about a population. Secondly, the observed value of a statistic depends on the particular individuals chosen to be a part of the sample. Finally, if the research study is repeated over multiple times, there might be some variability in the statistics obtained.

Consider this example. We are interested in studying the prevalence of backache among farmers in the state of Maharashtra. This is our population of interest. For this purpose, we *randomly* chose 10 districts out of 35 districts in Maharashtra. It is found that 80% of the farmers report backache (study 1). Now, if we were to perform the same study and randomly chose 10 other districts (study 2), it is highly unlikely that the percentage of farmers with backache would be exactly 80%. This is because the second study will not have the same farmers as the first study. Even if we performed the study in the same districts as study 1 after a year, we might not end up with the same percentage; farmers might have moved to other districts or might be unavailable during study. New farmers might have moved to the sampled districts- there could be many reasons. It is only after repeating this study in number of samples that we could probably come closest to the exact percentage of farmers reporting backache in the state of Maharashtra.

Sampling or the method of choosing a sample is very important for reasons discussed above. There are certain advantages and disadvantages of sampling.

Advantages

- Sampling is cost effective as compared to recruiting each individual in the population of interest.
- Since the number of individuals in a sample is far less as compared to the population, field work and analysis of results is faster.
- Usually, most of the times student research projects involve use of samples, since data collection, and analysis can be done with minimal help.
- A study can be detailed and designed as per the interest of the student, if sampling is done. In population studies, detailed and specific information is difficult to obtain in a limited time-frame. Good quality research findings can be done using a sample.

Disadvantages

- The chances of errors in sampling are high, if proper methods are not followed. If the sample has lot of errors, we might not be able to obtain population parameters using such a sample.
- The advantages of sampling are more than disadvantages. Hence, sampling is considered the ideal way to perform research.

Methods of Sampling[3]

Sampling can be either random or non-random. Random sampling means every individual from the population of interest has equal probability of being selected in the sample. A non-random sample means every individual does not have an equal chance of being selected. In research, most of the times, random sampling is done. Each type of sampling is used based on certain characteristics of the population like enumeration of the target population, cultural and geographical characteristics, literacy levels, language issues, to name a few.

Types of Random Sampling

- ***Selection of simple random sample:*** A simple random sample can be selected using lottery method or use of table of random numbers. In lottery method, every individual is numbered on an identical piece of paper. These pieces are folded similarly and mixed well before a draw. There is a table of random numbers which can be used for simple random sampling.
- ***Systematic sampling:*** Consider this example. There are 500 farmers in a district in Maharashtra and we wish to take a sample of 100 farmers. So the sampling interval is 5 (500/100 = 5). This means every 5th individual will be chosen in the sample. A number is randomly chosen between 1 and 10. Suppose this number is 4, the sample will consist of the 4th, 9th (4 + 5), 14th (9 + 5), 19th and so on. It has been argued by few statisticians that this method, though convenient, is not completely random since it is the first individual that is randomly chosen. The rest are chosen depending on the first individual's number. Hence, this type of sampling is also called quasi-random sampling.
- ***Stratified random sampling:*** Stratified random sampling is used where the population is divided into groups and sub-groups and simple random sampling is done from each group. This type of sampling is commonly encountered in preventive and community physiotherapy. Consider the earlier example where we wish to study backache in farmers in the state of Maharashtra. The state of Maharashtra is divided into 35 districts. These districts form the strata. Now from each district, we can randomly select the required number of farmers.
- ***Cluster sampling:*** This type of sampling is the easiest. If we were to use cluster sampling for understanding the number of cases of backache in the farming profession in Maharashtra, we would randomly select few districts and include **all the farmers** in those districts. This method is less random as compared to stratified sampling. In addition, this type of sampling might not be as representative of the entire population as stratified sampling.
- ***Convenience sampling:*** Convenience sampling, as the name suggests, depends on the convenience of the physiotherapist who selects the sample. This is one of the easiest and most commonly used methods of sampling in community research. However, such type of sampling is not very representative of the population. Hence, it should be avoided.

Sample Size

In research, it is not always possible to know the population size which could help in sample size determination. In such cases, there are two ways to calculate the sample size.

- ***Use of estimates from previous research:*** New research usually arises from the unanswered questions from previous research. Thus, the sample size for a study which is an extension of the previous study can be calculated using the parameters or statistics from the previous research. Literature review also helps to understand the previous research done in the field of interest and most of the studies also use statistics and parameters from similar studies in other states or countries.
- ***Pilot study:*** In certain research, previous research studies may not contain the required parameters or statistics for sample size calculation. In such cases, it is always best to do a 'pilot' study or a mini-study to check the feasibility of the proposed study. For example, the number of cases of backache in farmers in Maharashtra can be piloted in one of the cities in the state among 20–30 farmers. Based on these

findings, the actual sample size needed for the proposed research can be calculated.

Designing a Study in Community Physiotherapy

Designing a study involves many steps. Firstly, a research statement or a hypothesis needs to be developed. This can be done based on experience or area of interest. During undergraduate studies, it is difficult to gain enough experience to develop a hypothesis. However, intensive reading of literature can help to arrive at a broad area of interest. For example, we are interested in studying the prevalence of musculoskeletal aches and pains in urban slum school children in India. A hypothesis can be developed based on this broad area. There is high prevalence of musculoskeletal aches and pains in urban slum school children in India.

The second step after developing a hypothesis is to calculate the sample size. After literature review, you will realize that there are hardly any published studies that have looked at this topic. So, we are left with no choice but to conduct a pilot study. For a pilot study, usually convenience sampling is used. So, you decide to visit the nearest urban school for slum children.

By far, most of the research in community physiotherapy starts with a questionnaire or focus group discussion. A questionnaire needs to be developed to be able to collect the required data. The data can be collected through surveys or direct observation (Table 6.1). Direct observation is however expensive and respondent bias is high. However, the success of data collection lies in the tool used for data collection. Hence, drafting a good questionnaire and conducting a focus group discussion are important. Certain points in this regard have been given as follows:

Drafting an Effective Questionnaire

- The success of a questionnaire depends on how well it is developed and the extent to which the willingness of the respondents is secured.
- The form and tone of the questionnaire should make up for the missing personal element, especially in self-administered questionnaires.
- It is necessary to take the respondents into confidence so that they furnish correct information. One of the ways to do this is avoid asking the name of the respondent in the questionnaire.
- Prior to drafting a questionnaire, the purpose of the research needs to be outlined and the ideal data that is to be obtained must be set out in detail.
- Number of questions should be less. This provides an incentive to the respondent to take part in the questionnaire study and return it back on time.
- The sequence of questions is important and should be done as per the purpose of the study and the nature of participants.
- Questions should be short and simple to understand.
- At first, the identification questions (age/sex/city/occupation, etc.) are asked followed by closed-ended questions (using yes-no options), finally ending with open-

Table 6.1: Survey methods for literate population

Type of survey	Advantage	Disadvantage
Postal survey	Easy to administer	Expensive; postal delay and no guarantee about entire coverage; low response rates; no face-to-face interactions
e-Mail	Low cost	Low response rate; no face-to-face interactions
Telephone	Higher and quick response [Cell phone technology]	Expensive than postal and e-Mail surveys; no face-to-face interactions

ended questions (what is your opinion about).

- Necessary instructions should be provided to the respondents so as to ensure easy understanding and more cooperation.
- Likert scale can be used in a questionnaire to test the frequency of a particular response.

Here are some examples:

For instance, a. Sensory/Perception, e.g. Kindly comment on the following statement: 'I feel good about my work on the job.' Do you--------i. Strongly agree, ii. Somewhat agree, iii. Neither agree nor disagree, iv. Somewhat disagree, v. strongly disagree; b. Motor Ability: e.g. Can you travel in a bus comfortably?, i. Always, ii. Frequently, iii. Sometimes, iv. Rarely, v. Never

Grading of answer depends upon positive or negative questions.

- Questions should be so framed that the answer is objective in nature. For example, instead of asking how do you travel to school and giving a blank space to respond, the same question can be reworded as:
  How do you travel to school? (Tick only one that is appropriate)
  School bus ☐
  Walk ☐
  Family vehicle ☐
  Other ☐
- Questionnaire should look attractive.
- If possible, one or more cross-checks should be introduced in the questionnaire to check for accuracy of replies.
- Questions requiring calculations should be avoided. For example, instead of asking the annual salary of a person, his monthly salary can be asked and later multiplied by 12 to obtain the annual salary.
- Sensitive questions for instance, about income, drug use and sexual activity, to name a few, should be put at the end of the questionnaire.
- *Questionnaire must be pre-tested.* A pilot study should be conducted with the questionnaire on a small group. This will help identify the lacunae and also increase the response rate, if the shortcomings of the questionnaire are addressed. Greater co-operation from the respondents in the actual survey can be ensured.

Focus Group Discussion[4]

Focus Group Discussions is used to gather data from a group of respondents usually with experiences in the field of interest. This is similar to a group interview, where the research physiotherapist has a list of questions that s/he wishes to get answers for. The major advantage of this type of data collection is that most of the times, the respondents give more information than is anticipated and this could lead to a better understanding of the problem. This is a limitation of questionnaire method since the respondent answers only the questions that are asked. Focus group discussions need a well-trained physiotherapist who can 'lead' the discussion so to avoid straying from the topic of interest. In addition, monetarily, these are costlier than questionnaires since there needs to be videotaping or audio taping of the session in order to note down the responses.

Focus group discussions usually have more open ended questions than close ended, as opposed to questionnaires that have more close ended questions. Depending on the hypothesis and the topic of interest, some researchers use both focus group discussions as well as questionnaire method, as opposed to either one.[5,6] For example, a pilot focus group discussion can be conducted in order to understand if musculoskeletal aches and pains are reported by urban slum children. If there seems to be a higher prevalence, then the data can be collected using questionnaires in the sampled schools.

To conduct a Focus Group Discussion, we need to first identify a target group. The group needs to be assembled together. For example, in a village, a festival day can be chosen to conduct the discussion or a monthly meeting day, when most villagers are anticipated to come. Once this is done, a local community member is required to be present during the discussion. Special consent needs to be taken from the respondents in case videotaping or audio taping is done. Once the Focus Group discussion ends, the data can be used to understand the topic of interest.

Process of Knowledge Dissemination

Once the tool is ready, we approach the sample, i.e. urban slum school children. Once the data is collected after seeking necessary permissions and ethics approvals, this data is used for analyses. Our primary purpose is to check the prevalence of self-reported cases of musculoskeletal aches and pains in these children. In this sample, we find that 75% of the students report backache and only 25% report neck pain. Based on the findings of this pilot study, we can narrow down the hypothesis to focus on backache or we might retain the broader question of studying all the musculoskeletal aches and pains in these children.

Once the pilot study is done, we pick a sampling technique. Since our population of interest is all slum children of school going age in India and India is already divided into states and union territories, we can perform stratified random sampling. Based on the pilot study, we calculate the sample size 'n'. There are 29 states and 7 union territories, giving a total of 36 strata. Now, in order to get a sample size of n, we randomly choose children from these 36 strata. Now the size of each stratum is different so the sampling has to be proportional. However, this is beyond the scope of this Chapter. Once we get our desired sample of *n* students, we perform the necessary statistical analyses to arrive at conclusions.

This same study can be done in one particular state of India, say Maharashtra using the same sampling technique. However, at state level, the strata will be districts. Similar approaches can be used for other community studies to be conducted at village levels with tribal communities or in cities with industrial cases and so on.

The end of research is knowledge dissemination. The findings from this study need to be disseminated through conferences and journal publications. Further, public awareness and patient education follows along with face-to-face interactions. Use of print and electronic media to disseminate results is also commonly used. In addition, outreach programs for intervention and follow-up can be done through rehabilitation camps.

Public awareness can be created through face to face interactions commonly undertaken by local governments, NGOs and educational institutes, especially for illiterate population. The response rates are very high and good for data collection involving complex matters. However, this method is very expensive. The commonly used modes for creating public awareness are:

1. Illustrated lectures
2. Meetings (e.g. FGDs)
3. Street plays
4. Group Discussions and Debates
5. Social gatherings/community functions
6. Door-to-door campaigns
7. Local self-governed meetings

Print media and publicity materials have been used for large populations. Although this mode is expensive and mostly limited to the literate, they have shown promising results. The commonly used modes of print media and publicity materials are:

1. Notices
2. Posters
3. Cartoons
4. Photographs
5. Exhibitions
6. Films
7. Documentaries
8. Short messages on leaflets
9. Tickets (bus and cinema)
10. Shopping bags

11. Banners
12. Displays at public and sport events

Electronic media like TV and radio, as well, have been used with good results. While it can reach the remotest population and repeated easily, responses cannot be judged.

Importance of Research in Clinical Practice (Evidence-based Physiotherapy)

The progress of any profession is dependent on research. The concept of evidence-based practice has become commonplace in physiotherapy. One of the most important components of evidence-based practice is clinical evidence tested through research. It has been seen that western physiotherapists use a mix of personal experiences and research in the treatment of their patients[7]. What is currently being practised in India is not clear as there is seldom research in this regard. However, once the research is done, the findings could be incorporated on a smaller scale into clinical practice to check for external validity. Once the positive outcomes are established, policy changes at the treating physiotherapy center can be done to make the research findings available to every eligible patient/community[8,9] (Fig. 6.1).

Let's consider the example of a potter who comes from a local community. He complains of neck and shoulder pain bilaterally. The treating physiotherapist gives him electrotherapy and exercise therapy and home exercises. He reports reduced pain within two weeks. After a month, he comes back with two other potters from the community with the same complaints. This is a clear indication that there is some external factor, probably an ergonomic-related problem and modifications at workplace might need to be done along with physiotherapy treatment at the hospital. The attending physiotherapist conducts a research study on two groups. Group 1 is given only physiotherapy exercises at the hospital and home exercises. Group 2 is given workplace modifications in addition to the same treatment as Group 1. If the research findings show that Group 2 has better outcomes than Group 1, then physiotherapy protocol for Group 2 is further applied to other potters in local community and checked for effectiveness. If found effective, this protocol is incorporated into the departmental treatment sheets so that any potter seeking physiotherapy treatment will be given a comprehensive management that is not merely restricted to therapy at the hospital.

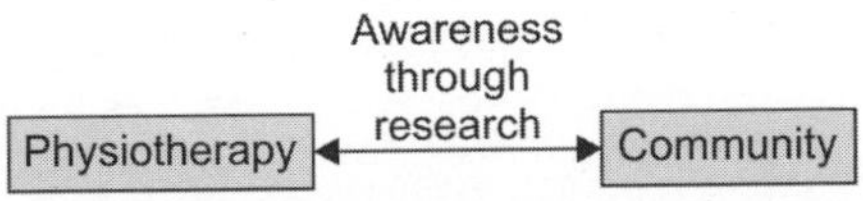

Fig. 6.1: Improved awareness between physiotherapy and community through research

This protocol could be presented at local and national conferences and wherever applicable, other treating centers could incorporate it into their regimen and check for effectiveness. Thus, a combination of personal experience and clinical evidence through research, also known as evidence-based physiotherapy, can help in better management and practice.

■ SUMMARY

This chapter gives a general understanding of the basic concepts of research in community health. Further, the need, importance and various methods of sampling commonly used in preventive and community physiotherapy research projects have been discussed. Designing a research study in community health and two important tools of data collection, namely questionnaires and focus group discussions are included in this chapter. In addition, the incorporation of research into clinical practice is described. After reading this chapter, the student should be able to conduct research in community health and practice evidence-based physiotherapy.

REFERENCES

1. Hassard TH. Understanding Biostatistics. United States of America: Mosby; 1991.
2. Beri GC. Business Statistics, 3rd edn. New Delhi: Tata McGraw Hill; 2011.
3. Gupta SP. Statistical Methods, 8th edn. New Delhi: Sultan Chand and Sons; 1976.
4. Rajan P. The application of focus group discussions and interviews in community physiotherapy. Disability, CBR and Inclusive Development. 2015;25(4):136-8.
5. Rajan P, Koti A. Musculoskeletal Health in Urban Underprivileged School Children in Western India. International Journal of Management and Behavioural Sciences. 2013;3:47-51.
6. Rajan P, Koti A. Cost effective rehabilitation: a cross sectional study on the underprivileged women and school children in the slums of Gujarat, India. International Journal of Advances in Management, Technology and Engineering Sciences. 2013;2(8:3):84-6.
7. Barnard S, Wiles R. Evidence-based physiotherapy. Physiotherapy. 2001;87(3):115-24.
8. WHO Commission on Social Determinants of Health. Closing the gap in a generation: Health equity through action on the social determinants of health. 2008.
9. Rose G. Sick individuals and sick populations. Int J Epidemiol. 1985;14:32-38.

PART III

Behavioral Key Components of Health and Wellness

7

Physiology, Strategies of Testing and Prescription of Physical Exercise

N Venkatesh

INTRODUCTION

The concept of exercise as the fundamental aspect of healthy lifestyle exists right from the time of ancient Greece. But in the current lifestyle, the physical inactivity prevails as a major public health risk factor. Physical inactivity leads paves way to cardiovascular diseases, Type-2 diabetes and certain types of cancers. Both physical activity and exercise play an important role in maintaining good health. Even though there is a lot of awareness about need for physical activity is present now, there is lack of translation of such knowledge while prescribing exercise as medicine by the health care professionals. Moreover, community level application such principles of training is sparsely prevailing and remains unknown.

Basic Concepts and Definitions

Physical activity: It is defined as bodily movements produced by skeletal muscles that results in energy expenditure.[1]

Physical activity can be further classified as:

1. Light
2. Moderate
3. Vigorous

Exercises are defined as planned structured and repetitive body movement in order to improve or maintain physical fitness.

Physical fitness is the ability to perform activities for a prolonged duration or specific task without experiencing physical stress or fatigue.

Parameters of physical fitness are as follows:

1. Cardiorespiratoryendurance
2. Skeletal muscleendurance
3. Musclestrength
4. Speed
5. Agility
6. Balance
7. Body composition[1]

Functional capacity: It is the exercise capacity equivalent to day-to-day normal routine activity (Activity of daily living) as measured using a standardized functional test such as six-minute walk test (6MWT) [American Thoracic Society (ATS) statement guidelines for the six-minute walk test].[2]

Exercise capacity: It is the power output of a person can sustain during an exercise tolerance test and is independent of any pathological symptoms and/or medical indications.[3]

Functional capacity evaluation: This evaluation is set of tests like six-minute walk tests, practices and observations that are combined to determine the ability of the evaluated to function in a variety of circumstances, most often employment in an objective manner.[4]

Types of Physical Exercise Training

Aerobic exercise: Aerobic exercise improves cardiorespiratory endurance and efficiency of aerobic energy production. Usually it is performed with large muscles in continuous or repetitive rhythmic motion mostly arms, trunk, legs are used either together or separately.

Aerobic exercises provide many health benefits like maintaining and reducing weight, reduction of fat, low-density lipoprotein (LDL), BP, heart-rate and respiratory rate. It increases high-density lipoprotein (HDL) on long-term the person gets efficient cardiorespiratory metabolic, muscular, endocrine and immune systems, and other overall general health benefits.[5] Resistance training improves muscle strength and power.

Resistance training: Muscle strength is defined as maximum ability of muscle to develop force as tension while muscle power is defined as to apply the force or tension at a given velocity. Resistance training is generally done using free weights, elastic bands, weight machines and medicine balls. Training can be in form of isokinetic, isometric orisotonic.

Flexibility training: Flexibility is the ability of the body tissues that determines the range of motion without injury to the joints.

Exercise Training at Patient and Community Levels

The components of physical fitness like balance, coordination, agility, motor power, muscle shape have to be handled with specific type of exercise according to the component requiring attention, e.g. agility is developed by practicing plyometric training. A normal person in a community needs cardiovascular endurance, muscle strength and endurance, ideal body fat composition, flexibility, agility and relaxation techniques.

In general, it is recommended that one should practice 3–5 times (per week) of aerobic exercises and 3 times (per week) of strength training and flexibility, and agility exercises daily. It is also recommended that one should do deep inspiratory and expiratory exercises and relaxation techniques and stretches to avoid muscle soreness.

EXERCISE PHYSIOLOGY

It is the study of physiology of exercises as acute responses and chronic adaptations. It covers biochemistry, bioenergetics, cardiopulmonary functions biomechanics, skeletal muscle physiology, cardiopulmonary function, neuroendocrine function and central and peripheral nervous system.[1]

Energy Expenditure

Human beings have high-capacity to utilize their energy for many hours. During resting state, the total energy expenditure is somewhere between 45–85 watts and for the muscle is 0.63 watts per kg.[6] During exercise and exertion muscle burns about 90 mg of glucose generating 24 watts of mechanical energy. Therefore, according to size, gender and age, the energy expenditure may vary from 2400 Calorie's to 3600 Calorie's.[7]

Acute Responses of Physical Exercise

Acute response of exercise influences the metabolic system

- Circulatory system
- Cardiorespiratory system
- Endocrine system
- Skin and temperature, immune system
- Physical and psychological well-being.

Influence on Metabolic System

Rapid energy sources during the initial high intensity exercise are derived from anaerobic metabolism within the muscle cells. Initially, the energy is provided by ATP (adenosine triphosphate) present the muscle glycogen followed by phosphocreatine system and then the blood glycogen which is broken down into 2ADP's (ATP and AMP). The whole of this activity takes place in conditions of hypoxia or oxygen less. The AMP (adenosine monophosphate) produced is activated by a protein kinase and supplies energy requiring for cell functions. As the glucose is utilized from blood, the liver starts converting initially carbohydrate and then fat into glucose by the process of gluconeogenesis (GNG). Thus the blood glucose level is constantly maintain in normal level during exercises, as the main organs of our body like our brains metabolism depends on presence of normal blood glucose.[6]

Therefore, during exercise initially it starts with anaerobic metabolism followed by aerobic-carbohydrate or fat metabolism. This depends on the ability of the body to convert lactate into pyruvate. The point at which one cannot convert lactate into pyruvate is called as onset of blood lactate accumulation/ anaerobic threshold/lactate threshold. An untrained normal individual can sustain exercises for 30–40 minutes only, after which later acid accumulates resulting into cramps and muscle soreness.[7]

Influence of Exercise on Circulatory System

As there is a high demand for blood supply by the muscles during exercises, the circulatory system responds with initial vasodilation which is governed by local J receptors present in muscles and joints, followed by cholinergic parasympathetic action. As a result of movements during exercises create vasomotion in arterial vessels which stimulates the endovascular endothelium which releases nitrous oxide, which can sustain vasodilation for 48 hours.

Normally, in untrained persons 60% of the capillaries are closed or inactive. Exercises opens all the closed capillaries and also produces new capillaries in the muscles and skin where the progenitor cells are present.

The area of vasodilation depends upon the area being exercised and the other areas will be in vasoconstriction. Hence, recruiting larger area of muscles during exercises results in vasodilatation to be dominant and there by reduces the after load to the heart. This also reduces the diastolic blood pressure to normal.[7]

Influence of Exercise on Cardiovascular System

The increase in blood supply to the working muscles due to increased vasodilatation by the circulatory system is augmented also by the increase in the cardiac output. The cardiac output increases by increase in heart rate and stroke volume. As a result of increase in heart rate, the systolic BP rises during exercises in linear relationship with the intensity of exercises. As the exercises strengthens the left ventricular muscle mass, in long-term exercises will normalize the systolic and diastolic BP and the heart rate lowers during rest. Moreover, the heart rate and BP response becomes more linear and stable responses are obtained at earlier point of time during exercises after training.[8]

Influence of Exercise on Respiratory System

As heart rate increases during exercises the respiratory rate also has to increase in order to oxygenate the excess blood required for muscle energy. The rate may increase to 30–40 or even more during exercise resulting in long-term increased lung volume, vital capacity and efficient thoracic cage pump.[8]

Influence of Exercise on Endocrine System

During the initial period of exercises, the fast acting hormones such as adrenaline of sympathetic system is secreted in order to maintain the central blood volume and prepare body for exercises. Gradually, the parasympathetic system takes over as exercise continues. But, at any time during exercises, the sympathetic system can provoke.

Insulin and glycogen on the other side act as slow acting hormone. Insulin pushes the glucose into the muscle and Glucagon producing glucose by gluconeogenesis in liver is pushed to the blood vessels to maintain optimal blood glucose in the blood

(Dr Cheatham Chapter 20 Exercise Physiology The Endocrine System: Organization and Acute and Chronic Responses to Exercise Western Michigan University).

Influence of Exercise on Skin and Excretory System

During intense exercise the skin becomes red, as a result of blood being directed to the skin through capillaries in order to lose heat as it comes to the surface. Intense exercise increases internal heat, thereby raising the core temperature which influences the hypothalamus to initiate sweating. Both of the mechanisms will cool down the internal body temperature by losing heat from the body.[9]

Influence of Exercise on Immune System

Immune factors like cytokines, interleukins and other inflammatory products are released during a bout of exercise. Initially, during exercise there is decrease in immune response, but in a long-term the immune response becomes more efficient.[10]

Influence of Exercise on Physical and Psychological Well-being

As a result of continuous physical exercises, all the components of physical fitness are kept in the optimal level and therefore the person feels healthy by shape, weight, muscle endurance, muscle strength, cardio-respiratory function, etc. This also gives him a psychological boost and a feeling of well-being.[11]

METHODS OF TRAINING

Aerobic Exercises

Activities such as long distance, slow running/walking which supply of enough oxygen to muscle, improves the cardiovascular and muscular endurance.[12]

Anaerobic Exercises

It is performed in short duration, high intensity, the heart cannot supply enough oxygen to the muscle and therefore the body utilizes anaerobic metabolic product like muscle glycogen, PC (**phosphocreatine**) system, lactate system which give energy without utilizing oxygen. (**Book Reference:** W Larry Kenny, Jack H Wilmore 2015. Physiology of Sports and Exercise 6th Edition, Human Kinetics, USA).

Weight Training

It is done by using weights to provide resistance to the muscles. Usually, 4–6 gross muscles are selected and 8–12 repetitions of 3 sets per session is done. After calculating 1 RM (repetition maximum) initially the training starts with 1/3rd of 1 RM, progressing to 2/3rd of 1 RM and then to 3/4th of 1 RM. The weight training is usually done after 48 hours. During weight training, micro tears occur in the muscle and it takes 48 hours to heal.

Circuit Training

It involves performing series of exercises,one by one in an order. Each activity takes place in a station and each participant changes from one station to another. Each station is designed for a particular ability of muscle like speed, agility, coordination, balance, muscle strength andendurance.

Continuous Training

It involves working for a sustained period of time without rest, e.g. long distance slow running in order to improve cardiovascular endurance.

Interval Training

It alternate periods of exercises and rest to improves speed and endurance.

Cross Training

It involves using another sports activity to improve fitness, e.g. cricketers playing football.

Fartlek Training

Playing/performing activities at different speeds and terrains designed by the coach/ trainer, it improves aerobic and anaerobic fitness.

Short-term and long-term benefits of exercise depends on intensity and duration of exercises.

SUMMARY OF ACUTE RESPONSES OF EXERCISES TRAINING

1. According to the type of training, the anaerobic and aerobic metabolism is utilized for energy consumption.
2. There is an initial sympathetic activation followed by slow onset of cholinergic activity.
3. The peripheral vasodilatation initially occurs through feed forward mechanism through J receptors of muscles and tendons.
4. After a short period of time a sustained vasodilatation occur as a result of sustained parasympathetic activation and also due to release of nitric oxide is endothelium of receptors.
5. There is a capillary recruitment in the normal body system is increased up to near 100% during exercise and the collateral circulation also comes into play during exercise.
6. As the muscle requires more blood supply, cardiac output increases, there is an increase in heart rate and stroke volume contributing to increase in cardiac output.
7. Because of increased heart rate, the systolic pressure increases, while the diastolic pressure remains normal.
8. The respiratory rate increases to provide more O^2 and removes CO^2.
9. The insulin and glucagon action enhances to maintain blood glucose level by process of gluconeogenesis in liver.
10. Exercises stimulate hypothalamus leading to more sweating, skin become red as blood moves to the skin surface to lose heat.
11. The immune system is at its low during exercise.[10]

LONG-TERM BENEFITS OF EXERCISES

1. The long-term effects of exercise can be seen in various body systems and there is an improvement in general fitness as well.[13,14]
2. The musculoskeletal systems changes due to long-term exercise performance include muscle hypertrophy, increased muscle strength and endurance, increase in bone density and increased capacity for glycogen storage.
3. The training threshold also changes as fitness improves and more efficient aerobic energy systems can be seen.
4. There is an increase in vital capacity and V02max (the maximum or optimum rate at which the heart, lungs, and muscles can effectively use oxygen during exercise, used as a way of measuring a person's individual aerobic capacity) this is due to efficient breathing, efficient gaseous exchange and stronger respiratory muscles.
5. Physical exercises also fatigue is reduced on along-term.
6. Long-term effects of exercises are particularly visible in cardiovascular system such as increased stroke volume, lower resting heart rate, increase in number of capillaries and increase in size of arteries.

7. These all effects in turn contribute to more efficient contraction of heart, O_2 transportation and reduced blood pressure.
8. The above effects also influence the recovery rate which seems to improve and also leads to increase in blood volume and quality.
9. Exercises also play a part in improving mental health and prevention of mental disorders.[14]
10. It also speeds up the process of metabolism and reduces weight.[13]
11. There is a decrease in low density lipoprotein and increase in high density lipoprotein. It also reduces cholesterol and triglyceride levels.
12. Exercise on long-term gives insulin like effect for glucose to enter directly into the cell requiring energy without insulin. **(Book Reference:** SA Plowman, DL Smith 2014, Exercise Physiology for Health, Fitness and Performance 4th Edition Wolter Kluwer Lippincott Williams and Wilkins, Baltimore).

EXERCISE TESTING AND PRESCRIPTION

Focused on Normal Population in the Community

Introduction

Basic principles of exercise testing and prescription are given in detail in ACSM guidelines [American College of Sports Medicines (ACSM's) guidelines for exercise testing and prescription 2013].[15] A pre-evaluation is required before exercise testing which include person's profile, previous medical illness (if any), patient's present condition in terms of body composition, cardiorespiratory fitness, muscular strength and endurance.[16] A thorough medical screening to avoid any red flags to exercise testing and prescription has to be done. Modifications has to be made in testing methods/prescription in special population having diseases like diabetes, obesity, cardiovascular disease, lung problems, etc. considering that this chapter focuses on general population, the exercise testing procedure is divided into three types based on the risk stratification derived from the above assessment. At the end of the assessment, he/she is classified as low risk, moderate risk or high risk.

Exercise Testing

Exercise Testing for High Risk Patients

Usually, minimal exercise testing using a six-minute walk test.[17] 12-minute walk test or 200 m walk test is done for high risk patients. The nearest to the gold standard is six-minute walk test which evaluates the person's functional capacity equivalent to his activities of daily life.[16]

Exercise Testing for Moderate Risk Patients

Usually, testing is done with a graded method using either a treadmill, ergometer, or incremental shuttle walk test.[18] These test are stopped at a predetermined end point according to the assessment the end points may be the patient's inability to continue, severe exertion, sweating, cramps, showing signs of angina or sudden changes in heart rate or BP.[19]

Exercise Testing for Low Risk Patients

Low risk patients are tested with maximal exercise testing using a treadmill, ergometer or field tests and they can go to maximal exertion.

After testing, a target heart rate and Rating of Perceived Exertion (RPE)[20,21] is calculated and used for exercise prescription.

Exercise Prescriptions

Exercise prescription is prescribed by principles of FITT:

- F—Frequency
- I—Intensity
- T—Time
- T—Type

While prescribing exercises, one should remember principles of adaptation, specificity overload and reversibility.

Exercise Prescription for High Risk Patients

High risk people are prescribed exercises sufficient to maintain their activities of daily living.

Exercise Prescription for Moderate Risk Patients

After exercise testing in a treadmill or ergometer, a Target Heart Rate (THR) for training is derived or can be done using Rating of Perceived Exertion (RPE). For starting the exercise program, one should start the training at 65% target heart rate or 11–14 in RPE scale [meaning a feeling of mild to moderate exertion with increased respiratory rate (Vivian H Heyward, Ann L Gibson, et al. 2014). Advanced Fitness Assessment and Exercise Prescription Human Kinetics USA].

Exercise Prescription for Low Risk Patients

As already discussed earlier, a combination of aerobic exercises, strength training, flexibility exercises, agility exercises, deep inspiratory techniques and relaxation techniques can be given. The aerobic training starts with 75% Target Heart Rate (THR) to 80–90% THR in normal population.[22]

SUMMARY

The community based exercise prescription may be based on risk stratification. Mostly other chapters will be discussing exercise testing and prescription for special population according to their need. In community after risk stratification and physical activity level during the whole day should be assessed by [International Physical Activity Questionnaire (IPAQ)] or [Global Physical Activity Questionnaire (GPAQ)] and the exercise prescription may be needed only for people with sedentary lifestyle. Quality of life may be assed using **WHOQOL-BREF** or **SF-36** Questionnaires. Heavy and moderate workers may need at an end of the day relaxation techniques.

Hence one should educate the need of 150–240 minutes' exercise per week. All components of exercise should be included aerobic exercise, strength training, flexibility training, jumping (not for geriatric and high risk group) deep breathing and relaxation exercises should be given.

FORMAT

Name: **Age:** **Gender:** **Previous Medical History:** **Current Medical History:** **Present Condition and Medications:**	
Work/Physical Activity Evaluation: **IPAQ Scores:** **Six-Minute Wall Test** **or** **Incremental Shuttle Test Report:**	
Quality of Life Score (WHO BREF QOL): **Risk Stratification:**	**Low Risk** **Moderate Risk** **High Risk**
Prescription of Exercises: Based on RPE/HR	**1. Frequency:** **2. Intensity:** **3. Type:** **4. Duration or Time:**
Evaluation: **Progression:**	

REFERENCES

1. Caspersen CJ, Powell KE, Christenson GM. Physical activity, exercise, and physical fitness: definitions and distinctions for health-related research. Public Health Rep.1985;100(2):126-31.
2. ATS Committee on Proficiency Standards for Clinical Pulmonary Function Laboratories. ATS statement: guidelines for the six-minute walk test. American Journal of Respiratory and Critical Care Medicine. 2002;166(1):111-7.
3. Granger CL, McDonald CF, Parry SM, et.al. Functional capacity, physical activity and muscle strength assessment of individuals with non-small cell lung cancer: a systematic review of instruments and their measurement properties. BMC Cancer. 2013;13:135.
4. Jetté M, Sidney K, Blümchen G. Metabolic equivalents (METS) in exercise testing, exercise prescription, and evaluation of functional capacity. Clinical cardiology. 1990;13(8):555-65.
5. Paffenbarger RS Jr, Hyde RT, Wing AL, et.al. Physicalactivity, all-causemortality, and longevity of college alumni. The New England Journal of Medicine. 1986;314(10):605-13.
6. Speakman JR, Selman C. Physical activity and resting metabolic rate. The Proceedings of the Nutrition Society. 2003;62(3):621-34.
7. Egan B, Zierath Jr. Exercise metabolism and the molecular regulation of skeletal muscle adaptation. Cell metabolism. 2013;17(2):162-84.
8. Golbidi S, Laher I. Exercise and the cardiovascular system. Cardiology research and practice. 2012.
9. Poortmans JR. Exercise and renal function. Sports Med. 1984;1(2):125-53. Epub 1984/03/01.
10. Pedersen BK, Hoffman-Goetz L. Exercise and the immune system: regulation, integration, and adaptation. Physiological reviews. 2000;80(3):1055-81.
11. Penedo FJ, Dahn Jr. Exercise and well-being: a review of mental and physical health benefits associated with physical activity. Current opinion in psychiatry. 2005;18(2):189-93.
12. Crane JD, Macneil LG, Tarnopolsky MA. Long-term aerobic exercise is associated with greater muscle strength throughout the lifespan. The journals of gerontology Series A, Biological sciences and medical sciences. 2013;68(6):631-8
13. Hall GM, Salmon P. Physiological and psychological influences on postoperative fatigue. Anesthesia and analgesia. 2002;95(5):1446-50.
14. Weir A, Jansen JA, van de Port IG, et al. Manual or exercise therapy for long-standing adductor-related groin pain: a randomised controlled clinical trial. Manual therapy. 2011;16(2):148-54.
15. Thompson PD, Arena R, Riebe D, et al. ACSM's new preparticipation health screening recommendations from ACSM's guidelines for exercise testing and prescription, 9th edn. Current sports medicine reports. 2013;12(4):215-7.
16. Fletcher GF, Ades PA, Kligfield P, et al. Exercise standards for testing and training: a scientific statement from the American Heart Association. Circulation. 2013;128(8):873-934.
17. Brooks D, Solway S, Gibbons WJ. ATS statement on six-minute walktest. American journal of respiratory and critical care medicine. 2003;167(9):1287.
18. Lewis ME, Newall C, Townend JN, et al. Incremental shuttle walk test in the assessment of patients for heart transplantation. Heart. 2001;86(2):183-7.

19. Gregoratos G, Abrams J, Epstein AE, et al. ACC/AHA/NASPE 2002 guideline update for implantation of cardiac pacemakers and antiarrhythmia devices: summary article: a report of the American College of Cardiology/American Heart Association Task Force on Practice Guidelines (ACC/AHA/NASPE Committee to Update the 1998 Pacemaker Guidelines). Circulation. 2002;106(16):2145-61.
20. Borg GA. Psychophysical bases of perceived exertion. Medicine and science in sports and exercise. 1982;14(5):377-81.
21. Pfeiffer KA, Pivarnik JM, Womack CJ, et al. Reliability and validity of the Borg and OMNI rating of perceived exertion scales in adolescent girls. Medicine and science in sports and exercise. 2002;34(12):2057-61.
22. Giné-Garriga M, Roqué-Fíguls M, Coll-Planas L, et al. Physical exercise interventions for improving performance-based measures of physical function in community-dwelling, frail older adults: a systematic review and meta-analysis. Archives of physical medicine and rehabilitation. 2014;95(4):753- 69.

Other References (from Books and Guidelines)

1. W Larry Kenny, Jack H Wilmore. Physiology of Sports and Exercise, 6th edn, Human Kinetics, USA, 2005.
2. SA Plowman, DL Smith. Exercise Physiology for Health, Fitness and performance 4th edn, Wolter Kluwer/Lippincott Williams and Wilkins,Baltimore.
3. A Report of the American College of Cardiology Foundation Appropriate Use Criteria Task Force, American Heart Association, American Society of Echocardiography, American Society of Nuclear Cardiology, Heart Failure Society of America, Heart Rhythm Society, Society for Cardiovascular Angiography and Interventions, Society of Cardiovascular Computed Tomography, Society for Cardiovascular Magnetic Resonance, and Society of Thoracic Surgeons, ACCF/AHA/ASE/ASNC/HFSA/HRS/SCAI/SCCT/SCMR/STS 2013 Multimodality Appropriate use criteria for the detection and risk assessment of stable ischemic heart disease. J AM Coll Cardiol.2014;64(4):380-406.
4. Vivian H Heyward, Ann L Gibson. Advanced Fitness Assessment and Exercise Prescription, Human Kinetics, USA,2014.

8

Movement Sciences in Indian Traditional Practices and Physiotherapy

Unnati Nikhil Pandit

Abstract: Both physical exercise as well as traditional practices like Suryanamaskara and Yoga are globally established modes to promote health and wellness. Both include various physical maneuvers but their concepts are totally different. Traditional practices are based on spiritual sciences; hence concepts have no link with any systemic physiological effect other than feeling of calmness. However, literature shows lot of evidence on their positive systemic effect.

This chapter compares the traditional practices and physiotherapy in terms of their concepts, types of various physical maneuvers including respective physiological effects. It also offers recommendations for further research in order to select physical maneuvers from traditional practices for the evidence-based clinical physiotherapeutic application in health and disease.

Keywords: Yoga, Asanas, Pranayama, physical exercises, breathing exercises, aerobics, Suryanamaskara, mobilization, health, wellness.

INTRODUCTION

'Health' is broadly defined by the Webster dictionary as 'State of being healthy, happy and prosperous.'[1] Good health results from perfect communication between each part of the body and mind; when each cell communes with every other. Health is not just freedom from disease but it is determined by the perfect equilibrium of the body and mind, intellect and soul, which is well endorsed by the definition of Health by the ***World Health Organization (WHO)*** which defines health as ***'a state of complete physical, mental and social wellbeing and not merely the absence of disease or infirmity.'***[2]

Various ***Physical maneuvers*** are incorporated in both the traditional practices as well as physical therapy but their basic concepts being totally different, the ultimate goal and objectives of obtaining specific beneficial effects are also different. However, the term **'exercise'** (substituting the term 'physical maneuvers') which is found to be commonly used in both the practices, creates a lot of confusion, whether similar looking maneuvers incorporated in both, also have similar outcome and vice versa. In fact, Christiane Brems (2016)[3] reported that Yoga is popularized as gym-based physical exercise in which the original yogic philosophy of self-discipline and living with purity is least endorsed.

Therefore for a physiotherapist it is very essential to understand basic concepts, methods of application and physiological outcome (based on the literature review) of the physical maneuvers used in traditional practices, so that he/she can develop an ability to select appropriate maneuver(s) from traditional practices as an adjunct or substitute maneuver to obtain desirable

Physiotherapeutic effect after establishing evidence.

COMPARISON OF BASIC CONCEPTS

Physiotherapy

It is an independent modern health science that deals with non-pharmacotherapeutic and nonsurgical intervention. Exercise therapy (Kinesiotherapy) is its major therapeutic mode, based on the principles of applied Anatomy (**Biomechanics and Biophysics**), applied Physiology (**Neuro-Exercise Physiology**) and **Biochemistry**. Exercise therapy includes wide range of physical maneuvers which are aimed to provide measures at all the three levels of prevention. In addition, these modes are also used for restorative intervention related to somatic pain or specific health conditions, encompassing locomotor, cardiopulmonary, metabolic and urogynecological systems.

Traditional Practices

'Yoga' is an ancient art based on the **concept of Philosophy and Spiritual Sciences**. It is an extremely subtle science that intends to unite body, mind and soul/spirit (Fig. 8.1), to achieve union of individual self or 'Jivatma' with the universal self or 'Paramatma'. Its philosophy is that, long-term practice of yoga can lead to a sense of peace and a feeling of being at one with his or her environment. Although yoga is essentially a spiritual science, it leads to a sense of physical and emotional wellbeing.[4,5] The World Health Organization (WHO) has recognized Yoga as a form of alternate medicine having its origins in India.[6]

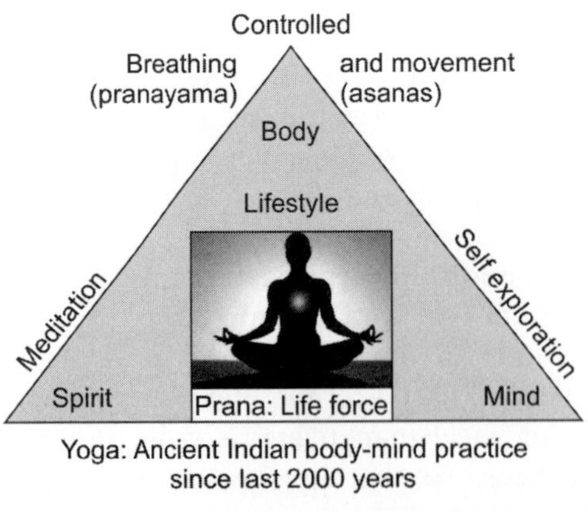

Fig. 8.1: Diagrammatic representation of Yogic concepts

Thus, Yoga traditional practice does not follow any applied anatomical or physiological/biochemical principles like physiotherapeutic physical maneuvers. Nevertheless, there are volumes of evidence documented about its positive effect on various physiological and biochemical health markers apart from desirable psychosomatic (calming) and cognitive (concentration) effect.

COMPARISON OF PHYSICAL MANEUVERS

Physiotherapeutics include following **three** types of physical maneuvers, all of which are to be implemented ***as per individual need.***

1. Active exercises (including active assisted and resisted exercises)
2. Breathing exercises
3. Passive movements and manual therapy.

Active exercises and breathing exercises are self-imposed physical maneuvers, whereas, during passive exercises and manual therapy modes, the subject rests in a specific position and the physiotherapist performs certain physical maneuvers. Passive movements are used to sustain joint mobility during paralytic or unconscious status. Manual therapy is a specialized physiotherapeutic mode used in musculoskeletal disorders in which, highly skillful physical maneuvers are performed in small ranges by the physiotherapist on the patient's affected body part to bring about relief of pain and/or improvement in the range of movement.

Traditional Maneuvers

They are self-imposed physical maneuvers, thus unlike physiotherapeutics, the concept of ***Passive maneuvers*** does not exist in the same.

Ashtanga Yoga, a traditional practice which was popularized by famous sage Patanjali more than 2000 years ago but as per the archeological survey reports, this practice is older than 3000 BC.[7] Patanjali described eight limbs of practice, i.e. Yama (moral behavior), Niyama (healthy habit), Asana (postures), Pranayama (breathing maneuvers), Pratyahara (sense withdrawal), Dharana (contemplation), Dhyana (concentration), and Samadhi (higher consciousness) (Fig. 8.2). Out of these eight limbs, only the ***third (Asanas) and fourth (Pranayama) limbs*** include ***physical maneuvers,***[8] which also incorporate sometimes, certain additional physical maneuvers called ***Bandhas*** (locks) and ***Mudras*** (poses) during the practice.[9]

Ashtanga yoga practices ***discourage isolated physical maneuvers*** and emphasize on the practice of entire package of all the eight limbs for attaining the final goal. However, there are various permutation-combinations of eight limbs of ashtanga yoga including certain additions/modifications forming various modified versions, with various connotations like *Hatha yoga, Vikram yoga, Power yoga, Kripalu yoga, Iyengar yoga,* etc.

Hatha yoga: It is the most popular form of yoga that is practiced globally, with a frequently used term just ***'yoga'***. This mode includes mainly physical maneuvers, i.e. Asanas and Pranayama but also includes meditation (Dhyana) sometimes.

In traditional practices the maneuvers are mostly performed slowly, however, there are certain exceptions such as, fast *Suryanamaskara* and *Bhastrika pranayama* or *Kapalbhati kriya,* etc.

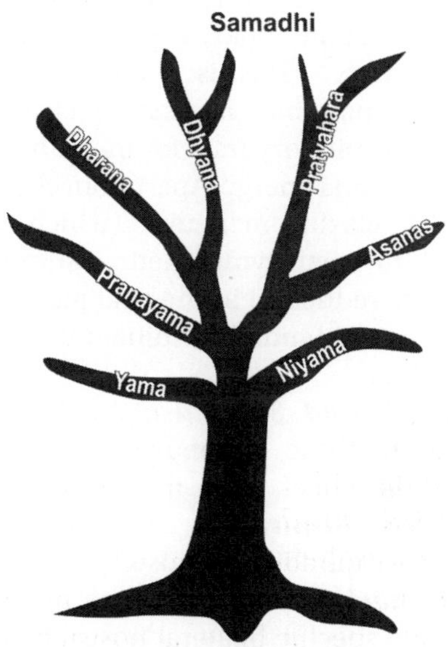

Fig. 8.2: Eight limbs of Ashtangayoga

COMPARISON OF BREATHING MANEUVERS

Natural breathing is a spontaneous maneuver, hence does not require any conscious effort but it can be stopped (breath holding) or its pattern can be modified voluntarily. Both Pranayama and Physiotherapeutic breathing exercises are consciously performed breathing maneuvers, hence need prolonged training of conditioning, so that they can turn into spontaneous breathing activity.

Spontaneous breathing includes two major phases in which, **Inspiration** is an active phase and **Expiration** is passive. **Breath holding** can be performed voluntarily anytime during the breathing cycle. However, it can happen spontaneously when intra-abdominal pressure has to rise while lifting-carrying heavy loads, straining during defecation and parturition (in women) or when nostrils touch water after diving (trigeminal reflex). Spontaneous breath holding is also observed during sudden emotional outbursts like when a child throws temper tantrums, or an adult reacts to a sudden shocking event.

Physiotherapeutic breathing maneuvers are termed as ***'Breathing exercises'***, which are totally based on pulmonary physiology. They are always slow and mostly sustain inspiratory: expiratory ratio as 1:2.

- ***Inspiratory exercises:*** They are used as primary and secondary prevention modes for healthy (incorporated in general fitness exercises) and in deconditioned persons (those under prolonged bed rest or in the postoperative status, etc.) respectively, focusing on improving vital capacity. They are also used as long-term tertiary prevention modes in those suffering from chronic inspiratory health issues such as post-pulmonary tuberculosis, bronchiectasis, cystic fibrosis, etc. Diaphragm being the main inspiratory muscle, diaphragmatic breathing is emphasized a lot during inspiratory training; nevertheless, it is avoided during first stage of labor to reduce labor pain.
- ***Expiratory exercises:*** They are specifically implemented in obstructive disorders such as asthma, chronic obstructive pulmonary disorders, emphysema, etc. In this method minimal resistance is offered to expiratory phase so that the back pressure can sustain the airways open and reduce their early collapse which is otherwise responsible for air trapping.
- ***Voluntary breath holding:*** It is generally not used as an exercise for clinical intervention in patient population, but its conditioning effect could be beneficial for those involved in singing or in underwater sports.

Pranayama (Prana-Ayama): It is the fourth limb of Ashtanga yoga which includes several breathing maneuvers but none of them have any concept that is linked with the health of pulmonary system. As per the yogic concepts, 'Prana' is considered to be the ***energy of life***, and 'Ayama' means to ***'control'.*** This can further be explained that, by practicing specific 'controlled breathing maneuvers' (by controlling respiratory mechanism), it is possible to control the body with mind first and then with the universal self.[10]

In the pranayama modes, in addition to the phases of inspiration ***(Puraka)*** and expiration ***(Rechaka)***, the breath holding ***(Kumbhaka)*** phase is considered to be ***extremely important*** which is very much in contrast with therapeutic breathing exercises. Yogic breathing maneuvers also include fast modes which are also in contrast with Physiotherapeutic breathing maneuvers. Nevertheless, as per our recent research outcome (article to be published), in spite of being fast, these maneuvers include a phase of Kumbhaka.

Variation in each ***Pranayama*** method is determined by its speed, resistance and specificity incorporated during inspiratory and/or expiratory phases as well as during breath holds (if any). The types of ***Pranayama*** maneuvers are briefed as follows:

Type-I: Slow Yogic Breathing Maneuvers

- ***Anulom-vilom:*** This is a slow and deep breathing maneuver performed via alternate nostril with recommended ratio of inspiration: hold: expiration as 1:4:2 respectively.[9] This is a 'Nadi Shodhan Pranayama' which is meant to cleanse the upper respiratory tract for the uninhibited flow of prana energy. Apart from cleansing, it is a relaxing maneuver (which occurs due to parasympathetic stimulation causing reduction in the vital parameters) and recommended to initiate pranayama practices.[11]
- ***Sheetali and Sheetkari:*** As the names suggest, these maneuvers also create ***'cooling'*** effect. Both include ***minimally resisted inspiration*** via mouth and passive expiration via nose.[9]
- ***Bhramari and Ujjayi:*** These maneuvers include specific bilateral nostril breathing to create ***acoustic effect*** (produce sound).

In ***Bramari***, which is similar to the concept of 'aum' chanting maneuver, the ***resistance*** is applied during ***expiratory phase*** which vibrates the vocal cords to produce 'humming' sound to bring about 'Relaxation' and soothing effect. In Bhramari Inspiration does not include resistance. Whereas in ***Ujjayi***, ***resistance*** is applied ***at the glottis*** during both-***inspiration as well as expiration*** which produces hissing sound.[9]

Type-II: Fast Yogic Breathing Maneuvers

- ***Bhastrika:*** A multiple benefits bestowing maneuver which involves rapid ***shallow*** breathing with ***active inspiration as well as expiration***.[9]
- ***Kapalbhati:*** This maneuver includes ***active expiration and passive inspiration***. Acceptance of its inclusion within YBM is unequivocal. In certain schools of thoughts, instead of being a pranayama maneuver, it is considered as one of the ***'Shuddhi Kriyas'*** that bring about cleansing effect on the visceral systems.[9]

There is a lot of documentary evidence on the positive effects of various pranayama maneuvers on pulmonary function in healthy[12-17] and in pulmonary disease.[18-27]

COMPARISON OF OTHER PHYSICAL MANEUVERS

Physiotherapeutics: Active exercises can be covered under the domain of neuro-musculoskeletal maneuvers. They include series of self-imposed physical maneuvers that are implemented involving either a part or the whole body, conducted under the supervision of a Physiotherapist and to be continued as home program as per the prescribed guidelines. The ***musculoskeletal types of active exercises*** mostly follow a specific dosimetry, in terms of intensity, speed, repetitions, frequency and most importantly, specificity. ***Dosimentry is determined according to individual need*** in health and disease, exactly the way it is determined in pharmacotherapeutic application for various health issues. In a person having difficulty in performing such maneuvers, 'Active assisted modes are used in which the assistance is offered manually or by using various aids, whereas, additional tools are also used to provide resistance for strength/power training. Active exercises are broadly aimed to improve physical fitness/independence or/and to provide secondary prevention when persons are involved in high impact competitive tasks like sports and dance or in immobilized/hypomobile status following injury or illness.' Active physical exercises can be subdivided as per their desirable effects as follows:

- ***Exercises based on biomechanics and muscle physiology:*** They are isometric, isotonic/dynamic or isokinetic exercises, which mainly focus of musculoskeletal performance focusing on strength, power, endurance, and flexibility.
- ***Exercises based on neurophysiology:*** They mainly focus on muscle tone (e.g. spasticity), motor control, coordination and balance.
- ***Exercises based on combination of physiological and biochemical (metabolic) principles:*** They focus on aerobic and anaerobic activities. Aerobics mainly focus on general fitness, weight/blood sugar control, and cardiopulmonary conditioning, with secondary psychosomatic effect of 'wellness.' Whereas, anaerobic activities mainly focus on high speed-short duration performance associated with sports or dance.
- ***Relaxation exercises:*** These are self-imposed highly subtle physical maneuvers used specifically for reducing stress related issues like tension headaches, or to induce relaxation after heavy exercise/activity. Jacobson's method of relaxation includes subtle rhythmic movements involving

small component of body at a time (such as, toe movements) for three to four times followed by 'let go' i.e. slow relaxation, which needs to be sustained throughout the session. This process is sequentially shifted from caudal to cephalad direction, finally reaching to a status of complete body relaxation.

Traditional Practices

Suryanamaskara and ***Asanas*** are the musculoskeletal maneuvers covered under the umbrella of traditional practices. Isolated practice of asanas is not known much.

- ***Suryanamaskara:*** It is a spiritually derived method of Sun salutation, hence its only objective is to worship the Sun-God. This traditional practice includes 12 cyclic sequential poses (including starting position), all performed in a sagittal plane involving entire body either slowly or with a maximum speed as per individual capacity. In this method, only sixth and seventh positions are attained once, whereas, the initial five positions are reversed sequentially from eighth to last/original position (Fig. 8.3). They are performed slowly with controlled breathing to induce similar effects like Yoga[28] or practiced as preparatory maneuvers prior to commencing with Yogasanas. Whereas, ***fast*** maneuvers of Suryanamaskara are known to create conditioning effects similar to ***aerobic exercise***[28,29] (see details below).

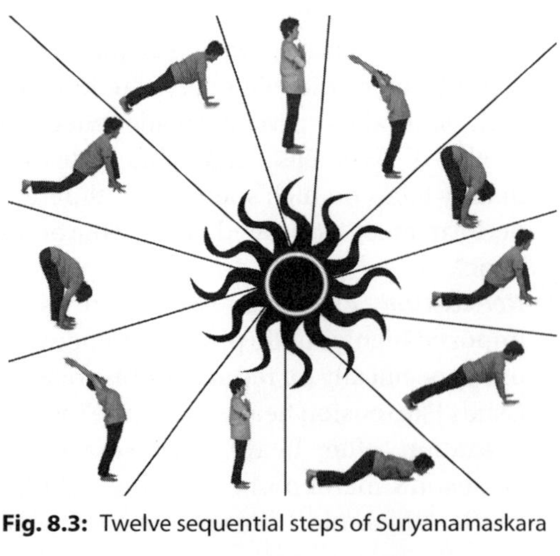

Fig. 8.3: Twelve sequential steps of Suryanamaskara

- ***Yogasanas*** are self-imposed very subtle, sequential physical maneuvers performed to attain a specific posture. After attaining the desirable posture, it is supposed to be sustained for a while during which conscious differential relaxation status (Prayatna-shaithilya) is attained.[30] The posture is then slowly unwound in a reversed sequence, back to original position. There is a long list of yogasanas which are to be performed as a package, using various starting positions.

Among various asanas only one asana that is meant for attaining ***complete body relaxation is*** **'Shavasana'** or the corpse posture which could also be attained step by step in a similar sequence like relaxation exercises. The only difference is that, there is ***no exercise/movement***, but the person has to ***just perceive*** the existence of a specific body part and should make a conscious effort to relax the same (prayatna shaithilya/differential relaxation).[30] Practice of Shavasana at the end of any yogasana session is a mandatory protocol, in contrast to relaxation exercise which can be used as an ***exclusive*** exercise mode for relieving anxiety, mental tension, etc.

Hathayoga/'yoga': As mentioned earlier, the current global concept or 'Yogic exercises' is a gym-based physical exercise program[3] clubbing both Asanas and pranayama.[31] A lot of documentary evidence is available on their positive physiological effect on the health markers[32-39] even though, basic concepts of Yogic maneuvers do not link with any positive physiological effect. However, unlike aerobic exercise, **dosimetry** quantifying intensity, duration, repetitions and frequency is ***found to be missing*** in the literature on ***yogic maneuvers.***[12]

Though there are various other styles of yoga practiced with different connotations, the choice of specific yoga style is not based on any specific desirable effect but based on individual preference or/and as per the availability of learning particular style.[40]

COMPARISON OF YOGIC PRACTICES (ASANAS + PRANAYAMA) AND AEROBIC EXERCISES (AE)

Difference between the two[30] in broad terms is documented as follows:

- Yoga is non-competitive and process oriented but AE is often competitive and goal-oriented.
- Yoga practices involves a rest period of few seconds after each cycle of a maneuver irrespective whether it is subtle/slow or fast (Bhastrika and Kapalbhati breathing maneuvers). AE are relatively rapid, continuous and strenuous physical maneuvers.
- Yogic maneuvers stimulate parasympathetic nervous system, hence reduce the vital parameters (e.g. respiratory and heart rate, blood pressure, body temperature, etc.) and end with relaxation, and rejuvenating feeling. Whereas, AE stimulate sympathetic nervous system hence raise vital parameters and end with fatigue/exertion.
- In yoga, awareness is internal (focus is on breath and the infinite) but in AE, awareness is external (focus is on reaching the goal as seen in sports or weight reduction, etc.)
- In yoga, subcortical regions of brain dominate in AE cortical region dominates.

Difference in Acute Effects

- Yogic maneuvers conserve energy, whereas, acute effect of AE increases energy consumption.
- Yogic practices under strict supervision never tax any vital parameters during acute exposure, in fact they reduce the respiratory/pulse rate and blood pressure which is parasympathetically mediated. Whereas, the parameters increase due to sympathetic stimulation in acute exposure to AE.
- In contrast with post-activity soreness or muscle fatigue observed after initial exposure to aerobic exercise, such effect is not seen in any yogic practices, unless any enthusiastic person overdoes any maneuver beyond capacity or does it wrongly. Nevertheless; as an only exception in yogic practices, the fresh learners often experience painful paraspinal spasm after practicing Bhastrika and Kapalbhati maneuvers. This is because, in both the maneuvers a posture of fully expanded chest (fixed with bilateral shoulder retraction after deep inspiration) needs to be adopted during which, the crura of the diaphragm lift the upper lumbar vertebrae causing increased lordosis and this posture needs to be sustained throughout each breath cycle by sustained isometric contraction of paraspinal muscles.

Conditioning Effects

- In yoga there are limitless possibilities for growth in self-awareness, whereas, in aerobic exercise there is generally no component of self-awareness.
- In both yoga as well as AE, similar positive conditioning effects are found in spite of different responses to acute exposure:
    - Basal values of vital parameters show reduction
    - Muscle soreness if any gets eliminated
    - Dietary intake gets reduced because of early stimulation of satiety center
    - Increase is seen in flexibility, vital capacity and perception of wellbeing.
    - Weight loss gets enhanced in both but the reasoning for the same is unequivocal, hence needs further research in this regards.

However, in their review of literature related to the health benefits of yoga and exercise, Alyson Ross et al. (2010)[41] reported that, yoga was equally effective, rather better than exercise at improving various positive health-markers in both healthy and diseased populations. In contrast, it is also documented that, conditioning effect of endurance exercise like swimming, is superior to yoga group in pulmonary parameters such as forced vital capacity (FVC), FEF 25-75% and maximum voluntary ventilation (MVV).[42]

Intergroup comparison between **yogasanas and Pranayam** in terms of pulmonary function, aerobic capacity and anthropometric assessment, the literature has shown significant improvement in lung function capacity in Pranayama group; whereas, aerobic capacity and anthropometric assessment was significantly superior in yoga group.[15]

Owing to its positive effects on various physiological parameters documented in the literature, yoga (Asanas + Pranayama) with/without other components such as suryanamaskara, om chanting, meditation, etc. is known to be utilized in clinical practice. Systematic review shows evidence on use of yogic maneuvers for the positive clinical outcome during cardiovascular and pulmonary, neurological, pediatric and geriatric rehabilitation; home health, oncology, and women's health.[7]

SIMILARITIES IN SPECIFIC PHYSICAL MANEUVERS

Certain physical maneuvers used in Physiotherapeutics and Yogasanas are similar though basic concepts differ between the two, e.g. Bhujangasana (Fig. 8.4) and one of the methods of 'Mckenzie's spinal mobilization' are similar even though Bhujangasana has nothing to do with spinal mobility. Both Kegal's exercises and 'Moolabandha' include isometric contraction of pelvic floor muscles (PFM). Moolabandha is to be applied while practicing any type of Pranayama with a purpose to prevent leakage of 'prana' energy.[10] Whereas, Kegal's exercises are mainly used for training pelvic floor muscles as preventive mode against high impact activities such as sports and dance or used in therapeutics for women with pelvic floor dysfunction.

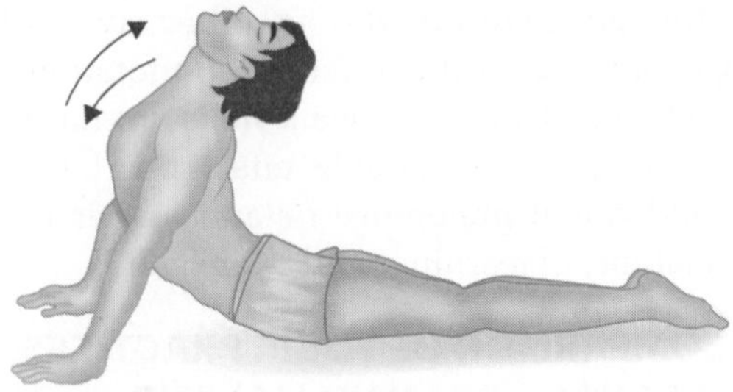

Fig. 8.4: Bhujagasana

Late (Dr) MG Mokashi is the first Indian Physiotherapist who linked Yoga with Physiotherapy in 1970's. With his number of international platform presentations, publications and with his own Doctoral thesis, he established the concept as to how certain maneuvers used in yogic practices offer efficacy in physiotherapeutic intervention in various aspects, e.g. he found yogasanas involving diagonal patterns such as Ardha Matsyendrasana (Fig. 8.5) useful in reducing spasticity in adult hemiplegic patients.

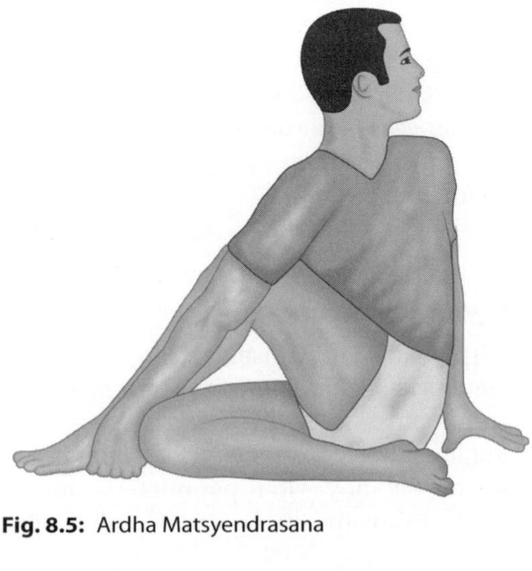

Fig. 8.5: Ardha Matsyendrasana

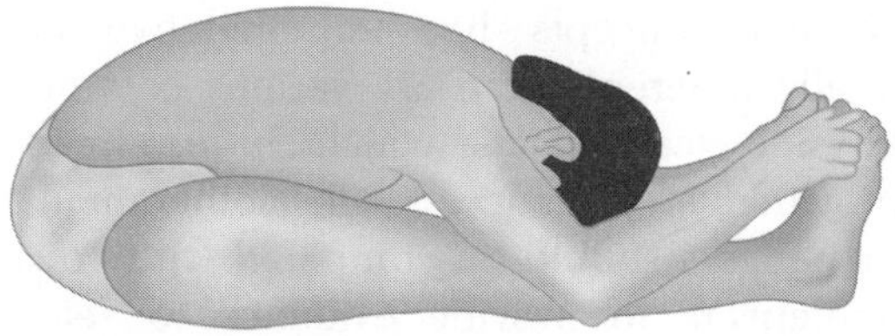

Fig. 8.6: Paschimottanasana

Dr Mokashi's latest research work as a PhD guide showed efficacy of Paschimottasana (Fig. 8.6) as a mode to mobilize sciatic nerve in subjects with radiating pain in lower limb with positive passive straight leg raise (SLR) test. This study provided evidence that, even though the concept of Paschimottanasana has no link with sciatic nerve, this posture could enable ***active*** mobilization of the sciatic nerve whereas, in Physiotherapeutics a ***passive*** mobilization (Butler's neural tissue mobilization) method is used with different physical maneuvers for the same purpose.

RECOMMENDATIONS

There is tremendous scope to utilize various physical maneuvers of traditional practices as adjunct or substitute to routine physical maneuvers used in Physiotherapy, after establishing the evidence on their outcome measures. Author's own doctoral study which incorporated a preliminary real time ultrasound analysis of Pranayama maneuvers on trained yogic practitioners opened Pandora's box. To quote an example: the author found lower values of diaphragmatic excursion during Shitali and Shitkari maneuvers, suggesting higher participation of other inspiratory muscles hence the study directed for further research in this aspect so that, in case this hypothesis is accepted, then these maneuvers could be utilized as specific Physiotherapeutic breathing exercises where apical or lateral costal breathing is advocated e.g. to minimize diaphragmatic excursion and distress the labor pain during first stage.

In the same research study it was also found that Bhramari Pranayama offered resistance during expiratory phase suggesting its therapeutic value in the treatment of obstructive pulmonary conditions. Evidence of its efficacy in treating such cases is already established.[23,43] Moreover, its efficacy in inducing relaxation by enhancing parasympathetic stimulation is also established.[44,45] Therefore dual effect of Bhamari pranayama would prove to be more beneficial than only expiratory type of breathing exercises, because those suffering from chronic obstructive pulmonary disorders are also likely to suffer from anxiety and depression. However, this hypothesis needs to be tested first by comparing physiological parameters between Bhramari pranayama and expiratory exercise.

Volumes of literature evidence is available showing positive physiological effects of yoga. The National Institutes of Health, USA (2008)[46] and National Health Services, UK (2015)[47] have also described yoga as a safe and effective intervention to increase strength, flexibility, balance, and treatment for high blood pressure, heart disease, aches and pains, depression, stress, and asthma. Therefore, even though practice of exclusive physical maneuver is not recommended in practices of asanas or Pranayama maneuvers, it ***is possible to utilize the same in Physiotherapeutics as an adjunct or substitute mode after establishing evidence***.

The aspiring Physiotherapy professionals thus have an ample scope (after establishing evidence) to develop a new trend combining Physical maneuvers of traditional practices with physiotherapeutic modes and offer a new connotation to this trend like 'Physiyoga' (already suggested by Dr Nilima Patel, Physiotherapist from Vadodara) or 'Physio-yoga' or 'Yogic Physiotherapy' or any other.

Nevertheless, taking into account the respective physiological effects, in case of combining yogic practices and aerobic exercises, yoga should always be conducted after aerobics to minimize the postexercise fatiguing effects.[48]

SUMMARY

The term 'exercises' creates confusion between the concepts of physical maneuvers included in traditional practices (Suryanamaskara, asanas and Pranayama) and Exercise therapy. Though concepts between the two are totally different there are various common Physiological effects which have already provided evidence. Physiotherapeutic maneuvers should be compared with yogic maneuvers to provide evidence to select appropriate yogic maneuver(s) that can be used either adjourned or substitute of specific exercises therapy maneuver(s) to achieve desirable physiotherapeutic effects.

REFERENCES

1. Merriam-Webster Dictionary Online at: htpp//www.m-w.com. Accessed December 10, 2004.
2. Catherine Rush Thompson. Prevention Practice: A Physical Therapist's Guide to Health, Fitness, and Wellness. Published in USA by SLACK incorporated. 2007.
3. Brems C, Colgan D, Freeman H, et al. Elements of yogic practice: Perceptions of students in healthcare programs. Int J Yoga. 2016;9(2):121-9.
4. Vivekananda S. Raja Yoga. 34th Impression. Advaita Asrama. 2007.
5. Madanmohan Role of Yoga and Ayurveda in Cardiovascular Disease. Available from: http://www.fac.org.ar/qcvc/llave/c039i/madanmohan.php.
6. http://www.wpro.who.int/health_technology/book_who_traditional_medicine_strategy_2002_2005.pdf 166.
7. Abigail Grover Snook, Ellenore Palmer, Sharon Richman. Yoga: Indexing Metadata/Description: Clinical Review. Cinahl Information Systems. 2016.
8. Pallav Sengupta. Health Impacts of Yoga and Pranayama: A State-of-the-Art Review. Int J Prev Med. 2012;3(7):444–58.
9. Sadashiv Nimbalkar: Pranayama: An effective means to mental health. Pub: Yoga Vidya Niketan, 2003.
10. Annapoorna K and Vasantalaxmi K. Practice of Pranayama: A Physiological Approach International Journal of Yoga and Allied Sciences. 2015:133-8.
11. Nidhi Jain, RD Srivastava, Anil Singhal. The Effects of Right and Left Nostril Breathing on Cardiorespiratory and Autonomic Parameters. Indian Journal of Physiology and Pharmacology. 2005;49(4):469-74.
12. Makwana K, Khirwadkar N, Gupta HC. Effects of short term yoga practice on ventilator function tests. Indian Journal of Physiology and Pharmacology. 1988;32:202-7.
13. Madanmohan, Thrombe DP, Bharathi B, et al. Effect of yoga training on reaction time, respiratory endurance and muscle strength. Indian J Physiol Pharmacol. 1992;36:229-33.
14. Madanmohan, Mahadevan SK, Balakrishnan S, et al. Effect of six weeks yoga training on weight loss, following step test, respiratory pressures, hand grip strength & endurance in young healthy subjects. Indian J Physiol Pharmacol. 2008(2):184-90.

15. Swati Dhingra, Biswas Manosree, Falak Pooja, et al. Effect of Pranayama on Selected Respiratory Indices and Body Composition. Journal of Yoga (JOY) Department of Post Graduate Studies and Research in Home Science, SNDT Women's University, Mumbai. 2010.
16. Ankad Roopa B, Ankad Balachandra S, Herur Anita, et al. Effect of Short Term Pranayama and Meditation on Respiratory Parameters in Healthy Individuals. International Journal of Collaborative Research on Internal Medicine & Public. 2011;3(6):430-7.
17. VS Shelke, AN Badwe, RG Latti. Effect of yogic breathing (Paranayam) on pulmonary function tests (PFT) and visual reaction time in healthy individuals. International Journal of Biomedical and Advance Research. 2015;6(05):438-42.
18. Xun-Chao Liu, Lei Pan, Qing Hu, et al. Effects of yoga training in patients with chronic obstructive pulmonary disease: a systematic review and meta-analysis. J Thorac Dis. 2014;6(6):795-802.
19. Yang ZY, Zhong HB, Mao C, et al. Yoga for asthma. Cochrane Database Syst Rev. 2016;4:CD010346.
20. Keshur A Karmur, Varsha S Joshi, Maulik S Padalia et al. Effect of ten weeks yoga practice on pulmonary function tests. International Journal of Biomedical Advanced Research. 2015.
21. Nagarathna R, Nagendra HR. Yoga for bronchial asthma: a controlled study. Br Med J (Clin Res Ed). 1985;291(6502):1077-9.
22. Singh V, Wisniewski A, Britton J, et al. Effect of yoga breathing exercises (pranayama) on airway reactivity in subjects with asthma. Lancet. 1990;335(8702):1381-3.
23. Tarun Saxena, Manjari Saxena. The effect of various breathing exercises (pranayama) in patients with bronchial asthma of mild to moderate severity. Int J Yoga. 2009;2(1):22-5.
24. Khue Ai Thi Hoang, Hung Manh Nguyen. The effectiveness of practicing Pranayama yoga on some respiratory in patients suffering from bronchial asthma. International Journal of Science Culture and Sport (IntJSCS). 2015:3(2):6-12.
25. Deepali S Jaju, Mohan B Dikshit, Jothi Balaji, et al. Effects of Pranayam Breathing on Respiratory Pressures and Sympathovagal Balance of Patients with Chronic Airflow Limitation and in Control Subjects. SQU Med J. 2011;11(2):221-9.
26. SudShushanth and SudKhyati S. Effect of Pranayama on pulmonary functions—An overview. International Ayurvedic Medical Jounal. 2013;1(2):1-6.
27. Navoday Raju NR, Deepika S, Kulkarni Pratibha, et al. Effect of Pranayama on respiratory system: Unique Journal of Ayurvedic and Herbal Medicines. 2015;3(4). Available online: www.ujconline.net.
28. Bhavanani AB, Udupa K, Madanmohan, et al. A comparative study of slow and fast suryanamaskar on physiological function. Int J Yoga. 2011;4(2):71-6.
29. Parag Javadekar and Manjunath NK. Effect of Surya Namaskar on Sustained Attention in School Children. Journal of Yoga and Physical Therapy. 2012.
30. Sadashiv Nimbalkar. Yoga for Health and Peace. Publishers Yoga Vidhya Niketan, Mumbai 2007.
31. Ramajayam Govindaraj, Sneha Karmani, Shivarama Varambally, et al. Yoga and physical exercise—a review and comparison. International Review of Psychiatry. 2016;28(3):242-53.
32. Savić K, Pfau D, Skorić S, et al. The effect of Hatha yoga on poor posture in children and the psychophysiologic condition in adults. Med Pregl. 1990;43(5-6):268-72.
33. Tran MD, Holly RG, Lashbrook J, et al. Effects of Hatha Yoga Practice on the Health-Related Aspects of Physical Fitness. Prev Cardiol. 2001;4(4):165-70.
34. Raub JA. Psychophysiologic effects of Hatha Yoga on musculoskeletal and cardiopulmonary function: a literature review. J altern Complement Med. 2002;8(6):797-812.

35. Galantino ML, Bzdewka TM, Eissler-Russo JL, et al. The impact of modified Hatha yoga on chronic low back pain: a pilot study. Altern Ther Health Med. 2004;10(2):56-9.
36. Clay CC, Lloyd LK, Walker JL, et al. The metabolic cost of hatha yoga. J Strength Cond Res. 2005;19(3): 604-10.
37. Narendran S, Nagarathna R, Narendran V, et al. Efficacy of yoga on pregnancy outcome. J Altern Complement Med. 2005;11(2):237-44.
38. Oken BS, Zajdel D, Kishiyama S, et al. Randomized, controlled, six-month trial of yoga in healthy seniors: effects on cognition and quality of life. Altern Ther Health Med. 2006;12(1):40-7.
39. Hagins M, Moore W, Rundle A. Does practicing hatha yoga satisfy recommendations for intensity of physical activity which improves and maintains health and cardiovascular fitness? BMC Altern Complement Med. 2007;7:40.
40. Cramer H, Lauche R, Langhorst J, et al. Is one yoga style better than another? A systematic review of associations of yoga style and conclusions in randomized yoga trials. Complement Ther Med. 2016;25:178-87.
41. Ross A, Thomas S. The health benefits of yoga and exercise: a review of comparison studies. J Altern Complement Med. 2010;16(1):3-12.
42. Gupta SS, Sawane MV. .A comparative study of the effects of yoga and swimming on pulmonary functions in sedentary subjects. Int J Yoga. 2012;5(2):128-33.
43. A Mooventhan, Vitthal Khode. Effect of Bhramari pranayama and OM chanting on pulmonary function in healthy individuals: A prospective randomized control trial. Int J Yoga. 2014;7(2):104-10.
44. Pramanik T, Pudasaini B, Prajapati R. Immediate effect of a slow pace breathing exercise Bhramari pranayama on blood pressure and heart rate. Nepal Med Coll J. 2010;12(3):154-7.
45. Kuppusamy M, Kamaldeen D, Pitani R, et al. Immediate Effects of Bhramari Pranayama on Resting Cardiovascular Parameters in Healthy Adolescents. J Clin Diagn Res. 2016;10(5):CC17-9.
46. National Institutes of Health. [online]. Yoga for Health. 2015. Available from: http://www.nccam.nih.gov/health/yoga/introduction.htm
47. NHS Choices: Your health, your choices. [online]. A Guide to Yoga. 2015. Available from: http://www.nhs.uk/livewell/fitness/pages/yoga.aspx
48. Boyle CA, Sayers SP, Jensen BE, et al. The effects of yoga training and a single bout of yoga on delayed onset muscle soreness in the lower extremity. J Strength Cond Res. 2004;18(4):723-9.

9

Nutrition for Exercise and Lifestyle Related Diseases

Monal R Velangi

Summary: This chapter discusses the concept of diet and nutrition, its impact on individual's health, alterations in dietary needs across the lifecycle and differences in needs as per activity levels and health condition, role of nutrition in management of good health, fitness and chronic degenerative diseases. This chapter defines the following points:

1. To define basic concepts of nutrition, nutrients and energy balance
2. To study variations in nutrient needs across life cycle
3. To understand importance of nutrition in exercise
4. To acquire an overview of dietary management in health and lifestyle diseases

Keywords: Nutrition, nutrients, balanced diet, energy balance, diet in life cycle, diet in exercise, diet in lifestyle diseases.

INTRODUCTION

Food is the primary requirement for survival of a human being. It comes first among the three basic needs of life for subsistence.

Let food be thy medicine and medicine be thy food.

Hippocrates

The word **'Nutrition'** was derived from the Latin word '*nutr-*' meaning nurture or to sustain. Nutrition is defined as the science of foods, nutrients, and other substances there in; their actions, interactions, balance and their relationship with health and disease. Nutrition science includes the study of ingestion of foods, its digestion, absorption and transportation and metabolism of the nutrients and excretion of wastes.

Good nutrition is necessary for energy production (ATP) for the functioning of human body, i.e. basal metabolism and physical activity, growth, maintenance and repair of the body and regulation of vital processes occurring in the human body.

Nutrients are constituents of food that are required in specific quantities for the optimal functioning and growth of the body. They are classified as–**macro and micronutrients**.

Macronutrients (required more than 10 gms per day): carbohydrates, proteins, fats, water and fiber. Carbohydrates give energy (kcals). Dietary fiber and indigestible carbohydrates present in plant foods which have health benefits in gut health and chronic degenerative diseases. Proteins are for growth, development and repair of all cells and tissues, hormones and immunity. Fats are for energy, protection of visceral organs and sex hormone synthesis and part of cell wall.

Micronutrients [usually in mg (milligram) or μg (microgram) less than 10 g/day]. They do not provide energy, but are essential for the metabolism and functioning of various systems in the body. They include vitamins and minerals as discussed in Table 9.1.[1,2]

Table 9.1: Vitamins and minerals[3,4]

Vitamins				
	Vitamins	Functions	Deficiencies	Food sources
Fat soluble	Vitamin A	Role in vision, growth, cell differentiation, gene expression, immunity, reproduction	Night blindness, conjunctival xerosis, Bitot spots, corneal xerosis, keratomalacia. Impaired growth, reproductive function and immunity	Animal foods–organ meats (liver), eggs, milk and milk products B-carotene is a precursor of vitamin A found in green, yellow orange fruits and vegetables
Water soluble	Vitamin B_1	Synthesis of coenzyme Thiamine pyrophosphate (TPP) essential for carbohydrate metabolism and production and function of neurotransmitter acetyl choline	Loss of appetite, depression, confusion, neurological changes: Beriberi, Wernicke's encephalopathy	Whole grains, organ meats, pork, liver, eggs
	Vitamin B_2	Synthesis of coenzyme FAD essential for metabolism, conversion of B_6 to folate and tryptophan to niacin. Production of adrenal gland hormones, formation of RBCs, glycogen production, fatty acid breakdown	Oral and tongue conditions (angular stomatitis, glossitis, cheilosis), seborrhoeic dermatitis, visual symptoms—photophobia, visual fatigue, burning, slow cognitive and motor skills	Milk and milk products, eggs, liver and green leafy vegetables
	Vitamin B_3	Synthesis of coenzyme NAD essential for metabolism	Pellagra: 4 D's Dermatitis, diarrhea, dementia and death	Whole cereal grains and pulses, nuts, meat
	Vitamin B_6	Coenzyme in macronutrient metabolism, formation of niacin and hemoglobin	Hypochromic, microcytic anemia, central nervous system disturbances, oral and skin lesions	Meat, fish, poultry, nuts, pulses and meat
	Vitamin B_{12}	Formation of RBCs, RNA and DNA	Megaloblastic anemia	Organ meats, liver, fish, milk and milk products
	Folic Acid	Formation of hemoglobin, RNA, DNA and choline	Megaloblastic anaemia	Fresh green vegetables, liver and pulses
	Pantothenate	Constituent of coenzyme A which is essential in carbohydrate and fat metabolism	Affects adrenal cortex, nervous system and skin	Liver, kidney, egg yolk, yeast, fresh vegetables, meat and milk
	Biotin	Cofactor in biosynthesis of fatty acids		Liver, soybean, egg yolk, whole cereals, legumes and nuts

Contd...

Contd...

Vitamins					
	Vitamins	**Functions**	**Deficiencies**	**Food sources**
	Vitamin C	Collagen Formation, Antioxidant, immunity, neurotransmitter synthesis, iron and cholesterol metabolism	Scurvy, capillaries burst, bleeding gums, delayed wound healing, poor immunity, halt in bone growth	Amla, guava, orange, lime, green leafy vegetables
	Vitamin D	Regulation of calcium levels in body. Role in bone formation and maintenance. Important for immune function, reproductive system and skin formation. Role in synthesis of endocrine hormones	Rickets, osteomalacia, osteoporosis	Sunlight for 10–15 mins between 11am–2 pm in India; cod liver oil, egg yolk, fatty fish, mushrooms, fortified milk and milk products
	Vitamin E	Antioxidant function-protects cells, PUFA, RBCs, LDL from oxidation. Role in synthesis of nucleic acids and heme	Neurological disorders, hemolytic anemia, retinopathy, platelet and lymphocyte malfunction	Vegetable oils-mainly wheat germ oil, whole grains and nuts
	Vitamin K	Role in blood clotting and bone formation	Prolonged blood clotting time and impaired bone formation	Mainly in green leafy vegetables
Minerals				
Minerals		**Functions**		**Sources**
Macro	Calcium	Role in bone formation, maintenance and muscle contraction	Rickets, osteopenia, osteomalacia, osteoporosis	Dried fish, milk and milk products, sesame seeds, green leafy vegetables
Micro	Phosphorus	Role in bone formation, maintenance and ATP regeneration	Rickets, osteopenia, osteomalacia, osteoporosis	Bananas, green leafy vegetables
	Iron	Hemoglobin formation and coenzyme in electron transport chain	Hypochromic, microcytic anemia	Organ meats, liver, chicken, dates, green leafy vegetables
Micro	Magnesium	Bone formation	Impaired bone formation	Green leafy vegetables
	Zinc	Antioxidant, reproductive system function, DNA synthesis, hair, skin and nail health, immunity, cofactor in metabolism of macronutrients	Impaired immunity taste and smell, decreased testo-sterone levels, impaired embryo formation, affects cell differentiation and metabolism	Oysters, meat, poultry, eggs, dairy products, whole grains and nuts
Trace	Selenium	Constituent of antioxidant enzyme, component of teeth and bones	Affects teeth and bone	Seafood, meat, dairy products, vegetables (based on presence in soil)

Table 9.2: Electrolytes[1,2]

Electrolytes	Functions	Deficiencies	Food sources
Sodium	Maintaining water–electrolyte balance, role in glucose absorption, muscle contraction and nerve impulse transmission	Water-electrolyte imbalance, impaired muscle contraction, affects nervous function	Salt and salted foods—papad, pickles, chutney, preserved foods
Potassium	Muscle contraction, role in glucose absorption, role in acid base balance	Affects cardiac muscle contraction and function, glucose absorption, acid base imbalance	Pulses and legumes, green leafy vegetables, fruits like banana, coconut water, fruit juices

Water and electrolytes (Table 9.2): Our body is made up of 60–70% water by weight—intracellular (ICF) and extracellular fluids (ECF). The water balance between these compartments is maintained by salts such as sodium, potassium and chloride. Good hydration (sufficient intake of water and salts) is required for structure, growth and functioning of cells and tissues, digestion, absorption, transport and metabolism of nutrients, excretion and maintenance of normal body temperature and regulation of blood pressure. Water does not provide energy (kcals).

Balanced diet is the diet providing all the nutrients in required amounts by including all food groups in correct proportions. Foods contain carbohydrates, proteins and fats in different proportions. However, each food is richer in any one or two macronutrients. Foods with similar nutrient profile are grouped together and hence there are food groups listed in Table 9.3. The diet should provide 55-60% of total kcals from carbohydrates, 15-20% of total kcals from proteins and 25-30% of total kcals from fats.[3]

ENERGY BALANCE AND REQUIREMENTS

Energy content of foods is reported in kilocalories (kcals), 1 kcal = 1000 calories. Carbohydrates and fats are sources of energy, while proteins are mainly for growth, repair, maintenance and act as may provide energy in case of inadequate carbohydrates till fats are metabolized to provide energy. **Carbohydrates give 4 kcals/gram, proteins give 4 kcals/gram while fats provide 9 kcals/gram.** The energy content of the foods is based on the quantity of macronutrients present in it.

Components of Energy Expenditure

- ***Basal metabolic rate (BMR):*** It is the amount of energy required over 24 hours to carry out all the involuntary functions of the human body performed by various organs.
- ***Thermogenic effect of food:*** It is defined as a stimulation of metabolic rate for 1-3 hours after food consumption due to the increased metabolic work of digestion, absorption, transport, storage or other metabolic conversion, and excretion.
- ***Physical activity:*** It includes the total energy required over 24 hours divided by BMR.

Based on age, body weight and physical activity, in consideration with body composition, an individual's energy requirements can be calculated as suggested by dietary guidelines by ICMR.[3,5] Table 9.4 denotes energy requirements per day based on physical activity of an individual.

Energy intake and energy expenditure both determine the energy balance, body composition, health and risk for diseases in an individual. If energy intake and expenditure are equal a person is said to have energy

Table 9.3: Food groups and foods[1,3]

Food groups	Examples of foods	Nutrients
Cereals	Rice, wheat, bajra, corn, maize and its products	High carbohydrates (more starch than fiber), moderate proteins, less of fats
Pulses and legumes	Whole pulses, *dals* and sprouts	High carbohydrates (more starch than fiber), moderate proteins, less of fats
Vegetables	Green leafy vegetables, cruciferous vegetables, yellow orange vegetables	High carbohydrates (more fiber than starch)
Fruits	Fresh fruits and dry fruits	High carbohydrates (more of sugars and fiber–varies in different fruits)
Milk and milk products	Milk, cheese, paneer, cream, curd	Good quality proteins, some saturated fats, cholesterol
Meat, fish, poultry	Eggs, chicken, fish, mutton, beef, pork	Good quality proteins, some saturated fats, cholesterol
Nuts and oilseeds	Nuts–almonds, walnuts, cashew nuts etc., oil seeds–flaxseeds, sunflower seeds etc.	Fats, proteins and carbohydrates
Fats and oils	Vegetable oil, ghee etc.	Fats
Sugars	Sugar, jaggery, honey and its products	Sugars

Table 9.4: Energy requirements of healthy individuals by ICMR[5]

Physical activity	Energy requirements (kcals/kg body weight/day)
Sedentary	25–30
Moderate	30–35
Heavy	35–40

Note: Requirements vary as per physiological status, health status and sports activity.

equilibrium. In case of intake exceeding expenditure-positive energy balance and if expenditure exceeds intake-negative energy balance.

NUTRITION THROUGH THE STAGES OF LIFE

With respect to the variation in age, life cycle, body composition and physiological conditions there can be variations in the nutrient requirements of individuals. Especially in vulnerable age groups—pregnancy, lactation, childhood, adolescence and elderly.

Pregnancy

During the 36 weeks of gestation, a woman may gain an average of 10–12 kgs of body weight due to increase in maternal tissues (placenta, uterus and mammary glands), increased blood volume and weight of the fetus. During pregnancy there are many physiological changes in blood volume and composition, cardiovascular and pulmonary function, renal function and gastrointestinal function, demanding an increased energy and protein needs.

Dietary guidelines: Additional 350 kcals to the total energy requirement/day, additional 23 g/day of proteins during pregnancy. However, care must be taken to choose good quality carbohydrates, protein, fats, fiber and water. There might be some concerns such as morning sickness, hyperemesis gravidarum, increased body fat, insulin resistance, pregnancy-induced hypertension, pre-eclampsia, eclampsia, heartburn, constipation, mild pedal edema, leg cramps and vaginal infections. Increased needs of iron (35 mg/day) and folate (500 µg/day) and calcium (1200 mg/day). Hence, supplementation of proteins, calcium, iron, and folic acid; Vitamin E and C, B6, zinc and antioxidants are essential. Even iodine is important. Omega 3 fats (EPA and DHA) and folate are crucial during pregnancy, its deficiencies might affect brain development and cognition, might cause neural tube defects in fetus respectively. They are especially required in case of poor dietary intake (especially in case of nausea or aversions), strict vegetarians, and multifetal pregnancy. Certain food items like, raw or semi-ripe papaya, methi seeds and soybean should be avoided during pregnancy as they might increase estrogen secretion, might stimulate uterine contractions.[1,7,8]

Lactation

Lactation is the period of breastfeeding, which begins just after the birth of the infant, continues till 2 years of age. Breast milk is the mammary secretion from nursing mother. It is fresh, sterile with high nutrient bioavailability, rich in whey, immunoglobulins, several enzymes, hormones and growth factors. Exclusive breastfeeding is complete source of nutrition for the infant for the first 6 months. First 3–5 days postpartum highly, thick and yellowish in color breast milk is produced called ***colostrum***—rich in protein, zinc and sodium and immunoglobulins. The process of lactation is nutritionally demanding, especially for the mother who nurses her infant.

Dietary guidelines

- During lactation, there is an increase in requirements of energy (additional 600 kcals/day during 0–6 months and additional 520 kcals/day during 6–12 months), protein (additional 19 g/day during 0–6 months and additional 13 g/day during 6–12 months), good quality fats and fluids, vitamin A (950 µg/day), folate (300 µg/day), vitamin C (80 mg/day), calcium (1200 mg/day) and zinc (12 mg/day), vitamin B_{12} (1.5 µg/day) are essential for production of good quality breast milk.
- Small frequent meals, calorically dense, protein rich meals are essential.
- Milk production is increased with higher infant demand (suckling), use of galactogogues (e.g. shatavari) and positive attitude and family support.
- Stress, poor maternal nutrition, use of oral contraceptives and feeding of infant formula or other foods affects breast milk formation.

Breastfed babies are less likely to be overfed and develop obesity, due to regulation of feed by infant demand, are healthy with good immunity and have better cognition and are leaner in later life. Breastfeeding provides benefits for lactating mothers such as faster recovery after delivery, contraceptive effect, weight reduction, and protection against breast cancer.[7,8]

Childhood

It is the period between infancy and puberty that can be divided into three stages of growth and development: toddlers (1–3 years), pre-schoolers (4–6 years) and school-going children (7–12 years). Childhood is a 'latent period' of slow and steady growth but significant development in cognitive, social, and emotional area; changes in body composition are observed. High metabolic rate and rapid nutrient turnover, set increased nutrient requirements. Hence as per Recommended Dietary allowances (RDA) nutrients must be provided in adequate amounts in relation to the age group of the child.

Dietary Guidelines

- Regularity of meal times, variety in food and cooking methods as per food and flavor preferences of the child, interesting and attractive food combinations, and a pleasant and peaceful atmosphere;

introducing family foods in small plates, finger foods, to encourage self-eating etiquettes.

- School-going children should have family meals that are: frequent and regular, quick to eat yet nutritious, and offering variety in color, texture, taste and flavor.
- Cereal snacks, sandwiches, sprouts, soups, boiled and sautéd vegetables, and extra liquids and salts may be included for children.
- Emphasize on calcium-rich milk and milk products, whole grain products, high-fiber fruits and vegetables, along with slightly seasoned foods and finger foods such as carrots and peas.
- Tea, coffee, sugary foods, and foods difficult to chew (sticky, hard) should be restricted.[7,8]

Adolescence

It is the period between 13 and 21 years of age. During puberty, there is physical transformation of a child into a young adult, and biological changes such as: sexual maturation, building of skeletal mass, increase in height and weight, and changes in body composition. Due to hormone influences, there are significant sex differences: boys show greater increase in lean body mass (LBM), while girls show greater increase in body fat. Adolescence is the second growth spurt, which is usually fastest for boys between 10–13 years and for girls between 12–15 years. Adult stature is attained between 18–20 years but bone mass continues to increase up to age of 25. Adolescents may have damaging food habits such as: irregular meal timings, skipping meals, imbalanced dieting, excessive snacking or eating away from home (especially fast-food), addictions such as smoking, alcohol and drug abuse; this may be due to peer pressure, media and advertising, body image, working parents, social eating, ignorance of health and nutrition, easier availability of junk food than healthy food, and perception barriers to choosing healthy foods. It leads to poor nutritional status and high-risk of eating disorders: anorexia and bulimia.

Dietary guidelines

- ***Adolescents have increased requirement of energy:*** Especially as slow-absorbed high-fiber carbohydrates, and good quality fats such as MUFA and omega-3 fats.
- Protein requirements are increased to 1.2–2 gm/kg body weight due to the growth needs and pubertal changes, especially in boys who have greater increase in LBM.
- ***Calcium:*** RDA: 800 mg per day, required for bone growth, and calcium retention to support increase in bone mass, adolescents with low bone mineral density are prone to osteoporosis later in life; iron: RDA for boys (13–15 years): 32 mg/day and (16–17 yrs): 28 mg/day, RDA for girls (13–15 years): 27 mg/day and (16–17 years): 26 mg/day, Especially important for girls: to make up for menstrual losses, If lost iron is not replaced, it predisposes to iron deficiency anemia.
- It will vary with the level of physical activity and participation in sports.
- Include adequate well-balanced nutritious foods; small and frequent, tasty and attractive meals; and healthy calories from: slow-absorbed carbohydrates, first-class protein, good quality fats.
- Include calcium-rich foods and iron-rich foods (in non-vegetarians chicken for heme iron, dates, watermelon, chickoo for non-heme iron); fruits and vegetables rich in antioxidants, vitamins, minerals and fiber; along with physical activity and sports participation.
- Avoid eating out, especially empty-calorie foods, junk foods and foods high in fat, sugar and/or starch due to high risk of adolescent obesity and related diseases in later life.[6,7,8]

Elderly

It is the period beyond 60 years of age. There are physical and physiological changes of aging may range from: wrinkling of skin, gray hair to decreased sensations, reduced gastrointestinal function, decreased cardiovascular function to other metabolic effects: impaired glucose tolerance, and decreased immunity. There may be reduction in lean body mass and metabolic rate, and increase in body fat due to high catabolism, protein-deficient diets and reduced physical activity. Priority should be given to improving body composition (increase LBM and reduce body fat percentage) rather than gaining or losing weight.

Dietary guidelines

- Energy requirements will depend on the individual's metabolic rate, body type, current body composition and level of physical activity and/or exercise. Protein intake of about 1 gm/kg body weight may be needed to increase anabolism over catabolism.
- Include first-class protein, slow-absorbed high-fiber carbohydrates and good quality fats. Minimize or exclude sugars, starches and fats to preventing insulin resistance, diabetes, obesity and related conditions.
- Water and fiber are important to maintain health, prevent constipation and related conditions such as cancer.
- All vitamins and minerals are of vital importance—especially calcium, iron, antioxidants (vitamins C, E, A, zinc, selenium, chromium) and B-vitamins such as folic acid and vitamin B_{12}. They may require to be supplemented.
- Health problems in old age obesity or underweight, diabetes, renal disease, heart disease (especially hypertension and stroke), cancer, sarcopenic obesity, sedentary death syndrome, sensory losses: loss of taste, smell, tooth loss, use of dentures, dry mouth, gastrointestinal problems and increased risk of deficiency diseases, neurological conditions: such as dementia, alzheimer's and parkinson's disease, osteoporosis.
- Soft and easily chewable, easily digested, calcium-rich foods; small, frequent meals; and adequate fluid intake in the form of plain water, coconut water, butter milk, lime juice and soups. Caffeine-containing foods, sugars and sugar contain foods are to be restricted.
- An anti-aging approach requires: a regular routine of resistance training, aerobic training and flexibility, along with a balanced diet that is rich in anti-aging nutrients: protein, water, omega-3 fatty acids, antioxidants and protective vitamins and minerals.[6,7,8]

ASSESSMENT OF NUTRITIONAL STATUS OF INDIVIDUALS

WHO defines ***Health*** as a state of physical, mental and social well-being and not merely an absence of disease or infirmity.[9] A healthy lifestyle refers to health behaviors aimed at reducing one's risk of disease and accidents, achieving optimal physical health, as well as maximizing emotional, social, intellectual and spiritual health.

Nutritional status of an individual is assessed using anthropometric measurements (weight, body mass index, waist and hip circumference, waist to hip ratio), biochemical parameters (complete blood count, fasting and postprandial sugars, serum protein levels lipid profile, serum vitamin levels or urine markers), clinical signs and symptoms (e.g. paleness, hair fall, fatigue in iron deficiency) and dietary intake (recall of food intake). It is also essential to consider physical activity of an individual, which is important to understand their nutrient needs.[10]

Human body composition is divided as a two compartment model—lean body mass (muscles, tissues, organs and fluids) and body fat (adipose tissue and essential fat). The extent of weight gain and the nature of body composition change (greater gain in lean body mass or body fat) depends on body type, i.e. tendency for muscle gain vs. fat gain, body weight and body composition of the woman prior to conception, clinical conditions—insulin resistance, diabetes or heart disease, physical activity levels and lifestyle factors, nutrient composition (quality and quantity) in the diet, and eating patterns. Hence, it is important to consider body composition of an individual to determine the dietary needs.[11]

NUTRITION FOR EXERCISE

Exercise is a condition of physical stress and hence nutrient requirements increase to support activity and to reduce catabolism. However the amount of nutrients required would vary from individual to individual which is calculated considering the athlete's or exercising individual's height, weight, BMI, body composition (body fat, LBM), any history or presence of clinical conditions.

Sources of energy and energy systems: ATP is readily available in muscle but in small amounts, hence other sources are needed to support energy needs. In anaerobic activities—ATP regeneration occurs via ATP-CP system, metabolism of carbohydrates via anaerobic glycolysis, whereas in aerobic activities it occurs by metabolism of carbohydrates and fats via aerobic glycolysis and B-oxidation. There is a shift in the fuel sources used as the exercise progresses—increased duration and lowered intensity from carbohydrates towards fats. Carbohydrate are energy currency for the body, protein is the 'back-up energy source' when carbohydrate supply falls short. Fat acts as the 'emergency energy store' of the body, reserved for use in case of emergency. They are metabolized via energy systems as discussed under energy balance depending on the activity type, intensity and duration. Hence depending on the activity its essential to make wise choices for providing optimal nutrition for good performance.[10]

Also, adequate proteins, vitamin and minerals must be provided to support growth, maintenance, repair and functions of human body.

- ***Pre-training nutrition:*** To provide a high amount of energy and ensuring sustained energy throughout the training. Complex carbohydrates with moderate fiber, slow absorbed carbohydrates, e.g. whole cereals (wheat, ragi, bajra, oats, etc.) provide sustained energy but are not too heavy for digestion, low fat foods. Slow-release first-class protein, e.g. casein, skim paneer or whey in milk provide slow sustained release of amino acids for energy, B-complex vitamins or a multi-vitamin-mineral.
- ***During training/event nutrition:*** To maintain hydration and provide some energy depending on the intensity and duration of training.
  - Short duration or light training (<1 hour): Plain cool water
  - High intensity weight-training or cardiovascular training (1–1.5 hours): ORS (electrolytes)
  - Endurance/Athletic training (>2 hours): Sports drink (6–8% carbohydrates, electrolytes). 20–30 minutes before exercise: 500 mL. During training: 150 mL every 10–15 minutes. After training: replace water as 1.25 to 1.5 liters per 1 kg of body weight lost. To avoid gastric distress and heavy digestion athletes should not consume solid foods, concentrated sugar drinks, very high fat or very high protein meals in pre-exercise meals.
- ***Post-training/event nutrition:*** To replenish glycogen stores; muscles repair and recovery. Immediately simple, fast absorbed carbohydrates: e.g. glucose are fastest absorbed, spike up insulin

(for delivery into muscles) and trigger glycogen synthase enzyme (for glycogen replenishment) glucose powder, medium-size bananas or fruit juice. After 10–20 min: Fastest-absorbed first class proteins, rich in branched chain amino acids, extremely light to digest, e.g. Whey (mixed in water) or egg whites + 1 yolk. Antioxidants such as Vitamins C and E along with β-carotene, zinc, selenium and chromium.[11]

However with modern lifestyle and nutrition transitions, it has been observed that across all the age groups we can observe some form of malnutrition like undernutrition or overnutrition or specific nutrient deficiencies. This can further lead to what we know as chronic degenerative diseases/lifestyle related disorders.

NUTRITION IN LIFESTYLE DISEASES

Modern lifestyle characterized faulty eating habits, sedentary lifestyle, increased exposure to stress and pollution have been risk factors for chronic degenerative diseases, generally called as lifestyle oriented disorders such as obesity, diabetes, heart disease, bone and joint disorders, affecting quality of life. Nutrition can have a crucial role in prevention and delaying progression of these diseases.

Malnutrition

Malnutrition can be overnutrition (excess intake of energy or nutrients) or undernutrition (poor intake of energy or nutrients)

Overweight and Obesity

A person with BMI higher than 25 is considered overweight and above BMI 30 is obese. While body fat more than 20% in males and 25% falls is considered to be higher fat percentage, these people need fat loss. **Causes:** Genetics, sedentary lifestyle, faulty eating habits fad diets, very low calorie diets, empty calories. **Aim:** To maintain ideal body fat and desirable body weight range. **Management:** It is essential to understand the cause and manage accordingly. Diet, increasing physical activity and exercise and stress management together proves beneficial in obesity manage. However pharmacotherapy and weight loss surgeries would be advised in case of morbid obesity.

Dietary Management

- Small frequent meals at the gap of 2–3 hours are a must, have regular eating habits, avoid skipping meals.
- ***Energy:*** 20–25 kcals/kg IBW/day. It should be low calories (up to 1500 kcals/day).
- ***Carbohydrates:*** 55–60% of total caloric intake. Include more of whole grain cereals, 4–5 serves of fruits and vegetables for dietary fiber which gives satiety and aids in weight loss. Carbohydrate rich fruits like bananas and mangoes and refined sources of carbohydrates like white rice and rice products, refined flour are to be restricted depending on the condition. White sugar which provides empty calories and its products should be avoided.
- ***Proteins:*** 0.8 to 1 gm/kg bodyweight/day, good quality first class proteins animal source protein chicken, fish, eggs and milk and milk products. Requirements would increase in exercise. However since these sources are also high in sodium they must be judiciously used under the prescribed sodium allowance.
- ***Fats:*** 20–25% of the total calorie intake must come from fat. The ratio of SFA: MUFA:PUFA = 1:1.5:1 or 1:2:1 and the omega 6:omega 3 ratio of 2:1 needs to be maintained. Sources of omega 3 fatty acids need to be provided in adequate amounts to handle the inflammatory state, e.g. flaxseeds, fish and walnuts, oils like: flax oil, canola oil, olive oil etc. Fish oil supplements can also be recommended. Trans fatty acids are to be completely avoided as they raise the LDL cholesterol levels and lower the HDL cholesterol levels. Trans fatty acids are found in fried foods,

commercial baked goods (donuts, cookies, crackers), processed foods, foods made with hydrogenated oils and margarines.

- ***Vitamins and minerals:*** To manage the low grade inflammation, appropriate amounts of antioxidants such as vitamins—A, C, E and minerals—Zn, Cu, Se. Vitamins B for energy metabolism.
- ***Fluids:*** 2–3 liters/day, with healthy kidney function.
- Avoid addictions like smoking and drinking alcohol, eating junk food, unhealthy fast food.
- ***Behavior modification:*** No TV while eating, small portion sizes, storing healthy snacks, reading nutrition labels and making informed choices.
- ***Physical activity:*** A combination of resistant training 3 times a week for 45 mins alternated with cardio exercises 3 times a week is most effective in fat loss.

In case or morbid obesity pharmacotherapy, i.e. weight loss drugs can be suggested doctors depending on patient's history and current medical issues or Bariatric surgeries (stomach resection) may be suggested.[8,12,13]

Undernutrition

If a person has BMI lower than 18, then he is underweight and undernourished and needs prompt attention to improve his nutritional status.

Dietary Management

Additional 500 kcals to total energy requirement based on present body weight. Proteins: 2 g/kg present body weight per day. Good quality fats up to 35% of total energy requirement day. It is essential to focus more on calorically dense foods starch rich—potato and sago, good quality fats form rice bran oil/groundnut oil, walnuts and almonds, first class proteins from eggs, lean meat, milk and its products. Cheese, cream can be used but in restricted amounts to keep SFA within limits.[8]

Chronic Degenerative Diseases

Diabetes

There are raised blood sugar levels, are higher than normal, i.e. above 110 mg/dL in fasting and above 140 mg/dL 2 hours after lunch as per American Diabetic Association Guidelines. The person experiences severe weight loss, polydipsia, polyphagia and polyuria, frequent night urination. **Causes:** Genetics, lifestyle factors, obesity, insulin resistence etc. are the risk factors of diabetes. **Aim:** To maintain euglycemia (normal blood sugar levels). **Management:** Oral Hypoglycemic Agents (OHA's), insulin, diet and exercise. Diet and exercise have proven to play a great role in management of normal blood sugar level and reducing the risk of future complications. In addition to dietary guidelines same as discussed under obesity management in case of obesity being a risk factor.

Dietary Management

- Energy from carbohydrates accounts for 55–60% from the total energy intake using sources such as vegetables, fruits, beams and whole grains as it improves the insulin sensitivity independent of body weight and ability to secrete insulin adequately to overcome insulin resistance.
- Carbohydrate is the nutrient of concern. Although both the amount (grams) and type of carbohydrates in food influence the blood glucose levels, monitoring total grams of carbohydrates, whether by use of carbohydrate counting or exchanges, remains a key strategy in achieving glycemic control.
- Glycemic Index (GI), Glycemic Load (GL) and carbohydrate counting is essential to be considered in diabetes. GI is the rate at which blood sugar rises on consumption of a carbohydrate containing food. Insulin resistance needs to be managed by low GI foods and lowering of total carbohydrates, i.e. GL has proved to be

beneficial. Fiber rich polysaccharides, low GI carbohydrates show positive effect in lowering the blood glucose levels. Roots and tubers are calorically dense foods. Salads, whole pulses lowers the glycemic index of the meal. Hence, include more of low-moderate GI whole grain cereals and whole pulses, fibrous fruit and vegetables.

- Avoid sugar, jaggery, honey and sugar based products like cakes, jams etc. Non-nutritive sweeteners can be used instead of direct sugar and high GI, low fiber fruits, fruit juices and vegetables. FDA approved aspartame and sucralose based sweeteners can be used.[8,12,13]

Hypertension and Cardiovascular Diseases

It is high blood pressure, dyslipidemia causing atherosclerosis and heart diseases (ischemic heart disease, cardiac failure etc.). Since both obesity and hypertension are potential risk factors for coronary artery disease, it is important to manage both.

Dietary Management

- ***Low fat diet:*** Energy from fats accounts for 20–25% from the total energy. Maintain good quality fats: The SFA: MUFA: PUFA recommended is 1:1.5:1; Omega 3 fatty acids are beneficial in the treatment of dyslipidemia because of its anti-inflammatory effects. Sources of omega 3 are fatty fish salmon, mackerel, herring, tuna and fish oil, olive oil, flaxseeds, walnuts, canola oil. Restrict cholesterol rich foods from the diet like beef, pork, egg yolk, organ meats and margarine. It is important to read the nutrition labels in order to check out for high saturated fat, cholesterol and trans fatty acid content in the food. Trans fats should be avoided because of its atherogenic property.
- ***Sodium restriction:*** It is essential to manage hypertension. 2–3 g of Na is usually recommended for hypertensives. Severe restriction of up to 500 mg Na is recommended for very high BP patients however, in this case the food becomes unpalatable. Avoid salty and preserved foods include papads, pickles, chutney etc.
- Include more of fibrous fruits and vegetables
- Antioxidant vitamins and minerals to reduce the inflammation.
- Functional foods like garlic, cinnamon, isoflavones in soybean, flaxseeds are useful in these conditions for dyslipidemia and hypertension management.[8,12,13]

Musculoskeletal Health and Disorders

Nutrition is very essential in maintaining bone health at different stages of lifecycle, the bone nutrients of concern are proteins, vitamin D, vitamin K, calcium, phosphorus, zinc, vitamin C, vitamin A, magnesium, silicon, boron.

Osteoporosis

This is a condition in which there is low bone mass density. Increased incidence is observed with aging and in menopausal women with drop in estrogen levels.

Causes: Inadequate intake, malabsorption and reduced assimilation of bone nutrients, increased excretion, hormonal imbalances in menopausal women, increased consumption of carbonated drinks which increase bone resorption. Vitamin D is essential for calcium absorption and maintaining calcium homeostasis in human body, its deficiency affects calcium absorption, in turn causing calcium deficiency and further increasing bone resorption and lowering bone mineral density which leads to osteopenia and further to osteoporosis making the bones more prone to fractures. **Aim:** To improve and maintain bone mineral density. **Management:** Bisphosphonates, bone nutrient rich diet and resistance training.

Dietary Management

- Include balanced diet, correct deficiencies if any.

- Emphasize on increasing intakes of protein, vitamin D, calcium, phosphorus rich foods (Ca:P ratio 2:1) in case of deficiencies.
- Include antioxidant vitamins and minerals.
- Resistance training to emphasize on bone remodeling and maintenance.[8]

Arthritis

Osteoarthritis is a degenerative joint disease involving the loss of habitually weight bearing articular (joint) cartilage. The loss can result in pain, swelling, loss of motion and changes in the joint shape, in addition to abnormal bone growth, which can result in osteophytes. **Aim:** To delay progression, control symptoms of pain, inflammation, stiffness, maintain healthy body weight and improve functional abilities/quality of life. **Causes:** Obesity, imbalanced diet, smoking, genetics, over use of joints, aging etc. **Management:** non-steroidal anti-inflammatory drugs, pain killers to control pain and inflammation, physical and occupational therapy, strengthening exercises, aerobic fitness also helps psychologically, joint replacement surgery in severe grades.

Dietary Management

- Small, frequent meals are advisable. Ingestion of more calories at a time can cause hyperglycemia.
- Obesity and injury are the two greatest risks for OA. Weight loss of 5 kg will reduce risk of development of knee osteoarthritis by 50%. Hence, obesity management is must as discussed under nutrition in weight management.
- Include more of bone protective nutrients—proteins, antioxidants (large doses of dietary antioxidants, including vitamin C, the tocopherols (vitamin E), beta-carotene, and selenium) are beneficial in OA management, bone formation nutrients—vitamin D: low serum levels of vitamin D, leads to progression of OA. Calcium and vitamin D: lower consumption of dairy products, calcium and vitamin D has been observed among OA patients. In case of deficiencies, vitamin and mineral supplements include B complex vitamins and iron for improving the basic metabolic rate. Glucosamine and chondroitin sulfate supplementation based on the severity of the disease as suggested by dietitian or orthopedic expert.[13]

Rheumatoid arthritis is debilitating, crippling, autoimmune, systemic, inflammatory. Inflammation of the synovium (lining of the joint) with accumulation of lymphocytes may affect any joint—back, knees, fingers, upper and lower limbs commonly and leads to loss of functions. Rheumatoid factors formed produces immune complexes with complements which furthers inflammation. Aim is to reduce pain, inflammation, stiffness and improve the ability to perform activities of daily living. **Causes:** Genetic/hereditary: autoimmunity or some hormonal issues, imbalanced diets—high Omega 6 PUFA which produces proinflammatory cytokines. Due to poor intake, absorption and utilization of nutrients, increased losses rheumatoid cachexia (Alterations in appetite, biochemical profile, weight loss) is observed. **Management strategies:** Surgery: synovectomy, tendon reconstruction, joint replacement, **Medicines:** NSAIDs, methotrexate, steroids to control pain and inflammation, **Exercise:** Physical and occupational therapy, strengthening exercises, aerobic fitness.

Dietary Management

- Detailed assessment of nutritional status, allergies, foods that trigger symptoms, metabolism, ability and independence to self-feed.
- Adequate consumption of bone building nutrients.
- High energy and high protein in active disease (protein-1.5-2 gms/kg bodyweight)
- Weight control required in obese individuals.

- Omega 3 fatty acids in fish oil, flaxseeds and evening primrose oils are beneficial in reducing inflammation. MUFA rich oils–olive/rice bran/groundnut oils should be included more in the diet. Gamma-linolenic acid (GLA) helps to reduce joint tenderness and pain.
- Antioxidants to reduce the free radical damage and reduce the burden of oxidative stress and inflammation. Zinc, copper, selenium, vitamin E are recommended.
- Turmeric, green tea, glucosamine have reported to have beneficial effects in arthritis management.[13]

Pulmonary Diseases

Chronic obstructive pulmonary disease (COPD). This includes emphysema, bronchitis and cor pulmonale. **Aim:** To prevent exertion while breathing, improve and maintain lungs function.

Dietary Management

- ***Mode of feeding:*** In acute cases, tube feeding can be given in case of patient anxiety, labor to perform, and cost. Complications of tube feeding, decrease in oxygen consumption during sleep must be considered. It must be understood that the patient's nutritional status may be improved as long as enteral nutrition is continued but will revert if and when supplementation is discontinued, later move onto a modified oral diet.
- Eating small portions of nutrient-dense foods, and planning expectorant medication use apart from mealtimes. For many patients using oxygen at mealtimes, eating slowly, chewing foods well, and engaging in social interaction all can enhance food intake, nutrient metabolism, and enjoyment of the experience. Special caution must be given to proper sequencing of breathing with swallowing as well as to proper sitting posture during eating to prevent aspiration.
- Total energy requirements are 35–40 kcals/kg bodyweight per day.
- Determination of a specific patient's macronutrient needs is made on an individual basis, with close monitoring of outcomes. Requirements are determined as per the stage of lung disease, oxygen therapy, medications, weight status, and any acute fluid fluctuations also metabolic side effects of malnutrition and the role of individual amino acids is necessary.
- A balanced ratio of protein (15 to 20% of calories) with fat (30 to 45% of calories) and carbohydrate (40 to 55% of calories) is important to preserve a satisfactory RQ from substrate metabolism use. Protein: 1.2 to 1.7 g/kg of dry body weight is necessary to maintain or restore lung and muscle strength, as well as to promote immune function. Modifications are essential in case of presence of other diseases like diabetes, heart disease etc. Adequate exercise, fluids, and easily chewed dietary fiber enhance gastrointestinal motility.
- Vitamin and mineral requirements depend on the lung pathology, other concurrent diseases, medical treatments, weight status, and bone mineral density. Smokers and tobacco consumers have high antioxidant vitamin C requirements. Vitamin D, K, calcium, magnesium and phosphorus are essential for bone mineral density. Calcium is required muscle contraction and relaxation, phosphorus for ATP regeneration hence essential in lung function. In case of cor pulmonale and fluid retention sodium and fluid restriction is essential. Depending on the diuretics prescribed, increased intake of potassium may be required.[13]

Public Health Nutrition

Government in conjunction with epidemiologists and public health nutritionists has launched numerous policies and programs to improve the nutritional status at national level. National nutrition policy was an initiative taken under which various schemes and programs were started such as Integrated Child Development Scheme, Mid-meal Program, Iron Deficiency Control Program, National Goitre Control Program, Vitamin A Deficiency Control Program, Janani Suraksha Yojana. However, still India needs a lot of vigilant attention in the area of public health nutrition as its one of the leading countries with 1 billion population as reported in 2016 census. Hence, there is wide scope of research studies to assess nutritional status and ascertain and implement solutions with an aim to improve National Nutritional Status, thereby improving country's health index.[14]

Researches and Opportunities

Nutrition is an emerging science and has applications in various fields such as Clinical Nutrition, Sports Nutrition, Public Health Nutrition, Food Science and Technology, Food Safety, Food Processing, Functional Foods, Nutrigenomics. Novel researches are conducted in basic and experimental researches at various institutes, known institute is National Institute of Nutrition (NIN), Hyderabad, India, Indian Council of Medical Research (ICMR). Food and nutrition softwares and applications are developed but still needs to be explored to avoid the lacunae.

Nutrition is a major concern not only at individual level, but also at national level and ultimately having an impact at the global level. Hence, it is essential to make people aware of good nutritional practices-good quality food choices at right time in right amounts in congruence with adequate exercise; and empower them to make right choices in their daily life by developing healthy habits, to promote a healthy lifestyle by keeping diseases at bay and thereby improving quality of life of people. Good nutrition and adequate exercise are main keys to healthy life.

QUESTIONS

1. Define nutrition and dietetics.
2. What are macro and micronutrients?
3. Discuss the functions and sources of vitamins and minerals.
4. Define balanced diet and its importance in health.
5. What is energy balance? Discuss three components of total energy expenditure.
6. How many calories do macronutrients provide?
7. Discuss the dietary guidelines for:
   (i) Pregnancy
   (ii) Lactation
   (iii) Childhood
   (iv) Adolescence
   (v) Elderly
8. What are the nutrient needs pre, during and post training?
9. Which are the nutrients of concern in following conditions:
   (i) Diabetes
   (ii) Hypertension
   (iii) Osteoporosis
   (iv) Arthritis
   (v) COPD
10. Enlist public health nutrition based schemes and programs for improving nation's nutrition status.

REFERENCES

1. Whitney EN, Rolfes SR. Understanding Nutrition, 9th edn., Wadsworth/Thomson Learning, Belmont, CA, 2002.
2. Bamji MS, Rao NP, Reddy V. Textbook of Human Nutrition, Oxford and IBH Publishing Co Pvt Ltd, New Delhi.
3. Srilakshmi B. Nutrition Science, 3rd edn., New Age International Pvt Ltd Publishers, New Delhi, 2008.
4. Gopalan C, Rama Sastri BV, Balasubramanian SC. Nutritive Value of Indian Foods (NVIF), National Institute of Nutrition, ICMR, Hyderabad, 2000.
5. Guthrie HA, Picciano MF. Human Nutrition. St. Louis, MO: Mosby-Year Book, Inc., 1995.
6. Nutrient Requirements and Recommended Dietary allowances for Indians, Indian Council of Medical Research (ICMR), 2010.
7. Brown JE. Nutrition through the life cycle, 5th edn., Wadsworth Cengage Learning, USA, 2013.
8. Srilakshmi B. Dietetics, 3rd edn., New Age International Pvt Ltd Publishers, New Delhi, 2008.
9. World Health Organisation (WHO) report, The Asia-Pacific perspective: Redefining obesity and its treatment, 2000.
10. McArdle WD, Katch FI, Katch VL, Exercise Physiology–Energy, Nutrition and Human Performance, 5th edn., Lippincott Williams and Wilkins, USA, 2001.
11. McArdle WD, Katch FI, Katch VL. Sports Nutrition, Lippincott Williams and Wilkins, USA, 2001.
12. Williams SR. Nutrition and Diet Therapy, 6th edn., Times Mirror/Mosby College Publishing, 1989.
13. Mahan LK, Escott-Stump S. Krause's Food, Nutrition and Diet Therapy, 12th edn., USA, WB Saunders Company, 2008.
14. Vir S. Public Health Nutrition in Developing countries Part 1, Woodhead Publishing India Pvt Ltd, New Delhi, 2011.

10

Rest and Sleep

Shailaja Sandeep Jaywant

Rest is an important part of a healthy life, it rejuvenates your body and mind, regulates your mood, and plays role in maintaining memory function. Lack of rest can lead to problems as decreased memory, increased stress level etc.[1]

We can get good rest during sleep. **Sleep** is a naturally recurring state of mind characterized by altered consciousness, relatively inhibited sensory activity, inhibition of nearly all voluntary muscles, and reduced interactions with surroundings. Sleep helps to protect your mental health, physical health, quality of life, and safety. Many suffer from sleep disorders and 60% of adults report having sleep problems a few nights a week or more. Lack of good rest or sleep may lead to stress.[2]

INSOMNIA/SLEEP DISORDER

A normal functioning adult requires about 7–9 hours of sleep per day. Every individual's need for sleep is different. Any deviation from normal pattern of sleep can lead to a number of sleep disorders.

The common disorders in children are dysomnias like sleep onset difficulty, snoring etc. Parasomnias such as sleep walking, night terrors, rocking, head banging etc.

One of the major disorder which can result from stress is INSOMNIA, a medical, psychiatric disorder characterized by a persistent difficulty falling asleep and/or staying asleep or sleep of poor quality. It can be seen in children as well as adults, but common in geriatric age group. Insomnia is typically followed by functional impairment while awake. Insomnia can occur at any age, but it is particularly common in the elderly. Insomnia can be short-term (up to three weeks) or long-term (above 3–4 weeks). Common symptoms of insomnia include: fatigue, low-levels of concentration, difficulty thinking clearly, irritability, lack of enthusiasm, excessive sleepiness in day time, anxiety, irritability and depression, which may lead to disturbed public health. Sleep loss has shown to have direct effects on health and daily functioning.[3]

Insomnia can be classified as transient, acute, or chronic—Details shown in Table 10.1.

A sleep deficit can make you feel mentally slower and more emotional, which can exacerbate your experience of stress. Dealing with lasting insomnia can cause stress too which can lead to more stress-related insomnia.[4]

Stress is a collection of physical and emotional changes that are felt in response to perceived challenge or threat. Disturbance in self-regulatory capacity leads to wear and tear of the body over time. In Indian scenario stress has become significant due to dynamic social factor and changing needs of lifestyles. Stress is man's adaptive reaction to an outward situation which would lead to physical, mental and behavioral changes.

Table 10.1: Classification of insomnia[4]

Type of insomnia	Duration	Symptoms
Transient insomnia	Lasts for less than a week	Can be caused by another disorder, by changes in the sleep environment, by the timing of sleep, severe depression, or by stress. Its consequences–sleepiness and impaired psychomotor performance
Acute insomnia	A period of less than a month	Difficulty initiating or maintaining sleep or when the sleep that is obtained is non-refreshing or of poor quality. It is also termed as stress related insomnia
Chronic insomnia	Lasts for longer than a month	People with high levels of stress hormones or shifts in the levels of cytokines are more likely than others to have chronic insomnia. Its effect may include muscular weariness, hallucinations, and/or mental fatigue. Chronic insomnia can cause double vision

Too little stress can lead to boredom. Eustress is a term for positive stress—stimuli that push us to act, take on challenges, meet deadlines, when at peak performance level is described as 'Eustress', some amount of stress is desirable to increase productivity in human beings. Too much stress described as 'Distress', is negative stress, dangers, seemingly insurmountable problems. This leads to various undesirable psychophysiological symptoms and can lead to various functional problems.[5]

In today's world, the degree of stress increased owing to urbanization, globalization is an inescapable part of modern life (Fig. 10.1).[7]

COMMON STRESSORS AND CAUSES OF SLEEP DISORDERS

Any agent or circumstance capable of triggering a stress reaction is called stressor.

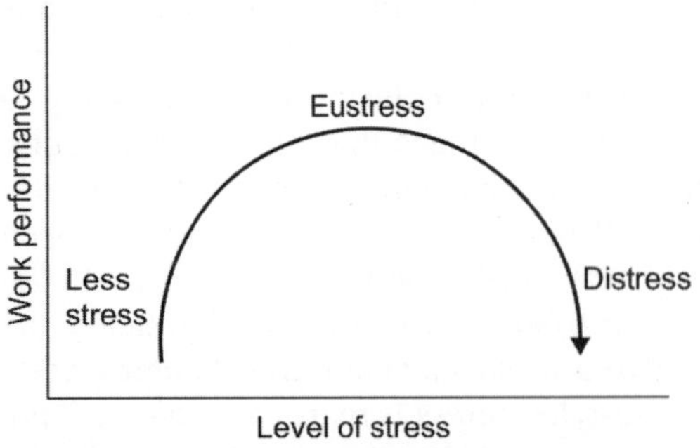

Fig. 10.1: Relationship of stress and performance level[6]

It is important for us to be aware of various stressors and etiological factors of Insomnia to be able to help our clients.

Potentially stressors fall into three categories: They are: external physical stressors, internal physical stressors and social environment stressors.[8-12] They have different effects on body depending on severity of impact and personality as shown in Table 10.2 and Figure 10.2.

PATHOPHYSIOLOGY OF STRESS AND INSOMNIA

Pathophysiology of Insomnia

Loss of sleep leads to its effect on heart rate, skin reactions and most significantly on sympathetic arousal affecting hypo-thalamus-pituitary-adrenal axis activity. Brain metabolism is raised in non rapid eye movement sleep (NonREM sleep). Irregularities are seen in reticular activating system in hippocampus, the amygdala and anterior singulate nucleus. This can lead to hormonal imbalance which further disturbs regulatory systems in the body.[14] Increased level of cortisol in the evening leads to insomnia.

Pathophysiology of Stress

There are two systems that react to stress within the body: the sympathomedullary pathway and the pituitary-adrenal system. Both systems are at work as soon as stress

Table 10.2: Classification of different stressors and their effects[8-12]

Types of stressors	Different components	Their effect
External physical	Crowding, poor lighting, inadequate ventilation, noise, environmental pollutants such as chemicals	Eye irritation, headaches, high blood pressure, nausea, drowsiness in workers leading to insomnia[8]
Internal physical	Internal neurobiologic environment like individual's biorhythm, brain hemispheric lateralization, susceptibility to stress, disrupted circadian rhythm[9] and chemicals ingested like caffeine such as tea, coffee, cocoa etc. and nicotine[10]	Two types of personalities to react to stress. **Stress Prone**—perceive change as stress, feels helpless, sense of alliniation about their lives **and stress resistant**. Perceive change as challenge have control over environment and have sense of commitment. Caffeine, nicotine sympathomimetic effect exhausts the nervous system to cope with stressors
Social environmental	Major life changes that alter social roles relationships—marriage, divorce, job change, serious illness, death of loved ones.[11] Minor changes in life such as misplacing, losing the things, being concerned about changed physical appearance, having too many things to do, unemployment, poverty, lack of clear job description, relationship problems, caring for a disabled family member or friend, difficulties at work, bad housing, noisy neighbors	Insomnia and increase susceptibility to stress

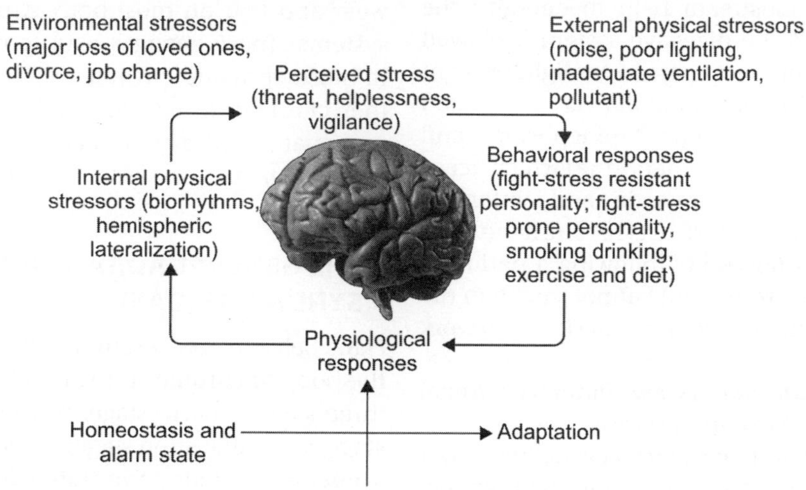

Fig. 10.2: Central role of the brain in the behavioural and physiological response to stressor[13]

occurs but have different functions in helping us to combat stress and prevent its adverse effects (Fig. 10.3).

Sympathomedullary pathway reacts to acute (immediate) stress.

Sympathomedullary pathway is activated without any conscious control. It involves a higher brain structure called the hypothalamus which acts like a thermostat. Once a need is detected it alerts the pituitary gland,

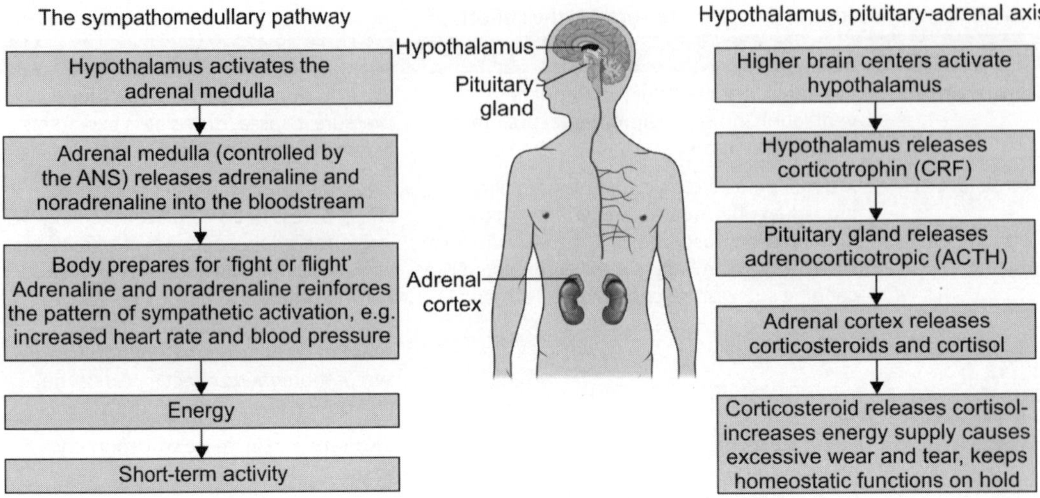

Fig. 10.3: Bodily responses in stress and sleep disorders[16, 17]

it throws the autonomous nervous system (ANS), the sympathetic and parasympathetic nervous system (SNS and PNS) into action. It increases heart rate, respiratory rate and blood pressure, sugars and fatty acids are released into the bloodstream help to energize the muscles and the digestive system is slowed down. This prepares person for fight or flight reaction. Adrenal medulla is stimulated to produce adrenaline (epinephrine) and noradrenaline (norepinephrine) which act as arousal hormones supporting and reinforcing the SNS response. PNS acts to return the body to a state of normality following a period of sympathetic arousal but cannot maintain the level of functioning for long, designed to work short-term.

Pituitary-adrenal system: Pituitary-adrenal system reacts to chronic stress.

Hypothalamic-pituitary-adrenaline axis activity emphasizes on continued energy production system activated by the hypothalamus, once a situation is assessed as stressful. It releases corticosteroids in bloodstream facilitating release of cortisol by adrenal cortex. This raises sugar and breaks down fats to release more energy blood, helps the body combat chronic stress by maintaining energy levels. It is designed to work long-term. Cortisol also suppresses immune systems and places most homeostatic functions on hold including digestion and cell replenishment and repair. Cortisol has long lasting effect on body and brain, eventually cause excessive wear and tear on most body structures and systems. These changes lead to disturbance in biorhythm and circadian cycle which further can lead to loss of sleep, insomnia. In menopausal women levels of estrogen are decreased, this can also lead to decreased sleep.[15]

THE GENERAL ADAPTATION SYNDROME (GAS)

Hans Selye in 1956 examined the reaction of the body to chronic stress. He classified it in three stages: Alarm stage, resistive/adaptive stage, and exhaustion stage; he called this the 'General Adaptation Syndrome' (GAS).

1. ***Alarm stage:*** The alarm stage enables the body to respond at speed and with energy to the potential problem it faces can only be short-term as it is highly demanding.
2. ***Resistance stage/adaptive stage:*** Stress resistant people continue to work hard to maintain energy so that its resistance to stress is maintained as much as possible.

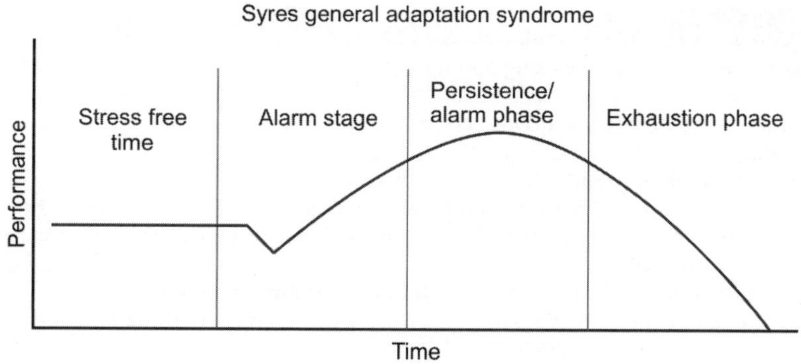

Fig. 10.4: Work efficiency of a person in several of adaptation stages of stress[18]

Stress prone persons may not be able to return to this phase, they get stuck in alarm phase, until their body enters in exhaustion stage. People who are able to reach the adaptive phase may later enter in exhaustion phase if there are too many stressors in their lives.

3. ***Exhaustion stage:*** Selye thought that chronic stress could eventually exhaust hormone reserves so much that the body would be unable to maintain its resistance, therefore, stress related illnesses such as insomnia, high blood pressure, ulcers and mental health problems might manifest themselves.[11] This different stages also affect the work efficiency of the person under stress.

The work efficiency shows variations in different stages as shown in Figure 10.4.[18]

Chronic Stress

The constant physiologic demands of chronic stress have been linked to many diseases or disorders.[18]

If the stress sustains for longer period it can lead to many diseases such as insomnia, hypertension, arteriosclerosis, myocardial infarction, migraine, headache, intestinal ulcers, inability to concentrate, neglect of responsibility, inability to learn and retain new information, irritability, nameless fears, feeling of hopelessness, loss of sexual drive, loss of self-esteem, communication problems such as finding it difficult to talk to others, sleep disorders.[5]

Stress management programs are offered for many clients those with insomnia, cardiac ailments, mental health disorders and neurologic and pain problems.

SLEEP DISORDERS MANAGEMENT

Sleep disorders can be successfully addressed by occupational therapists using various measures. Interventions focus on promoting optimal sleep performance. These interventions include educating clients and caregivers on sleep terminology, misconceptions, and expectations. The most effective intervention is lifestyle modifications such as encouraging smoking cessation, reduced caffeine intake, a balanced diet, adequate exercise, etc. establishing routine can also be one of the effective intervention in sleep disorders as shown in Box 10.1.[19,20] For addressing and treating sleep disorder—insomnias it is important to teach various stress management and coping techniques to the patients.

MANAGEMENT OF STRESS

These techniques are learned behaviors that interrupt the nervous system's stress reactions. The different techniques work at different levels.[21] **Table 10.3** shows different

Box 10.1: Shows strategies for establishing routines in sleep disorders

- **Sleep hygiene-regular times** for waking and sleeping, for several weeks of strict adherence, especially in children.
- **Implement age—appropriate incentives** or by **developing a 'contract' that** offers increasing flexibility of bedtime schedule on non-school nights in adolescents.
- Stimulus control techniques, sleep restriction, and biofeedback.
- Consistent stepwise advances of bedtime and waking time by 10 to 15 minutes nightly. Progressive delays in bedtime and waking time, until desired effect is achieved by a process also known as **chronotherapy**.
- **Managing** pain and fatigue.
- **Addressing activities** of daily living, particularly for **bed mobility and toileting**.
- **Establishing individualized sleep hygiene** routines, e.g. habits and patterns to facilitate restorative sleep.
- **Restricting** only sleep activities in the bed.
- **Avoiding** use of **technology** in bed.
- **Teaching** self-management or caregiver management, refraining techniques.
- Better **self-control**.
- **Modifying** the **environment**, including noise, light, temperature, bedding, and technology use **while in bed**.
- The therapist also takes care of **discussing the importance** of maintaining **work schedules** for self and **public safety**.[19]

stress management techniques according to level of nervous system on which they have highest impact.

Some of the stress management techniques are given in brief here, other resources may be used for detailed information.[22-43]

Aerobic Exercises

Aerobic exercises involves slow, repetitive, rhythmic contractions of large muscles of legs and arms including jogging, swimming, cycling, walking, gardening, and dancing, have been proved to reduce anxiety and depression. It plays an important part in memory formation as well as in mood and motivation.[20] This also improves stress resistant behavior.

Aerobic training program should be started after physician's complete check-up, started gradually and should work slowly towards increased difficulty.[11]

Progressive Relaxation Exercises

Progressive muscle relaxation (PMR) is a deep relaxation technique that has been effectively used to control stress and anxiety, relieve insomnia, and reduce symptoms of certain types of chronic pain. **Jacobson's progressive relaxation** technique involves systematically contracting and relaxing the muscles to make you feel calmer. The technique teaches difference between muscle tension and muscle relaxation by exaggerating the contrast between two extreme tone states. This deep muscle relaxation technique is a two-step process that involves:

1. Tensing individual muscle groups
2. Relaxing the muscle groups and feeling the tension subside.

Learning sequence for this technique is (1) systematically tensing and relaxing muscle groups to verbal cues (2) Systematic relaxing to muscle groups on verbal cues (3) relaxation of muscle groups by autosuggestion.

In this technique 11 sets of muscles are progressively tensed and relaxed in following order Hands–Elbows–Arms–Lower Back–Shoulder girdle–Back Neck–Face–Front Neck–Stomach and Chest–Leg–Foot.

This requires mental discipline and daily practice for several months.[22] This technique decreases amount of cortisol, thus decreasing stress, it is not recommended for clients with upper motor neurone lesion and spasticity, also for clients with hypertension and cardiac disease.[23] Preferably recorded commands and suggestions by therapists

Table 10.3: Stress management techniques[11,24-28,34-43]

Nervous system level/Stress function	Stress management techniques and their mode of action	
Cortex (Interpretation of events, control of emotional reactions, planning of behavior)	Autogenic training, cognitive behavioral therapy (Hypnosis)	Blood pressure, heart rate, body temperature brought under control, on loads unpleasant experiences interfering neurophysiological activity, allows brain directed self-regulatory mechanism
	Communication skills	Helps in solving problems, modifies behavior
	Biofeedback, mental imagery	Interrupts habitual stress
	Verbalization, journalizing	Analyze thoughts and brain storming to manage stressful situation
	Time management	
Hypothalamus (Autonomic nervous system and parasympathetic nervous system)	Deep breathing	Decrease heart rate, BP and increases nitric acid levels
	Laughter	Stimulates release of *endorphins*, brain endogenous opiates, thereby helping to alleviate pain and stress.[11]
	Meditation, yoga, brahmavidya	Adrenal glands produce less cortisol, activates anterior hypothalamus, controls parasympathetic nervous system. Your mind ages at a slower rate, and your immune function improves
Reticular activating system (Alertness level)	Aerobic exercises	It stimulates communication of the HPA axis with several regions of the brain, including the limbic system, amygdala and hippocampus which controls motivation and mood
	Vestibular stimulation, yoga	It modulates somatosensory perception and inhibits both hypothalamic–pituitary-adrenocortical (HPA) and sympathetic adrenomedullary (SAM) axis and decreases cortisol level and heart rate and blood pressure within normal limits and brings to stressless condition
Peripheral nervous system	Aerobic exercises	As above
	Progressive relaxation exercises	It prevents the development of serious tension melody, to use bodily energy more effectively. Relieves autonomic, cardiovascular and other systems

should be avoided. Jacobson relaxation technique mainly aims at self-awareness about tensed body parts and thus increasing the mental awareness.[24]

Yoga

Yoga—a mind-body practice is considered one of many types of complementary and integrative health approaches. KN Udupa suggests, a combined practice of physical postures, breathing exercises and meditation in a sequence to reduce anxiety and relax the person. *Shavasana* (corpse pose) provides the perfect training ground for relaxation. Training the body to respond to the request for relaxation on a muscular level and breathing deeply create a habit of relaxation that can be very helpful in turning off the stress response.[25] Studies show that yoga decreases levels of salivary cortisol, blood glucose, as well as plasma renin levels, and 24-hour urine norepinephrine and epinephrine levels. Yoga has an immediate quieting effect on the SNS-HPA axis response to stress. Yoga significantly decreases heart rate and systolic and diastolic blood pressure. Yoga reverses the negative impact of stress on the immune system by increasing levels of immunoglobulin A as well as natural killer cells.[25]

VESTIBULAR STIMULATION

Rocking is soothing because it is similar to the movements in uterus. Vestibular stimulation promotes sleep by relieving pain and reducing stressor. Rocking chair used after aerobic exercises gives positive effect on relaxation. This can be best used to promote sleep.[25]

Deep Breathing

Deep (Diaphragmatic) breathing involves slowly inhaling and exhaling to slow down general pace and work off tension. This technique involves quiet concentration on a rhythmic body function, it is also form of meditation. The process begins with focussing on normal breathing in quiet and comfortable place. This is followed by a period of deep inhalation and slow exhalation. This can be effective just before sleep time in insomnia patients. It can be practiced anywhere as long as the person is able to ignore outside distractions. It can be practiced anytime in a day. It is not recommended for clients with Chronic Obstructive Pulmonary Disease (COPD).[22]

Laughter

Laughter has the healing power of humor. Purposeful laughter can show significant increase in several different aspects of self-efficacy, including self-regulation, optimism, positive emotions, and social identification. Purposeful laughter is a realistic, sustainable, and generalizable intervention that enhances' morale, resilience, and personal efficacy beliefs.[26] It is a popular methods followed in the urban areas in India.

Meditation

It is the deep breathing technique combined with concentration on breathing. Your mind also clears and your creativity increases.[27] Meditation requires considerable discipline and can take many months to learn. There are many types of meditation which are as follows:

Transcendental meditation (TM) technique is a simple, psychophysiological stress reduction procedure. It is the ancient vedic tradition of India. The TM technique is simple and easily learned, requiring to be practiced for 20 minutes twice daily while sitting with eyes closed and repeating a mantra, a meaningless sequence of sounds specific to each individual, to promote a natural shift of awareness to a wakeful but deeply restful state. TM is taught through a 7 step course of instruction by a certified TM teacher.[28]

Brahmavidya is another practice which uses cognitive behavioral technique. The first step is to recognize the true sources of stress in your life, have positive attitude and halt stress in its track, do not get overwhelmed. It is done through spiritual breathing and meditation. This is a very ancient system of spiritual practice or sadhana. It is mainly based on concept of upanishad. The upanishad mainly explains the structure of Om, aspect of its sound, its placement, its beginning and end, and the significance of the Laya.[29]

Tai chi is another form of meditation. In the West, tai chi is practiced as a moving meditation to gain greater self-control. Using breath and balanced moving postures, practitioners facilitate the flow of chi (life force energy) to restore internal balance and harmony. Many of the movements are influenced by and derived from the natural world. It may enhance one's coping ability and potentially impact neuroendocrine responses.[30]

Mindfulness meditation is a form of meditation also known as Mindfulness-based Stress Reduction (MBSR) technique. MBSR teaches 'mindfulness,' which is a focus only on things happening in the present moment.

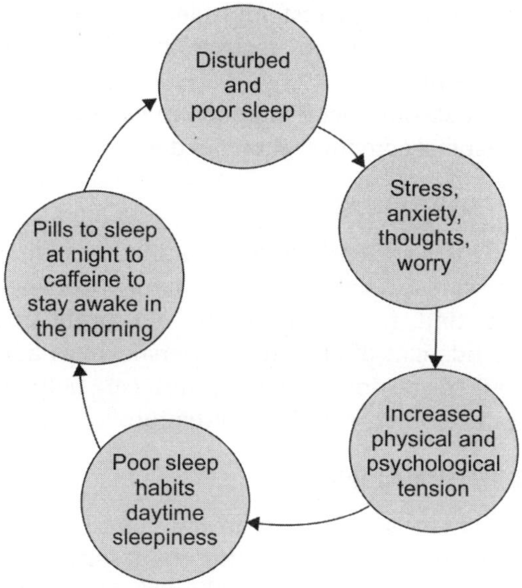

Fig. 10.5: Vicious cycle of insomnia[32]

Mindfulness is a time to purposefully pay attention and be aware of your surroundings, your emotions, your thoughts, and how your body feels. By training your mind to focus only on the present, you learn not to get lost in regrets from the past or worries about the future. Letting go of such thoughts may help you worry less and accept things as they are. Mindfulness teaches you to be in control of your mind so that your mind does not control you.[31] Mindfulness-Based Cognitive Therapy (MBCT) gives the client the opportunity to heal themselves by interjecting positive thoughts. MBCT is useful in breaking vicious cycle of sleep disorders.[32,33]

Sleep disorders become chronic due to a vicious cycle developed during the process as given in Figure 10.5.

Autogenic training: It uses cognitive behavioral therapy. It can be effective in training for sleep disorders as well as stress management. Autogenic training is meditative process that uses self-suggestions or **self-hypnosis** and mental imagery and verbal cues to achieve relaxation.

Table 10.4: Stages of visual imagery intended to resolve insomnia[34]

Step 1	Imagine spending time in your relaxation place until you become tired
Step 2	Imagine going to sleep, and notice how you become tired and can fall asleep more easily as you watch yourself falling asleep
Step 3	Imagine a master control room in which there are switches or levers that control everything that you do
Step 4	Find the control panel for your sleep
Step 5	Change the control panel slowly towards the sleep position, and notice how you become sleepy as this occurs
Step 6	While you are in hypnosis, tell yourself that you are becoming sleep

It involves six steps which go through achieving mental stance to stage of cardiac regulation to cooling down and visual imagery leading to sleep peacefully. It is very useful in acute insomnia. Stages of visual imagery, self-hypnosis are shown in Table 10.4.

Self-hypnosis is found to be very useful in sleep disorders. Most people who attempt self-hypnosis use a script that has already been written or recorded for them. And most scripts use a combination of visualization and body self-awareness. This is not recommended for clients who are agitated or hallucinating.[34]

BIOFEEDBACK

Biofeedback is the technique of using equipment (usually electronic) to reveal human beings some of their internal physiological events, normal or abnormal, in the form of visual, auditory signals in order to teach them to manipulate these otherwise involuntary or unfelt events by manipulating the displayed signals. Biofeedback helps to change characteristic body response to the stressors.[11,35]

COMMUNICATION SKILLS

Stressful situations are caused by misunderstanding. One of the technique to improve communication is transactional analysis. It helps in solving the problems that create stress. Information from this is used to change person's behavior or modify reactions to the behavior of others.[36,37]

MENTAL IMAGERY

Imagery is a potent method of stress reduction, especially when combined with physical relaxation methods such as deep breathing. Mental imagery techniques use both active and passive daydreaming to interrupt habitual stress. This can be effectively **used with hypnosis** in sleep disorders. By allowing you to rehearse mentally, imagery also allows you to practice in advance for anything unusual that might occur, so that you are prepared and already practiced in handling it.[22,38] This technique is contraindicated in hallucinating patient.

TIME MANAGEMENT AND LIFESTYLE MODIFICATION

Time management technique includes:

1. Identify your best time of day, realistically scheduling and organizing the time
2. Setting limits. Try not to do too many things at once. Accepting that everything cannot be done at once
3. Make a list of things you have to do setting priorities about task accomplishments.
4. Try to vary your tasks in a day, changing schedules or daily routine to avoid the stressful situation.
5. Exercise regularly by bicycling, walking, hiking, jogging, or working out at the gym. Your body can fight stress better when it is fit.
6. Avoid alcohol and recreational drugs. And do not smoke and eat healthy, well-balanced meals.
7. Get enough rest and sleep. Your body needs time to recover from stressful events.
8. Seek out social support, involve in pro-social activities when needed.[40]

VERBALIZATION

Talking to friends and acquaintance about stressors can help to ventilate pent up feelings and find new solution to old problems. Friends can offer different perspectives and new suggestions. This support can help to come out of the problem situation.[11]

JOURNALING

If a client is waking up in the night because he/she cannot stop thinking about something that causes stress during the day, journaling can be helpful. Journaling is the act of writing disturbing thoughts which cause stress and analyze them later. The act of journaling can help you clear your mind, help you process strong emotions that are causing you to lose sleep, and help you brainstorm and construct plans that can help you manage the situations that are causing you stress. It is most beneficial in adult INSOMNIAS.[41]

STRESS MANAGEMENT IN INDIAN INDUSTRIES

Increasing competition in the global market has compelled Indian organizations to deal with stress management issues on a priority basis. Organizations employ various methods to manage stress among their employees. Such methods include providing:

- Healthy and hygienic work environment
- Fair compensation
- Flexible work schedules. Lifestyle modifications
- Proper feedback mechanism
- Insurance options
- Proper leaves and holiday options
- Training and job security so that employee feel motivated to work

- ***Stress audit:*** Teaching person causes of stress and its impact on them

Some organizations employ counselors to deal with stress related problems of employees. Activities like picnics, outdoor sports, stress management seminars and lectures, spiritual programs are also undertaken by organizations to reduce stress levels among their staff.[42]

ASSESSMENT FOR STRESS AND FOR INSOMNIA

DSM-5 gives diagnostic criteria of insomnia (Box 10.2). Sleep history in past month also provides important information. Numerous self-report instruments exist for the assessment of sleep disturbance. Among the most widely used are the epworth sleepiness Scale (ESS), Pittsburgh Sleep Quality Index (PSQI), which provides a global assessment of sleep. Some other subjective scales, i.e. patients perception about their wakefulness are Stanford Sleepiness Scale (SSS), Visual Analoge Scale (VAS) of Alertness/Sleepiness, Karolinska Sleepiness Scale (KSS) and the Insomnia Severity Index (ISI).[43,44]

Guided self-assessment of individual stressors and stress reaction is the first step of ideal stress management program. Stress management questionnaire can help to identify stress.[45]

The Holmes and Rahe Stress Scale/Social Readjustment Inventory—Understanding the impact of long-term stress-series of 43 life-events in the previous two years is evaluated in this scale.[45] The Standard Stress Scale (SSS) is used for measuring stress in the life course and has 11 items. It can be used in chronic stress.[46,47]

Other forms are available to identify physical, emotional and behavioral stress responses such as Perceived Stress Scale (PSS), remains a popular choice for helping us to understand how different situations affect our feelings and our perceived stress. **Stress coping resources inventory:** A self-Assessment of stress is also useful to assess use of coping skills in a person.[48] Formal stress scores should be interpreted carefully. Work, play, balance in life and daily activities along with time management plays important role in life.

General factors for choosing the appropriate technique for intervention of stress and sleep disorders.

Some general factors should be considered in suggesting stress management techniques—learning style of the client and the technique demands (concrete or abstract), financial and interpersonal resources required, lifestyle and daily routine of client, time available to learn new technique, e.g. for a patient with insomnia due to acute stress, referred to you. Time management, advice about sleep hygiene can be the techniques of priority over the other techniques.[11]

Box 10.2: Diagnostic criteria for insomnia

DSM-5[2] Criteria for insomnia disorder

- Dissatisfaction with sleep quantity or quality, associated with difficulty initiating sleep, difficulty maintaining sleep, or early morning awakening with inability to return to sleep.
- Sleep disturbance causes clinically significant distress or impairment in social, occupational, educational, academic, behavioral, or other important areas of functioning.
- Sleep difficulty occurs at least three nights per week.
- Sleep difficulty is present for at least 3 months.
- Sleep difficulty occurs despite adequate opportunity for sleep.
- Insomnia is not better explained by another sleep-wake disorder, a coexisting mental disorder, or the physiological effects of a substance.

Case Study 1

A 55-year-old female patient was referred to occupational therapy department for improving social skills. She had come with complains of disturbed sleep, unexplained fears, difficulty in concentrating at work, inability to complete household chores in time, scared to go out of her house, feeling of helplessness, decreased appetite since a year, worsened now. She also had complains of uncontrolled hypertension. She was on anti-hypertensive and antianxiety medicines.

Assessment: Patient had scored moderate anxiety level, i.e. 49 on Zung Self-Rating Anxiety Scale. She revealed difficulties in completing Instrumental Activities of Daily Livings (IADLs). In narrative interview it was revealed that, she is on antihypertensives since 10 years. But had uncontrolled hypertension since last years, after her son had met with a road accident and is bedridden since then. She exhibited above symptoms since this episode. Patient did not reveal any gastrointestinal abnormalities on investigations.

Interpretation: Her premorbid personality was anxious. She had these symptoms secondary to her heightened anxiety levels. She may have uncontrolled hypertension due to this stress. Her symptoms may have worsened as left untreated till now. Along with pharmacological treatment, she needs to get trained for some stress management techniques such as, autogenic training for bringing down her anxiety. This may resolve her social problems.

Intervention: Patient was counseled for the various methods of treatment. Her basic personality was analyzed and individualized program was planned for her. After getting her consent she was first treated with daily Jacobson's Relaxation Technique sessions. After 3 weeks she reported decreased fearfulness and reduced hypertension. Her anxiety level has come down on Zung anxiety scale.

Later she was taught mental imagery techniques. She was advized to use it especially before sleep time and/or before she has to set to go out. Her sleep pattern is gradually improving, can venture out without fear, but still requires known person with her. Due to this she has started participating actively in managing household chores.

Later she will be counseled for identifying stressful situations and can be taught deep breathing techniques on anticipation of stressful situation. This may benefit her in coping with the stress.

Thus use of stress relieving techniques should be decided after careful evaluation of patient's personality and causes of stress.

A case study done in Occupational Therapy Department, LTMM College and General Hospital, Sion, Mumbai.

SUMMARY

Stress is perceived differently by each individual depending on the personality of the individual. The stress can lead to various physical and psychological symptoms, including sleep disorders. Stress management program can be individualized or group activity. Various stress management techniques mainly aims at reducing the stressors or teaching a coping techniques. These different strategies act on different levels of nervous system. The techniques used for stress and sleep disorders should be chosen after evaluation of individual causes of stress and personality of the client. All clients may not need formal stress management techniques training.

Stress management techniques should be learnt from trained personal or psychologist or occupational therapists. Choice of stress management technique depends on professional judgment of the person. One style of training does not fit all. Managing stress can help client to achieve maximum functional independence.

REFERENCES

1. The Importance of Rest and Relaxation, (Internet) (Place-Unknown). (https://www.washington.edu/admin/hr/benefits/publications/carelink/tipsheets/rest-relax.pdf).
2. Why sleep is so important? (Internet) American Psychological Association. (http://www.apa.org/topics/sleep/why.aspx).
3. Cognitive Behavioral Therapy in Insomnia. National Sleep Foundation, (Internet). (https:/sleepfoundation.org/sleep-news/cognitive-behavioral-therapy-insomnia).
4. Ruth Benca. The Impact of Stress on Insomnia and Treatment Considerations: Association Between Stress and Insomnia, Medscape Multispecialty, (Internet) (Place Unknown). (http://www.medscape.org/viewarticle/557651_2).
5. Jagdish Parikh, Eds. Stress Management and Self-development, Managing Yourself, Management by Detached Involvement: Blackwell, India book distribution Basil, 1991;pp 44-50.
6. Work Life Balance, Human Function Curve (Cited: 18th February 2016), (http://mysmallroom.blogspot.in/2008/02/work-life-balance.html).
7. A Study on Stress Management and Coping Strategies with Reference to IT Companies, Uma Devi T, Journal of Information Technology and Economic Development, 2011; 2(2):pp 30-48. (http://www.gsmi-ijgb.com).
8. Raloff. Building illness, Science News, (1981 a, b), 120, 316.
9. Geschwind N and Galaburda A. Cerebral Lateralization: Biological Mechanism, Association, and Pathology: A Hypothesis and Program for Research, Archives of Neurology, 1985;42:pp 428-459.
10. Kobasa, Hilker and Maddi. Who stays healthy under stress? Journal of Occupational Medicine, 1979;21:pp 595-98.
11. Elizabeth Blesedell Crepeau, Ellen S. Cohn, Barbara A, et al. Eds. Willard and Spackman's Occupational Therapy, 8th edn., Wolters Kluwer/Lippincott Williams and Wilkins, Baltimore, Philadelphia, 2003;pp 588.
12. Lazarus RS. Little hassels can be hazardous to your health, Psychology Today, 1981;15:pp 58-62.
13. McEwen RS. Physiology and Neurobiology of Stress and Adaptation: Central Role of the Brain; Physiological Reviews, 2007;87(3):pp 873-904.
14. Pigeon WR. Diagnosis, Prevalence, Pathway Consequences and Treatement of Insomnia, Indian J Med Research, 2010;131:pp 321-32. Available from: (www.icmr.nic.in).
15. Elizabeth Blesedell Crepeau, Ellen S Cohn, Barbara A Boyt Schell. Eds. Willard and Spackman's Occupational Therapy, 11th edn., Wolters Kluwer/Lippincott Williams and Wilkins, Baltimore, Philadelphia, 2009; pp 718.
16. Bodily responses in Stress and Sleep Disorders (Image). (http://intranet.tdmu.edu.ua)
17. Bodily responses in Stress and Sleep Disorders (Image). (http://www.simplypsychology.org)
18. Martin Fortin, Maud-Christine Chouinard, Tarek Bouhali, et al. Evaluating the integration of chronic disease prevention and management services into primary health care, BMC Health Services Research, 2013;13:132. Available From: (http://bmchealthservres.biomedcentral.com/articles/10.1186/1472-6963).
19. Occupational Therapy's Role in Sleep; (Internet) (Place: unknown). (http://www.aota.org/about-occupational-therapy/professionals/hw/sleep.aspx).

20. Timothy F Hoban. Sleep and Its Disorders in Children, Semin Neurol. 2004;24(3), Available From: (http://www.medscape.com/viewarticle/491438_7).
21. Guszkowska M, Effects of exercise on anxiety, depression and mood, Psychiatr Pol, 2014; 38(4):611-20, Pub Med; Cited by Ashish Sharma, Vishal Madaan and Frederick D. Petty. for Exercise for Mental Health, Primary Care Companion J Clin Psychiatry, 2006;8(2):pp 106.
22. Jonathan C Smith, Eds. Stress Management: A Comprehensive Handbook of Techniques and Strategies, Springer Publishing Company, 2002;4:pp 48-51.
23. Cyndi Courtney and Barbara Escobedo. A Stress Management Program: Inpatient-to-Outpatient Continuity, American Journal of Occupational Therapy, 1990;44:pp 306-10.
24. FJ McGuigan and Paul M Lehrer. Progressive Relaxation: Origins, Principles, and Clinical Applications, Stress Management Methods. (http//www.bodypsychyoga.com/ Downloads_BCMT/Progressive Relaxation.pdf).
25. Ellen Serber. Stress Management through Yoga, International Journal of Yoga Therapy, 2000; 10(1):pp 11-6. (http://iaytjournals.org/doi/abs/10.17761).
26. Kumar Sai Sailesh, Archana R and Mukkadan J K. A Controlled Vestibular Stimulation: A Physiological Method of Stress Relief, Journal of Clinical Diagnostic and Research; 2014;8(12) :pp 1-6. (www.ncbi.nlm.nih.in).
27. H Beckman and N Regier. Judy Young Effect of Workplace Laughter Groups on Personal Efficacy Beliefs. The Journal of Primary Prevention, 2007;28(2):pp 167-182.
28. RC Deshpande. A healthy way to handle work place stress through yoga, meditation and soothing humor, International Journal of Environmental sciences, 2012;2(4). (www.ipublishing.co.in).
29. Liza Varvogli and Christina Darviri. Stress Management Techniques: Evidence-based procedures that reduce stress and promote health: Health Science Journal, 2011;5(2):pp 74-89. (www.hsj.gr).
30. Vihangam yoga (Internet) (Place –unknown). (https://en.wikipedia.org/wiki/Vihangamyoga).
31. Song R, Lee EO, Lam P, et al. Effects of Tai Chi Exercise on Pain, Balance, Muscle Strength, and Perceived Difficulties in Physical Functioning in Older Women with Osteoarthritis: A Randomized Clinical Trial; Journal of Rheumatology; 2003;30(9):pp 2039-44.
32. Marchand WR. Mindfulness-based stress reduction, mindfulness-based cognitive therapy, and Zen meditation for depression, anxiety, pain, and psychological distress, J Psychiatry Pract, 2012;18(4):pp 233-52.
33. Sipe WE and Eisendrath SJ. Mindfulness-based cognitive therapy: Theory and practice, Can J Psychiatry, 2012;57(2):pp 63-9.
34. RD Anbar and MP Slothower. Hypnosis for Treatment of Insomnia in School-Age Children: A Retrospective Chart Review, BMC Pediatrics, 2006;6:23.
35. Harry Mills, Natalie Reiss and Mark Dombeck. Hypnosis and Autogenic Training for Stress Reduction, 2008, (Place unknown). (https://www.mentalhelp.net/articles/hypnosis-and-autogenic-training-for-stress-reduction)
36. Jane B Lemaire, Jean E Wallace, Adriane M Lewin, et al. The Effect of a Biofeedback-Based Stress Management Tool on Physician Stress: A Randomized Controlled Clinical Trial, Open Med, 2011;5(4):pp e154–e165.
37. Transactional Analysis and Communication (Internet) (place unknown). (www2.hull.ac.uk/ifl/docs/UFA-TransactionalAnalysis.doc).

38. Communications and Stress Management, (Internet) (place-unknown), Rev. Fall 2011-Level I Communications and Stress Management 10-1; (cited20th Feb2016). (http://www.tmcec.com/public/2010.pdf)
39. Imagery-Mental Stress Management, (Internet) (place Unknown), Comprehensive Behavioral Healthcare. (www.cbhcare.com).
40. Jonathan C Smith. Stress Management: A Comprehensive Handbook of Techniques and Strategies, Springer Publishing Company; New York: ABC Relaxation, 2002;12:pp 219-26.
41. Elizabeth Scott MS. Stress Related Insomnia: How To Deal With Stress-Related Insomnia, 2014, (Place unknown). (http://stress.about.com/od/otherconditions/a/insomnia.htm).
42. Uma Devi T. A Study on Stress Management and Coping Strategies With Reference to IT Companies, Journal of Information Technology and Economic Development, 2011;2(2);pp 30-48. (http://www.gsmi-ijgb.com/Documents).
43. Bastien CH, Vallières A and Morin CM. Validation of the Insomnia Severity Index as an outcome measure for insomnia research, Sleep Med, 2001;2(4):pp 297-307. (http://www.ncbi.nlm.nih.gov/pubmed/11438246).
44. M Johns. Rethinking the assessment of Sleepiness, Sleep Medicine review, 1998;2(1):pp 315. (Epaworth sleepiness scale.com).
45. International Stress Management Questionnaire by International Stress Management Association UK-2013:S. (www.isma.org.uk).
46. The Holmes and Rahe Stress Scale/Social Readjustment Inventory. (https://www.mindtools.com).
47. The Standard Stress Scale. (https://www.neps-data.de).
48. Matheny KB, Aycock DW, Curlette WL, et al. The Coping Resources Inventory for Stress: A Measure of Perceived Resourcefulness, J Clin Psychol, 1993;49(6):815-30. (http://www.ncbi.nlm.nih.gov/pubmed/8300870).

11

Leisure Activities for Mental Health

Odette M Gomes

Abstract: Bundy (1993) stated 'we must actively and systematically promote play and leisure in our clients' lives and in our intervention sessions.[1] People benefit from participation in leisure activities that are safe, meaningful and associated with successful performance. This is perhaps especially critical to those with mental illness. It is essential that as occupational therapists we partner with our clients to achieve this goal. Full participation and engagement in occupations that hold meaning and value is the intended outcome of successful occupational therapy intervention.

Keywords: Leisure activities, burn out, work-life balance, occupational balance, occupational performance model, leisure in treatment, mental health.

'All work and no play makes Jack a dull boy' is a well-known saying'

In today's fast paced life where one is constantly on the move, be it a school going child, a young working adult or even an elderly person. The twenty four hours in a day are just not sufficient enough. Before one day ends, the chores, duties, stressors of the next day are already upon you. Days merge into weeks, weeks into months and lo and behold the year has come to an end. Another year has gone by.

When was the last time you had time for yourself doing things that you really enjoy? This is something you probably may not even remember, owing to the fast-paced life. With work taking priority in the lives of many, people have very little time for any kind of leisure activities. No matter how busy you are with work, there comes a time when your body and mind start signaling to you for some much needed break, so much so that you feel like running away to some isolated, quite, and far off island. And that's when you should definitely listen to both and take a break from the daily hustle-bustle. At the other end of the spectrum—the retiree–one who has retired from active service, does not quite know what to do with himself/herself. The fact of the matter is that we are raised with a strong work ethic. In today's world, the hectic pace of our jobs reinforces our work ethic. With what seems like more and more work to do along with fewer and fewer people to do it. When we retire we may leave the job behind, but we don't necessarily leave the work ethic with it. Often a 'burn-out' is seen in workaholics. The secret is to find a balance between work and leisure during both your career and retirement.

In both cases—the young worker as well as the older retiree have been subjected to the stresses and strains of daily life which in turn have had an adverse effect on one's physical as well as mental health.

All wellness gurus advocate that one should maintain a good work-life balance. Maintaining an occupational balance is a domain of 'Occupational therapy'.

Occupations are 'the chunks of culturally and personally meaningful activity in which humans engage'.[1] People create or orchestrate their daily experiences through planning and participating in occupations. Occupational Therapy generally considers work, self care, leisure, play and rest to be the major occupations of people. Since the inception of the profession, Occupational Therapy has always valued a balance of these occupations.

The science behind this lies in the Occupational Performance Model which consists of Performance Areas, Performance Components and Performance Context.[1]

Performance Areas are further divided into (a) Activities of Daily Living, (b) Work or Productive Activities and (c) Play or Leisure Activities.

Performance Components are divided into (a) Sensorimotor components, (b) Cognitive intigration and cognitive components and (c) Psychosocial skills and Psychological components.

Performance Contexts are divided into (a) Temporal aspects and (b) Environment.

Mary Reilly (1974) describes play along a continuum leading to work and leisure.[1] Children learn skills and develop interests through play that later affect choices and success in work and leisure.

The term play and leisure are often used interchangeably and are usually differentiated by age, in that children play and adults engage in leisure activities.[1]

Throughout a person's life, the amount of time spent in activities defined as play, work or leisure varies. In early childhood, most of the time is spent in play. As children mature, time is divided between school and free time, later work and non work. In older adults, leisure time predominates.

Play and leisure are important parts of life and like all activities take place within a sociological context.[2] Childhood play and adult play, i.e. leisure, are both important for overall health.

As Indians, we do not give importance to getting involved in active leisure time activities. And how important it is to cultivate hobbies/active leisure time activities as adults that in turn help later on in life. Older adults/retirees invariably face boredom which is a leading cause of depression. Leisure activities where individuals engage with other people also help in developing a sense of belonging to a group.[3] The adult's predominant use of time is in work and rasing a family. Multiple factors affect leisure patterns in adulthood, such as age, sex, marital status, work roles etc. Single adults take part in a wider variety of activities outside the home than married people and in particular physical recreation or social activities vary between man and woman of different ages.

Leisure activities are those in which the individual participates in order to socialize, relax or pursue interests and hobbies.[2] Play or leisure activities are intrinsically motivating activities for amusement, relaxation, spontaneous enjoyment or self expression.[1] Recently the emphasis has been more on play and leisure as an experience or state of mind and this seems more helpful when considering a balanced life. Cultivating a hobby in one's younger days is a useful activity. This gives one a headstart as an adult to fall back on and catch up with, in one's 'spare time'.

Leisure or play usually occurs outside of the obligations of one's work and provides opportunities for enjoyment, relaxation, recreation, personal growth and personal achivements.[1] Leisure is driven by internal motivation, implies freedom of choice and is not usually done within time constraints.

The functions or characteristics of leisure or play can be described as (1) personal development, (2) enjoyment, (3) entertainment, (4) interaction with others, (5) free choice, (6) relaxation, (7) challenge and (8) goal achievement.

The way a person approaches the activities in his or her daily life may be more important to health and life satisfaction than the activities themselves. If a person really enjoys and is challenged by a task, be it work or play, satisfaction and a feeling of well being ensures.

Leisure persuits meet different needs. Sometimes people want to do something different or exciting or creative or competitive. Other times they just want to relax. Studies have shown the same leisure persuit often met different needs for different participants. What is the importance of Leisure? Leisure activities are important to bring about a positive flow of energy in a person, physical and health benefits and aids positivity.

LEISURE IN TREATMENT[1]

People are usually referred when their participation of daily occupations has been altered as a result of injury or illness. However, practitioners are also involved in prevention and wellness programs when there is the potential for disruption of occupation. A major goal is to help the individual achieve a balance of meaningful activities in daily life.

Activities that are usually ascribed to leisure are also used by practioners to achieve specific goals. Crafts and recreational activities provide opportunities for active involvement on the part of the client and can be adapted to meet therapeutic goals. With adults, as with children, it is important to use activites that are both meaningful to the person and are therapeutic.

Examples of Leisure Activities: These are examples of types of leisure activities you can choose from. Active leisure activities include energetic activities that even require one to use mental strength. You can learn to dance (or pick up where you left off). Currently 'Line Dancing' is a popular 'seniors' form of dance in our city as is all over the world. Listening to music-devotional or other, learn to play a musical instrument or even join a singing class. Yoga an ancient Indian art is ideal as an activity for mental wellbeing. The breathing techniques as well as some simple asanas can be performed even by the elderly. Yoga is known to be a great de-stresser. Healthier individual could do some keep fit exercises, join a laughter club or just go for a walk-individually or with someone. Another leisure activity that also helps keep fit is swimming. Social activities by joining a neighborhood club/group, volunteer work at the community center too is a good option. Sharing one's expertize with the young ones, be it cooking or teaching, reading or telling stories to the children is a rewarding leisure activity. On an individual level playing remedial or cognitive games, doing puzzles, even travel helps keep mind and body relaxed. One cannot emphasize enough on the benefits of needlework, gardening, walking, cooking and even pet care.

Passive leisure activities are all about relaxation and can even mean watching a movie with friends, reading, taking a stroll in a park or on the beach, or even visiting a spa. Even if you want to sit at home and do nothing, it's completely okay! That's just another way to spend some quality time with yourself or your family. It will help strengthen the bond with your family members.[4] Both play and leisure are considered areas of occupation, therefore performance concerns related to exploration and participation in these areas are addressed. Participation in play and leisure has many benefits for people across the life span regardless of the conditions they may experience.

Leisure is believed to positively influence health, enhance well being, improve coping skills, buffer stress and provide a means to augment self identity and development.

Having leisure occupations available and accessable enhances quality of life. These are critical issues for persons with mental illness.

SUMMARY

Bundy (1993) stated 'we must actively and systematically promote play and leisure in our clients' lives and in our intervention sessions.[1] People benefit from participation in leisure activities that are safe, meaningful and associated with successful performance.[3] This is perhaps especially critical to those with mental illness. It is essential that as occupational therapists we partner with our clients to achieve this goal. Full participation and engagement in occupations that hold meaning and value is the intended outcome of successful occupational therapy intervention.

Case Study 1

Mrs P, a 72-year-old lady—a case of depression, was referred to OT. She came from a middle socioeconomic strata of society. History showed that she had been caring for her ailing husband for the past 8 years and was recently widowed. Her children were living in another state and she was on her own. As she had been busy with looking after her ailing husband for a while, she had lost touch with her friends and her social interaction had diminished.

She was assessed keeping the OP Model in view, her problem areas were in ADL, Productive activity and Leisure activity from the performance areas and temporal and environmental aspects from the performance context. Her strengths were she loved reading, children and was a helpful person.

The therapist devised the following program for her. An activity scheduling was done so she had a structure for the day, a timetable of sorts–earlier her schedule revolved around her ailing husband. She was encouraged to look after herself, her dressing, perhaps get a hair cut too. This would help increase her self esteem and self worth. Since she loved reading, she was encouraged to read or tell stories to the children of the building. She lived in–at least once a week. A volunteer from the local ladies group was asked to accompany her on walks or to the market and gradually involve her in the group/community activities. To keep the memory of her late husband, it was suggested to her to plant something to keep in her balcony/windowsill and nurture its growth.

Performance context-at times, the placement of a particular piece of furniture (a chair or the bed) used by the deceased can be a constant and sometimes painful reminder. If required a change or rearrangement of the furniture in the room, may help.

In course of time, Yoga in groups was started. Subsequently, she was able to run errands more confidently, her self esteem was brighter and she was able to face the world with a lot more positivity.

Case Study 2

Mr X, a 80-year-old gentleman from an upper middle socioeconomic strata of society, living with his wife, son, daughter-in-law and two grandchildren, showed affectation in his performance areas of ADL, productive activity and leisure activities. He felt his self worth diminish as he was no longer being a useful part of society. He was home bound.

His strengths were, he had worked as an officer in a bank, loved music and was a sportsman. The program planned was. Activity scheduling to give a structure to the day. Simple exercises with yoga deep breathing and asanas to limber up (considering he was home bound for a while). To occasionally help the building society in the office matters (as a consultant), gave him a purpose and usefulness in life. The yoga at home and his involvement in the building management gave his self esteem a helpful boost. This led to him being invited to be the chief guest at a building society function, at a later date. He began taking walks along with the other seniors in the area, helping the young ones in banking matters, learnt a couple of board games like scrabble, Uno, chess and was an 'honorary grandpa' to those little ones around, playing ludo and snakes and ladders with them.

In course of time, his health and general well being showed a sharp incline and the family too were happy with the change.

REFERENCES

1. Neistadt ME, Crepeau EB. Willard and Spackman's Occupational Therapy, 9th edn.
2. Turner Ann, Foster M, Johnson SE. Occupational Therapy and Physical Dysfunction, Principles, Skills and Practice, 4 th edn.
3. Helen L Hopkins. Willard and Spackman's Occupational Therapy, 8th edn.
4. Catana Brown, Virginia C Stoffel. Occupational Therapy in Mental Health: A Vision for Participation, 2011.

RECOMMENDED ADDITIONAL REFERENCES FOR FURTHER READING

1. Jennifer Creek, Lesley Lougher. Occupational Therapy and Mental Health, 4th edn.
2. AOTA: A Curriculum Guide for Occupational Therapy Educators. Rockville MD, 1974.
3. AOTA: Uniform Terminology for Occupational Therapy, 3rd edn, American Journal of Occupational Therapy. 1994;48:1047-54.
4. AOTA: The Roles and Functions of Occupational Therapy Personnel. Rockville MD, 1973.
5. Miller RJ, Sieg KW, Ludwig FM. Six Perspectives on Theory for Practice of Occupational Therapy, Rockville MD, 1988.
6. Rosemary Hagedorn. Occupational Therapy: Foundations for Practice: Models, Frames of Reference and Core Skills, 1992.

12

Yoga and General Fitness

Sabir Shaikh

INTRODUCTION

Yoga is essentially a Practice and Experience. It is not an exercise. Yoga is a journey towards inwardness by incessant practice of various techniques leading towards silent meditation; it is the experience of perfect calmness of mind and self knowledge. Yoga is an Art, a technique for achieving the purest form of self awareness devoid of all thought and sensation. Such knowledge of self has the power to destroy illusions about our nature and the world, and thus release us from the bondage of fear and ignorance. Yoga is the highest wisdom; it is the most perfect form of self expression.

Yoga is an art of life. Art achieves practical results through both theory and practice. Art as technique needs conceptions and ideas to guide it in the achievement of its goal. Yoga, as the art of living, has its formulations, its interpretations of life, based upon subtle perceptions gained through concentration. These interpretations are not the supreme ultimate silent truth that is beyond speech and mind, but they do give us a picture of the subtle realities of life and help us to live intelligently. They are conceptions which illuminate our life and moral sense, our activity and spiritual aspiration, our quest for truth, goodness, beauty and perfection. They provide the deepest insight into the profound mystery of existence and guide life to its fulfillment.

History of Yoga dates back almost 5000 to 6000 years, we find its techniques explained in Vedas. The Upanishads are the original source books of Yoga. Yoga teachings are to be found in many sections of the great epic, the Mahabharata. The Gita which forms a small part of this work gives the fundamental concepts of Yoga. Yoga teachings were later presented in organized form by many different schools. One of the comparatively late books, which have been regarded as the outstanding compilation of Yoga principles and practice, of Yoga psychology, ethics, metaphysics and practice of concentration, is known as *The Yoga Sutras of Patanjali*. This work is attributed to second century BC. The method of Yoga advocated by Patanjali is popularly known as *Raja Yoga*.

Later from 6th century to 18th century many Hatha Yoga texts came into existences which were more focused on achieving the Raja Yoga of Patanjali with different perspective. Hatha Yoga is a system of health and hygiene involving both body and mind. It aims at the whole man for his full development and self-realization. It takes into account not only the proper growth, strength and tone of the different muscles of the body but also the efficiency and function of the basic factors of constitutional health, namely the inner organs and the glands. Finally it emphasizes emotional balance and a mature outlook on life, for in the long run the health which is not mental health is no health at all.

The Hatha Yoga Practices were first developed as a preparation for the Yoga of contemplation (Raja Yoga); yet in later times elaborate techniques and methods of health and hygiene were evolved which could be followed for their own sake apart from any high spiritual motive. The purely physical aspect of Yoga thus came to be known as the Ghatastha Yoga (*Gheranda Samhita*) or the Yoga of physical body.

The original meaning of Hatha Yoga is not the yoga of force or physical violence but the physical and vital control of the body by physiological means for purposes of higher concentration according to individual's ability and capacity. Later on, the word Hatha came also to symbolize the two bio-motor processes of the body, the energy-consuming and the energy-acquiring, which are called respectively the Sun (Ha) and the Moon (Tha) principles. According to this explanation, Hatha Yoga aims to balance and harmonize these two forces by means of breath control, which again is accessory to higher contemplation.

From the earliest times the Yogis emphasized balance–balance between body, mind and spirit. An all-round development of personality is not possible without constitutional health. An ancient Yoga text declares: *The Self of man cannot be attained by the weak; the aspirant after yoga must be disciplined, strong, firm and intelligent.*

Proper attention to body is a spiritual act. It helps to free the mind from physical bondage. Many so-called spiritual teachers who look suspiciously at Hatha Yoga but who are often preoccupied with their bodies, relying so easily and quickly on drugs and surgery, are thoughtless. They would be better physically and spiritually if they had practiced a little bit of Hatha Yoga.

A brilliant intellect in a sick body devoid of the capacity for strong feeling and sensation, and a superbly developed physique with a dull mind and without subtle perceptions are, neither of them, idle or desirable conditions.

Hatha yoga is based on a body of empirical knowledge built up in the course of centuries. Long, continued observation and experiment enabled the yogis to build up a system of health and hygiene eminently fitted not only to keep the body healthy, supple and strong but also to prolong youthfulness, delay aging and decay, and to make the body resistance to disease.

Evolvement of Hatha Yoga

Hatha Yoga has continued to be practiced in India by several groups who have passed their knowledge from teacher to pupil without disruption for tens of centuries. A few dedicate themselves exclusively to mastering and improving its techniques, while many others, whose work and interests do not permit such exclusive concentration, follow it along with other pursuits, thus invigorating and enriching their life far beyond ordinary measure.

The various techniques and theories of Hatha yoga have evolved through the practice and experience of a large body and teachers over many hundred years, during which time the effects of these exercises upon different kinds of individuals has been under continuous observation. This serves to assure us that hatha yoga is, in every respect, a superior method of physical hygiene and culture, more reliable than modern systems which have not gone through the test of time and which are partial and external in their outlooks and application.

Hatha yoga techniques and theories came to be formulated, organized and presented in a number of texts. Not many of the ancient texts are available today. Of those which are in existence, many are still in manuscripts form, held by the libraries of different institution. Only a few have been printed and published, of which the best known are *Hatha*

Pradipika, Siva Samhita, Goraksha Samhita, Gheranda Samhita. All have been translated into English. None of these books are very old, the earliest only dating back to thirteenth century. These books are short, cryptic and often full of hyperbolic claims. They cannot be properly appraised, understood and followed without expert guidance.*

Hatha yoga is a rational and comprehensive system of health and self-culture. It is not the acrobatics or vulgar performance to which some tend to reduce it. Practice of various techniques of yoga no doubt gives one extra ordinary power over the body, but character, serenity of mind and even health in the long run cannot be attained by mere physical postures. Those who preach, mislead others.

Diverse types of physical exercise were developed in ancient India. The encyclopedia of Indian Physical Culture, published in 1955, records and illustrates many of them; weightlifting, discus and javelin throwing, exercises with bars, rings, poles and maces, wrestling and so on. But hatha yoga was not evolved to build bulky specialized muscles for aggressive purpose but to assure constitutional health, and a well-proportioned, firm, and flexible body, to retain youthfulness, to delay age and decay, and above all to develop the kind of body essential to a life rich and meaningful in content.

THE TECHNIQUES AND THE GENERAL FACTORS OF HEALTH

The hatha yoga techniques are collectively known as *Nadi-Shuddhi* process, i.e. processes for purifying the nerves and vitalizing the body. Purity in Yoga means calmness or balance, while impurity stands for dullness and restlessness. There are four broad divisions of these techniques which are: 1. Postures (Asana and Mudra), 2. Breathe control (Pranayama), 3. Dynamic exercises (Sandhi Chalana, Suryanamaskar), 4. Cleansing, special control and locking practices (Shatkarma, Bandha and Mudra). Of these the Asanas or postures, and the Pranayamas or the breath regulations, are the most well-known and widely practiced.

Before going on to posture, breathing and other techniques by learning them under the guidance of a teacher, it will be of interest to consider the Hatha yoga exercises generally in relation to the basic factors of health. The efficiency of abdominal-thoracic structure, the internal organs and the glands, determine our health, youthfulness, vigor and longevity. This includes spine, thoracic and abdominal muscles, lungs, heart and endocrine glands.

Spine

A firm and flexible spine is essential for health and youthfulness. A man is as old as his spine. Age bends the spine. We are all familiar with the expression 'A man of strong backbone'. Doctors today realize the great importance of the spine in preserving health and assuring long life. The emphasis that Chiropractors or Osteopaths place on the spine is well known. If the spine loses its natural spring-like curvature, if the spinal bones are not properly aligned, or if they are burdened with calcium deposits, our health and efficiency are vastly reduced. Wrong alignment and stiffness of vertebrae impair the function of nerves which issue out of vertebral apertures and control the motor and sensory activities of the different limbs. An increasingly greater number of people are today suffering from various forms of back troubles, from weak vertebrae, slip discs and sacroiliac difficulties, which are so often due to bad posture and lack of specialized exercise. Wrong posture also interferes with the normal activities of various internal organs and reduces their efficiency.

The spinal, abdominal and respiratory muscles function as the fundamental muscles in all mammals, including man. The earliest means of locomotion and patterns of movement are connected with the spinal musculature.

An erect spinal posture is necessary for holding the thorax in the correct position. Weakness of chest muscles makes the thorax droop to the position natural for exhalation, which hampers normal breathing. On the other hand the high up raised barrel chest often develop through 'muscle-building' exercise, lifts the thorax to an inspiratory position also interfering with normal breathing. Erect trunk posture and proper development and tone of the chest and abdominal muscles are important conditions for proper breathing, healthy body function, concentration and high emotional level.

Hatha yoga is the only system which pays special attention to spinal culture. The spinal exercises make the backbone firm and flexible, hold the vertebrae in position and stimulate the sympathetic nerve chains which lie embedded in the muscles of the back along the spine. The various specialized spinal and abdominal movements of hatha yoga stimulate the fundamental nerve centers and the basic muscular movements of the body apart from producing other effects.

Breathing

Proper breathing habits are essential for health. It is the basic function of the body on which depends the proper functioning of every other organ. Regular and correct exercises and education for lungs are essential. In the living lifestyle of comfort today most of us use only a small part of our lung capacity. As a consequence of faulty and shallow breathing, the extreme areas of lungs remain un-exercised, becoming inelastic and atrophied like muscles which grow stiff and wither away from lack of use. As breathing becomes more shallow and rapid, the heart beats more often. There is a close relationship between the rate of breathing and the rapidity of heart beats. Faulty breathing puts a severe strain on the heart. The heart muscle rests only during the interval between the beats and if we shorten the interval needlessly by faulty breathing, we deprive it of its needed rest. It is like making a horse run continuously by flogging it. It can be expected to break down quickly from sheer exhaustion.

Regular and proper movement of the diaphragm is necessary for health of the various organs inside the abdominal cavity. Nature intended those organs to be stimulated by the rhythmic movement of the diaphragm which imparts to them a kind of massage. Without such stimulation, the functioning of organs is impaired and many troubles ensue. The proper and educated movement of the diaphragm and the abdominal muscles helps to ensure healthy periods and facilitates natural childbirth.

Proper breathing improves the form and structure of the body. Studies have proved how breathing controls the various functions, and how the proper structure of the body depends on proper breathing. Unless the lungs function well, the body, especially in the trunk and the shoulders does not have good form.

Yoga lays special emphasis on breathing techniques for both physiological and psychological reasons. Proper functioning of the lungs is essential for physical and mental wellbeing. One can prolong life and retard the aging process through breathing.

The lungs need to be fully stretched by special exercises to maintain their full efficiency. Untrained lungs run quickly out of breath and take an unduly longtime to recover, even after modest exertion. The air passages which remain stagnant due to poor breathing provide areas where bacteria find easy lodging and grow quickly. Lack of movement and faulty circulation in the lungs cause a good many colds and respiratory troubles.

Oxygen forms by far the major constituent of the body. Faulty breathing lowers vitality by depriving the body cells of their proper oxygen needs. Some researchers maintain that lack of oxygen in the tissues is a prime factor in causing cancer. They say that the body cells which are chronically cut off from oxygen supply go back to a primitive method of metabolism which causes cancerous growth. There is no doubt that faulty breathing wears out the body in many ways.

Age reduces the efficiency of bodily organs. Breathing capacity is progressively diminished with growing years. Being the key function of life, the loss of breathing power inevitably hastens the deteriorations of other organs and cell in the body. Breathing exercises retard such processes.

Slow and rhythmic breathing acquired through yoga practice slows down the heart and prevents both the unnecessary wear and tear on the body and the strain on the nervous system which come from irregular breathing. Ordinarily a man at rest breathes 15 or 18 times a minute. One who has practiced yoga-breathing faithfully breathes 8 to 10 times a minute. Such slow and deep breathing is restful to the nerves and cuts down the aging process.

Breathing and Psyche

The various psychic and physiological effects of regulated breathing are coming to recognized by doctors and psychiatrist throughout the world.

Breathing is a bridge between the voluntary and involuntary functioning of the body, between the conscious mind and the subconscious psyche, between body and spirit. A breathing reflects our state of mind; elation or depression, restlessness or repose. Through proper and regulated breathing, we can gain a large major of control over our emotions. By controlling and regulating our breath, we can do much to relax our nerves and develop powers of concentration.

Deep, rhythmic and controlled breathing has a profound effect on the whole nervous system and the psyche. Many doctors, psychiatrists and analysts today advise their patients to do some form of breathing to relieve tension. Persons have been relieved of heart conditions through regulated deep breathing. The yogis discovered long ago the physiological and spiritual benefits of educated and controlled breathing. They went deep into the subject and developed it into a great art.

Heart

Heart disease is the greatest killer in India today. The reason is both physical and mental. False values, false worship and estrangement from the deeper truth of our nature, the rush and hurry of the 'rat race', create tensions which attack the heart. Diet no doubt plays its part but its role has been overstressed. Overweight and lack of exercises also contribute to heart trouble, but emotional tensions plays by far the most important part in lowering vitality and causing damage to the heart. The yogis emphasize the importance of emotional balance for health. There cannot be any true integration and balance between the different demands and sides of our personality without a central purpose of life. This is the function of philosophy—to provide us with a scale of values and a perspective. Though ultimately thinking individual cannot be very healthy without a philosophical outlook, yet physical means are not to be neglected. Yoga breathing postures and exercises relax tension and improve the heart.

Glands

Glands, which control metabolism, growth and body functions are, as a whole, influenced by emotions. As heart disease is the greatest killer in the world today, arthritis is the greatest crippler. The faulty function of adrenal glands in an affluent and well-nourished society is due primarily to emotional difficulties.

Constant fear, resentment and anxiety, open or suppressed, deplete the glands which then fail to supply the hormones necessary to ward of arthritic attacks. Emotional trouble wears out the body so quickly that the old age with all its stiffness, aches and pains sets in early. Yogic hygiene, including mental outlook, diet, and exercises, especially certain breathings and postures, improves the functioning of the glands and restores prematurely lost powers.

The different yoga postures involve the body in diversified exercises, thus keeping it well-proportioned, slim and flexible. Yoga helps to reduce excess weight and tone up the muscles, especially those left untouched by ordinary strenuous exercises.

The control exercises and cleansing practices of hatha yoga are for higher breath control and breathe suspension. Of these only a few are suitable for those who are interested in physical health and hygiene. The others are for specialists and are not to be recommended to the general public.

Cleanliness, both outer and inner is an essential condition of health. Daily washings and baths, especially for persons living in warm climates and overheated rooms, keep the body free from troubles of various kinds. Much heaviness and dullness of the body and mind come from unclean habits and food. One begins to desire stimulants in order to be wakened from a feeling of torpor and sluggishness. Lightness of body and cheerfulness of mind, which stems from cleanliness, diminishes and stops the craving for strong drinks and tobacco.

Many of the intricate cleansing techniques of hatha yoga are difficult to learn; they need have no place in modern hygiene. Some results can be more easily and effectively achieved by modern methods. Further, the elaborate and intricate cleansing methods were prescribed originally for individuals who were preparing themselves for special techniques of body and nerve control and for those who has special health problems. It is not advisable for normal persons to do them either for health or spiritual progress.

Ordinary cleansing methods are important and can be easily followed by one and all.

The basic postures and breathing exercises of hatha yoga are easy to learn and follow. No instrumental or mechanical aids are necessary. They can be done by young and old alike. No matter what your age you can always improve by practicing some aspects of yoga.

There are thousands in the whole world today who keep themselves fit and vigorous by doing yoga. Yoga postures are being increasingly incorporated into the disciplines of various physical culturists and dance instructors for promoting health, control, flexibility and versatility of body movement.

Hatha yoga shapes the body on a slender, wiry pattern, capable of great exertion and endurance, and stresses a muscular development consistent with constitutional health and vigor. Overdeveloped and hypertrophied muscles, enlarged through wrong and strenuous method of exercises, prey like parasites on general vitality, hence succumbing to various health issues. In failing to train the lungs and heart for increased oxygen and fuel demands of overdeveloped body, such exercise programs bring about premature senility and death.

Its rational, psychophysical, integral approach makes hatha yoga the most suitable form of health culture for the civilized man.

■ FOOD, FAST AND ASCETISM

Food should generally be moderate. Yogis say that only half the stomach should be filled with food. Of the rest, a quarter should be for liquid and other for air. Unless there is enough space in the stomach, the muscles cannot work; the rest is indigestion. It is good as a general rule to leave the table a little hungry, especially for those who are past middle age.

Foods should be fresh and clean and as far as possible unprocessed. Domestic animals are often better nutritionists than many of us whose natural and healthy instincts have been blunted and corrupted by artificial flavoring and treatment of food. Animals avoid food which has been so processed by chemicals and other means as to have been deprived of its essential nutrients and vitamins, although it has been made alluring and attractive by color and scent which serve as decoys. Older people should avoid greasy and fried things which are hard on the liver.

One should reduce meat eating and give it up altogether, if possible, as one grows in years, especially if one lives in warm or hot climates. However, in considering dietary rules and changes, doctrinaire attitudes are to be avoided and attention should be given to the various factors which demand consideration, such as background, occupation, age, interest, etc. individuals differ in their metabolic machinery, in the production and utilization of different enzymes. They further differ in their need for and assimilation of different types of protein.

Periodic fasting, one day in a week or in a fortnight, is very beneficial for grownups. It cleanses the body and restores vitality. Take plenty of fluids in the form of diluted fruit juice or lemon water while you fast. If you feel hungry, take a light fruit or a vegetable meal in the evening.

Fasting and food regulations are also effective in curing many troubles, but they should be undertaken only under expert advice and observation.

Many persons who suffer from a variety of trouble and diseases have been cured of them while undertaking fast for reducing weight.

Modern nutritionists have discovered that animals who are a little underfed live longer and have more vitality than those whose intake is larger.

Yoga is often identified with asceticism (Sanyasa). Asceticism which is spiritual is not a kind of senseless and morbid self-torture. It is a self-disciplined, like that of an athlete, to train and organize the mind. It is positive in its aim like the breaking in of a vicious horse. It is for self-mastery and self-conquest and not for self-destruction.

We must master life and not to be made in victims. Though I see the absurdity of many traditional views and practices dogmatically followed, yet I perceive clearly and appreciate all the more, in surrounding of affluent society and a scientific civilization, the profound spiritual truth of our Indian heritage.

To return to the subject of food and fasting, food should be diversified as far as possible. If one keeps to the following varieties of food generally one can be sure of healthy diet. Fresh vegetables, including roots, stems, leaves and flowers, salads, fruits (seasonal), seeds and whole cereals, fresh fish (boiled and broiled), vegetable oil, yogurt (less butter, cheese and cream) and a lemon a day.

People very often take to wrong food and other improper means to reduce or control weight. Weight should be controlled by proper diet (natural), exercise and fasting. It is injurious to take pills or to rely on artificial foods. I have seen quite a number of scientific people without common sense. While counting calories people forget that they have teeth and digestive organs which need exercise. The liquid and soft foods which dispense with chewing are harmful for teeth. A doctor in a well-known hospital in Mumbai once told me how a friend of his damaged his teeth by depending on soft artificial food for some length of time. Dieting without exercise is unhealthy.

Fasting for grown men is very healthy practice, for both of getting rid of the morbid materials from the body as well as for improving the functioning of various organs. There is an old Indian medical saying to the effect that fasting is the supreme medicine. Full moon and new moon day are especially good for fasting, but people who work may find difficult to observe them. They can fast on weekends or on holidays.

GENERAL UNDERSTANDING OF YOGA EXERCISES

Yoga exercises are not competitive. Yoga insists that a man lives a life of his own dedicated to his wellbeing and happiness. The exercises however can be combined with other systems of physical culture and sports.

The Yoga exercises are suitable for all, especially for the needs of people past their youth. They can be done with benefit all through life.

The exercises are to be done slowly and deliberately with concentration. All jerky and bouncing movements should be avoided. The positions in the static postures are held for sometime. In the beginning the postures should be held only as long as one does not feel great discomfort. It is not advisable to go beyond these points without instructions.

The exercises should be done in a warm room filled with fresh air.

The best time for doing the yoga exercises is early morning as well as evening when the body limbers up naturally. The hour before lunch is also a good time. The exercises can be divided into: 1) Simple stretching in standing positions and breathing, 2) postures on the floor–supine and prone. The stretching, breathing and meditation can be done in the morning, while the postures can be practiced in the evening before dinner. Wait half an hour after the exercises before eating.

It is a good practice to take a warm shower after the postures. Turn the shower from warm to cool gradually. After drying yourself with a large towel take another and have a dry friction bath with it.

To learn to do the exercises in a proper manner, sequence and spirit, it is necessary to have the help of an experienced teacher. It is best to have individual lessons. Individual needs and requirements are different and much is lost in character and spirit in group lessons. Those who cannot have a teacher can follow the exercises given in various books of Yoga techniques by great teachers like Swami Kuvalyananda, Yogacharya Sadashiv Nimbalkar, etc. by carefully studying the instructions. Avoid hurry and proceed gently and slowly. Books will be more useful after one has studied with a teacher.

Misconceptions in Yoga

Yoga as a practice for physical fitness and spiritual growth has become a mainstream activity in today's global society; it is slowly becoming associated with a certain image. If you are a Yoga teacher, you may find yourself clearing up a lot of confusion. Many people have formed beliefs about yoga knowledge or yogic methodology that may or may not be entirely true. Some may think that yoga is only for young, it's only for people with flexibility who can contort their bodies into challenging postures. Others believe it's too complicated or advanced for a beginner to even try. Those who teach yoga best know that these ideas are erroneous and founded only in ignorance.

It is Not for Beginners

The concept of stretching and relaxing in a quiet, calm environment is often perceived as a threat. Many people feel like they would be judged upon stepping into a yoga class for the first time. They feel like they are not knowledgeable enough to participate in a class. It is not true. In fact, many classes are tailored to beginners, providing explanations and cues for each pose or breathing exercise. Whether an instructor is a recent yoga teacher training graduate or a seasoned teacher with decades of experience, it is our mission to make beginners feel welcome in our classes.

You Must Be Flexible

Some people might shy away from yoga because they feel like they need to be flexible to do it. Asana practice definitely improves flexibility, but it is not a prerequisite for beginning your practice. You can do any of the poses whether you are flexible or not because the idea is to stretch to the extent that your body will let you, not to stretch as far as the instructor or as far as the person next to you. Additionally, the postures are only one part of the many parts of Yoga technique.

Yoga is meant for Sadhus or Sanyasins

To practice Yoga you need not leave home and go to Himalayas or become a Sanyasi or get completely detached from regular life. In fact Yoga is a way of life where one discipline himself to lead life according to the need of society and self-development. Being in Grahastha Ashram, raising a family one can very well be part of Yoga and make Yoga as part of his or her life.

You Should Be Young and Healthy

Yogic practices are for all ages and types of people. Old and young alike will receive the benefits of a regular practice. People with chronic illness can benefit from yoga training by promoting the body to heal and releasing stress and anxiety. Even if you are middle-aged or older and have never tried, it's not too late to start. Asana, pranayama, meditation and relaxation will benefit anybody at any time in their life.

Yoga is for only Aged and Weak

Many a times the on the contrary it has been also observed people saying that Yoga is for old and weak and they should be doing more of Gym and aerobics but as clarified above it is equally beneficial for all. They feel that up to a certain age when one cannot do weight training in Gym he can join yoga for his physical fitness. The fact is yoga is complementary for other exercises and would be very helpful to enhance the benefit of the same.

You Shouldn't Practice If You're Injured

Asana can actually help an injured body heal. While there are certainly precautions that need to be taken when poses specifically affect an injured area, there is no reason to stop practicing when injured. In fact, there are gentle, therapeutic and restorative styles, which specifically address recovery from ailments, pain and injuries.

It's Only for Women

Perhaps the majority of the classes you have seen largely composed of women. If you look into the history of yoga, you'll find that all of the first yogis were men. Yogic techniques do not discriminate against either sex. Men and women can both reap the benefits that meditation, asana, pranayama and relaxation provide.

Yoga Belongs to a Particular Religion

People belonging to other religion feel that Yoga belongs to Hinduism and may bring in differences to their faith. Which is absolutely very vague thinking, on the contrary Yoga helps to develop better skills of concentration and contemplation observed in a particular faith.

Yoga is Therapy

Here I may be slightly controversial. Though today Yoga is practiced mostly to manage many disorders and ailments and even cures them but still the real aim of Yoga is self-realization, *kaivalya* or liberation. Healing happens due to the practitioners (sadhak's) return to basics and purification of the whole body and mind from the root. Yoga is an Art and Science of knowing the self and getting established in the SELF.

■ CONCLUDING REMARKS

I would like to make a few observations before concluding this section on Yoga, specifically Hatha Yoga per say.

I have not mentioned any yogic technique or exercises for practical purpose. Those who want to do yoga and go further and specialize will find the techniques of Yogic practices well explained in above mentioned books as also mentioned in the Bibliography at the end of the article useful. To attain thoroughness and mastery over advanced techniques the need for a teacher and dedication to the subject are indispensable.

If you are doing the yogic exercises described and illustrated in the suggested books with care, patience and regularity you will realize their benefits and be able to develop from within yourself standards of judgment for estimating the worth and usefulness of many things written on the subject.

I have seen marvelous results flow from regular practice of yoga exercises. I have seen diseases, defects and conditions of different kinds like cysts, colitis, backaches, menstrual disorders, partial immobility from paralysis, arthritis, respiratory and cardiac troubles, overweight, insomnia and tensions relieved from the following of yoga disciplines. Many maintain and improve their health and appearance through regular practice of yoga.

To reap results one needs seriousness, enthusiasm and application. But there are today, due to general climate of public relationships, an increasing number of eternal shoppers who are too wary to trust and be serious about anything or pursue any worthy object steadily and earnestly. Such people do not go far in life in the realization of any of its true values or profound experiences, whether it is love, friendship or spiritual knowledge. They play safe and save themselves from both bad and good, remaining always indifferent.

RECOMMENDED TEXTBOOKS FOR REFERENCE

1. 'Raja Yoga' by Swami Vivekananda
2. 'A Study of Yoga' by Jnaneshwar Ghosh
3. Hatha Yoga by Shyam Sundar Goswami
4. 'Yoga for Health and Peace' by Yogacharya Sadashiv Nimbalkar, 7th edn., Publishing Committee—Yoga Vidhya Niketan, 2007.
5. 'Yoga Asanas and Pranayamas' by Swamy Kuvalyananda

PART IV

Community Physiotherapy Related to Specific Contextual Factor

13

Health in Behavioral Context

13.1 LIFESTYLE RELATED ISSUES: OBESITY PREVENTION

Amita Anil Mehta, Mariya Prakash Jiandani

Obesity and lifestyle issues: Obesity in community is an obvious problem leading to low self-esteem and health issues. It requires judicious addressing of the problem and a very fine tackling of it with balancing of energy input and energy output. Energy input requires fine adjustment of nutrition filled calories, rich with fibers and water content. Energy output can be addressed by enhancing physical fitness with structured exercises and physical activities with active lifestyle and recreational activities.
Keywords: Obesity, Physical fitness, Structured exercises, Active lifestyle, Energy input, Energy output.

INTRODUCTION

Obesity is seen as the first wave of a defined cluster of non-communicable diseases called 'New World Syndrome,' creating an enormous socioeconomic and public health burden in poorer countries. The World Health Organization has described obesity as one of today's most neglected public health problems, affecting every region of the globe[1] contributing to 112,000 preventable deaths each year. Additionally, obesity is strongly associated with other metabolic disorders including diabetes, hypertension, dyslipidaemia, cardiovascular disease and even some cancers. Individuals with obesity have higher rates of mortality and morbidity compared to non obese individuals.[2]

DEFINITION AND OVERVIEW

Obesity is a surplus of adipose tissue-containing fat stored in triglyceride form resulting from an imbalance due to excessive energy intake relative to energy expenditure.[3] Overweight is defined as deviation in body weight from a standard or ideal weight and related to height. Body mass index expressed as weight in kilograms divided by height squared in meters has been adopted a standard for expressing body weight. Body Mass Index (BMI) is a simple index of weight-for-height that is commonly used to classify underweight, overweight and obesity in adults. Overweight was defined as a BMI ≥ 23 kg/m^2 but <25 kg/m^2 for both genders (based on the World Health Organization Asia Pacific Guidelines) with or without abdominal obesity (Table 13.1).

Distribution of fat in the upper body around the abdomen is known as android type or abdominal obesity and carries a greater morbidity and mortality than that around lower body (pelvis and hips) is known as gynoid obesity (Figs 13.1A and B). In Barrel type obesity the distribution of fat is equal in upper and lower body. This is also referred to as general obesity.

Table 13.1: Classification of Obesity: WHO Asia Pacific Guidelines

Classification	BMI (kg/m²)	Waist circumference	
		<90 cm (men)	>90 cm (men)
		<80 cm (women)	>80 cm (women)
Underweight	< 18.5	Low*	Average
Normal	18.5–22.9	Average	Increased
Overweight	>23		
At Risk	23.0–24.9	Increased	Moderate
Obese I	25.0–29.9	Moderate	Severe
Obese II	>30	Severe	Very severe

*Increased risk of other clinical problems

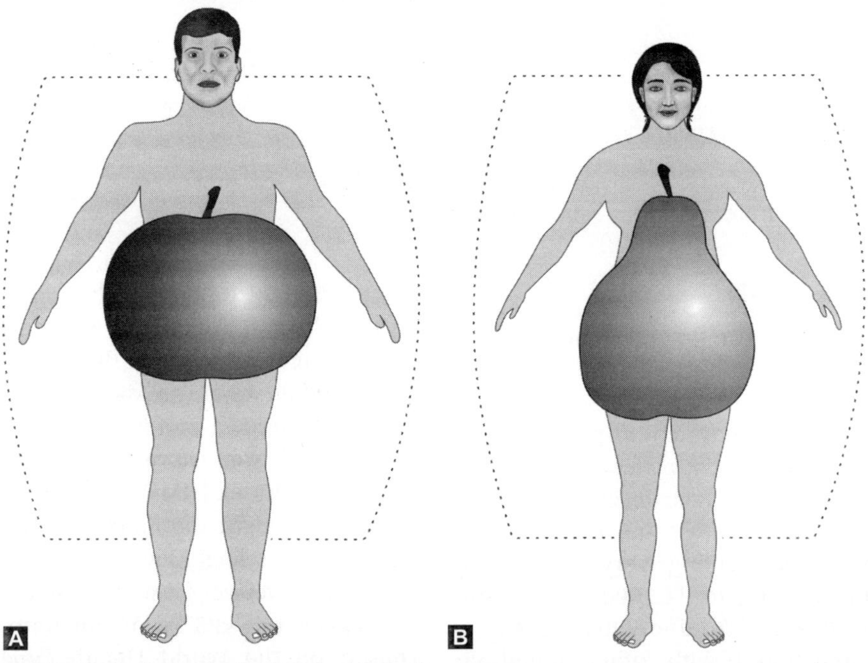

Figs 13.1A and B: A. Android obesity; **B.** Gynoid obesity

In 2011, the AHA published a consensus statement on how to assess adiposity.[4] It highlighted the relationship between excess adiposity and health concerns also citing waist circumference as a good measure of abdominal obesity. Waist circumference (WC) measured midway between rib and iliac (Figs 13.2A and B) provides an estimate for visceral adipose tissue which puts a person at risk for cardiometabolic disease [MenWC >than 102 cm (40 in) and women >88 cm (35 in)].[4,5] Waist hip ratio compares the ratio of waist girth to hip girth and is used to estimate body fat distribution. The measurement of waist hip ratio and waist circumference are strong predictors of cardiovascular risk than body weight or body mass index. WHO states that abdominal obesity is defined as a waist-hip ratio above 0.90 for males and above 0.85 for females.

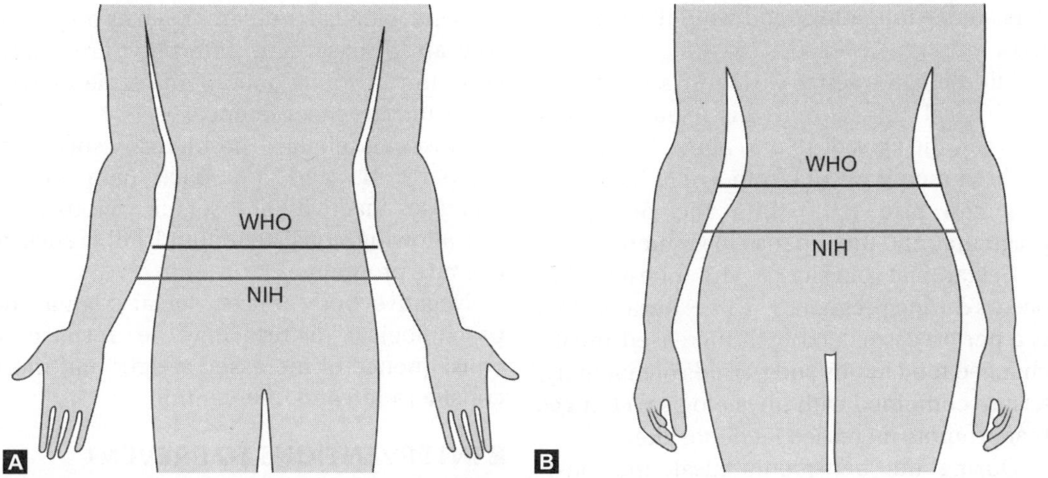

Figs 13.2A and B: Waist circumference measurement sites for men and women based on World Health Organization (WHO) and National Institutes of Health protocols

Note: Following the WHO protocol, the measure is taken midway between the highest point of the iliac crest and the bottom of the rib cage. Following the NIH protocol, the measure is taken at the highest pint of the iliac crest

Percentage fat and lean mass can be determined using simple methods like skin fold thickness and bioelectric impedance to measure body composition. The gold standard hydrostatic weighing requires sophisticated laboratory. Highly accurate measurements of abdominal adiposity is accomplished using computed tomography, magnetic resonance imaging (MRI) and dual X-ray absorptiometry (DXA) scan.[6] However they are expensive and not practical in clinical setting but can be used for research purposes. Waist circumference measurement is an inexpensive and time efficient way not only to measure abdominal obesity but also to assess the effects of intervention.

■ WHY IS THE COMMUNITY GETTING OBESE?

The community is dominated by obese people in urban area. Advanced technology at finger tips and food epidemic are the culprits.[7] There is street food and snacks available such as bread, biscuits and pasta. Noodles are known to one and all. All full of saturated fat and carbohydrates with no fibrrs in it, it has high glycemic value;[8] surges insulin levels high and shoots it down too. These spikes of insulin, leads to insulin insensitivity[8] and resistance in body leading to metabolic havoc, storing fats as adipose tissues, peripheral subcutaneous fat and central visceral fat. Metabolic syndrome as a result of high calorie, high carbohydrate with less fibers, less water intake which Saturated and minerals, antioxidants provokes hormonal disturbances and burdens body/this is provoked and further supported by varied stress levels of urban life. Where, starting from a newborn to new mother, school going children to teachers and principal, employee to employer and retired have various reasons for stress. Lifestyle modifications are designed understanding these backgrounds.

Childhood obesity occurs because of increased risk nutrition during fetal life that may contribute directly to the development of the size, shape and composition of the body of the fetus and also due to the metabolic incompetence of the child to handle macronutrients. The most important consequence of childhood obesity is its persistence into adulthood with all its health risks.

Middle age obesity is due to a reduction of physical activity and this usually occurs between the ages of 19 and above in females while in men it occurs from age of 30 years.[9] This can also fall within the period of pregnancy and menopause in women.

Gestational obesity is the obesity that occurs during pregnancy. This is because this is a period associated with increased meals, changed food habits and periods of inactivity, leisure combined with physiological changes that promote increased fat deposition.

During the peri-menopausal and post-menopausal period the hormonal imbalance associated with psychological issues are more than enough for an ascending ladder towards weight gain. The loss of cardioprotective effect post menopause increases the probability of suffering from cardiac event.

OBESITY ASSOCIATED DISEASES

Obesity affect's multiple systems of the body. Obesity has a strong association with coronary heart disease, hypertension, dyslipidemia and stroke. Obesity and physical inactivity are key contributors to development of endocrine disorders such as type 2 diabetes and metabolic syndrome. Adipose tissue dysfunction is thought to be responsible by altering the receptor sites and therefore reducing the ability of the body to effectively take up glucose.

Respiratory diseases, such as obesity hypoventilation syndrome, obstructive sleep apnea and pulmonary hypertension secondary to it are commonly seen in obese individuals. Children with BMI in 95th percentile are significantly more likely to suffer with asthma and wheezing.

Certain cancers (endometrial, breast, and colon) and liver and gallbladder diseases are commonly associated with abdominal obesity.

Gynecological problems such as polycystic ovarian disease and infertility are issues common in young obese females along with stress urinary incontinence.

Musculoskeletal problems such as osteoarthritis and low back pain further increases inactivity and sets in vicious cycle not allowing consistency and adherence to exercise programs.

Negative body image, social stigma and psychological distress may be a cause or consequence of increased weight and merit consideration and intervention.

INTERVENTIONS TO PREVENT LIFESTYLE RELATED DISEASE

Nutrition, exercise and behavior change are three key elements of weight control programs.

Lifestyle Education and Behavior Modification

Lifestyle and behavioral change are cornerstones to an effective treatment. It includes not only changing exercise and eating habits but understanding the relation between emotions and incidents that cause these (binging) habits and its consequential chain of events and feelings.

Parents may need nutrition education intervention to better understand how children can be guided in the selection and enjoyment of healthy diets and lifestyles. The importance of modelling healthy food choices and physical activity and the identification of personal and family behaviors that may be acting as barriers to change needs should be recognized. Access and exposure to a wide range of healthful foods, such as fruits, vegetables, low-fat dairy products, whole grains, and lentils, are important for the development of a preference for these foods. Children served large portions tend to eat more food than children served smaller age-appropriate servings. Fruit and vegetable tasting activities introduces the child to food they have never tasted and thus developing a liking to healthy food.

Behaviors such as stopping smoking, taking regular physical activity and eating a healthy diet promote health and have no known harmful effects. All individuals should be asked about their tobacco use and, where relevant, given advice and counseling on quitting, as well as reinforcement at follow-up. The percentage of population with young females smoking has been increased recently. Maternal smoking during pregnancy increases the childhood risk of obesity. Young children are exposed to these habits from school as a result of increased availability of resources, a means to combat stress and as a fad. Strict measures at school and parental counseling are equally important to prevent addictions to nicotine.

Changing the environment to make it more 'activity friendly' will be able to make more permanent change. There should be health conscious culture around the work environment to encourage and inculcate lifestyle changes. Sedentary behavior, such as television viewing, playing video games, mobile chats and sitting on the desk for prolonged period of time is associated with increased risk for overweight.

With growing concern in public and health professionals there is awareness but not acceptance towards changing behavior to healthy lifestyle. The health belief model assumes that people change behaviors when there is a perceived threat of disease or susceptibility of disease.

Barriers to lifestyle change have to be identified and a problem solving approach with acronym **'IDEA'**, i.e. **I**dentify the problem, **D**evelop a list of solution, **E**valuate the solution, **A**nalyze how well the plan worked needs to be adopted. Individual can be taught coping skills to overcome difficult situation and prevent negative reactions. Mental preparation and mental set up is extremely important to adopt lifestyle modification behaviors. These should be observed as pleasurable task rather than compulsory medical regime.

Energy Input-output Balance

Nutrition and physical activity are important to maintain the balance between energy input and output.[10] A cardioprotective diet should consist of a variety of foods, and should aim to achieve four major goals: a healthy overall diet, a healthy body weight, a desirable lipid profile, and a desirable blood pressure.

Physical activity improves endothelial function, contributes to weight loss, glycemic control, improved blood pressure, lipid profile and insulin sensitivity. The possible beneficial effects of physical activity on cardiovascular risk may be mediated, at least in part, through these effects on intermediate risk factors. Overall, the evidence points to the benefit of continued regular moderate physical activity, which does not need to be strenuous or prolonged, and can include daily leisure activities, such as walking or gardening.

Considerations for Energy Input

Energy input and Energy output equation balance is challenged and various diet and exercise programs bring about temporary change and soon it is nullified with weight gain again (relapse).[10]

Lifestyle modifications to which one can adhere comfortably and can be sustained lifelong is advocated. **Motivation and self-determination** is the key to begin change in obese person.[11] **Self-awareness and education regarding caloric dense food item** in the form of carbohydrate and saturated fat requires restriction and portion size control is must. Sugar filled beverages, bread, biscuits, pasta, noodles, roti and rice, sweets and fried foods are examples of same such food items. Also, intake of fruits juice which has carbohydrates without fibers is to be restricted. Foods with high thermic effect increases metabolic rate. They help burn fat as uses internal calories. Vegetables, whole fruits and water with high nutrient value are a key to health.

Apart from **type** of food and the **amount** of food, it is important to **time** the food. This is important for digestion in absorptive and postabsorptive phases. This also takes care of hormonal play by insulin and helps in controlling insulin levels and insulin sensitivity. This helps in turning the body into a fat burning machine. The calorie and hormonal play driven by insulin now can further be augmented along with exercise programs. **Maintenance of a food diary** to record caloric intake and recommend nutrition proportions also creates awareness to type, quantity and time of food consumed.

Considerations for Energy Output

Consistency, adherence and ***enjoyment*** rather than intensity or mode of exercise are the goals of exercise for weight control. Physical activity in the form of daily chores or a programed exercise protocol both uses calories. Simple bodily movements that promote activities of daily living, especially walking in sunlight helps to augment and adhere to the circadian cycle.[12] Thus aerobic activities are encouraged to be continued for long durations may be throughout the day. With emphasis on not assuming a sedentary, sitting[13] or lying position in the day time.[14]

How much weight loss in a week or month may be decided by individual health and physical capacity of the person. Target weight loss can be 5–10% of weight in initial 3–6 months. What is important is **steady continuous response** in terms of weight loss and health benefits. Choose activities that **match lifestyle and schedule**. Walking should be within tolerance limit of most obese people. The limiting factor more often is back pain and knee pain being reasons for attrition from exercise. Remember any exercise or activity is better than none. Becoming active can be difficult, tiring, and painful under the added workload of obesity. **Minimize discomfort and potential for injury**, including attention to appropriate clothing and footwear.

Rest, relaxation and **resistance** exercises are to be incorporated especially with body part resistance exercises and individual needs.[15] This helps to preserve muscle mass, increasing metabolic rate and adhere to dietary modifications further enhancing activities in the form of walking for long durations,[16] walking fast, walking uphill, walking with weights, walking on sand, climbing stairs, travelling, enhancing social interactions and contributing to welfare of self, family and community with changed lifestyle where modifications in the form of dietary changes in the type and time of food and daily activities becomes a natural lifestyle.

Physical activity is one of the ways of to maximize caloric expenditure (330–500 kcal/day). Non-weight bearing activities should be considered. One should emphasize an increase in duration rather than intensity (150-300 minutes/week).

Patients with severe or uncontrolled hypertension should add exercise to their treatment plan only after consultation with physician and being prescribed anti-hypertensive treatment. If resting systolic blood pressure is more than 200 mm Hg and or resting diastolic Blood pressure is more than 110 mm Hg, do not exercise. Valsalva maneuver should be avoided during resistance training.

Patients with associated dyslipidemia and taking lipid lowering medications have a potential to cause muscle damage may experience muscle weakness and soreness termed myalgia.

Current health recommendations state that all healthy individuals aged 18 to 65 years, need moderate intensity activity for a

Table 13.2: Recommendations to lower cardiovascular risk

- Quitting tobacco use, or reducing the amount smoked, or not starting the habit
- Making healthy food choices
- Being physically active
- Reducing body mass index (to less than 25 kg/m^2) and waist–hip ratio (to less than 0.8 in women and 0.9 in men)
- Lowering blood pressure (to less than 140/90 mm Hg)
- Lowering blood cholesterol (to less than 5 mmol/L or 190 mg/dL)
- Lowering LDL-cholesterol (to less than 3.0 mmol/L or 115 mg/dL)
- Controlling glycemia, especially in those with impaired fasting glycemia and impaired glucose tolerance or diabetes

minimum of 30 minutes on 5 days each week or vigorous intensity aerobic activity for a minimum on 3 days each week. Additionally, on 2 or more days a week you need muscle-strengthening activities that work all major muscle groups (legs, hips, back, abdomen, chest shoulders, and arms). Children should get at least 60 minutes of activity every day.[17.]

Participation in household activities and regular physical exercise will help in lowering the prevalence of overweight. Therefore, the role of physical activity, games, and sports should be emphasized, and facilities should be provided for outdoor games in schools, with compulsory hours of sports and games. Developing after school activities and nutritional programs that kids love is extremely essential.[18] Outside of home, schools and child care center's are key places for making a change. Rather than having them 'exercise' have them 'play'.

Children should be made a part of Games club, healthy food club, gardening and fit club to bring about a change in their knowledge, physical activity behaviors and attitude. Encouraging the demonstration of love, affection, and nurture with the use of non-food items avoids the gratification related to food.

The problem with gestational obesity lies in the belief of feeding two. The mother is fed with high fat laden foods to provide nutrition to the child in the antenatal period and for lactation in postnatal period,which only adds to the fat mass of the lady. The myth of 'do not exercise' after a 'C' section enhances the imbalance of input and output and leads to fast gain of weight and obesity. This along with the weak core and lax abdomen and pelvic floor leads to problems associated with women health at a later stage.

The key to success of a weight loss program and preventing cardiometabolic disease is

- Be sensitive to the excess weight and body image concerns
- Emphasize consistency and lifestyle activity
- Select the right exercise
- Maintain the risk markers within normal range (Table 13.2).

SUMMARY

Obesity is a growing public health concern involving complex interaction of various physiological, psychological, genetic and cultural factors. A comprehensive approach involving lifestyle and behavioral modification, physical activity, exercise and social support holds promise for lifelong result. Non consideration of special psychological and physical burdens of being overweight affects compliance. Aggressive work is needed to prevent relapse and potential psychological and medical consequences.

Case Study 1

Sunita, a 17-year-old college going student, c/o weight gain since 3 years with irregular menstrual cycle and mood swings. She feels shy to go out and does not socialize.

Her thyroid function are normal. She was brought by her mother to attend obesity clinic.

1. What are your goals?
2. What factors would you consider while planning program?
3. How would you implement the program?

Case Study 2

Mrs Joshi, 52 years Homemaker, diagnosed case of hypertension since 7 years controlled on medication. She visited physiotherapy OPD for complaints of weight gain in the past 2 years and to improve fitness. Her BMI is 35.7 kg/m^2 with waist circumference of 100 cm. She walks every day for 15 mins once.

1. What would be target weight loss schedule for her?
2. What factors would you consider while planning the program?
3. How would you calculate caloric expenditure for weight loss?

REFERENCES

1. Kalra S, Unnikrishnan AG. Obesity in India: The weight of the nation. Journal of Medical Nutrition and Nutraceuticals. 2012;1(1):37-41.
2. Pradeepa R, Anjana RM, Joshi SR, et.al. Prevalence of generalized and abdominal obesity in urban and rural India-the ICMR-INDIAB study (phase-I) [ICMR-INDIAB-3]. Indian J Med Res. 2015;145:139-50.
3. Swain DP, Brawner CA. ACSM's resource manual for Guidelines for exercise testing and prescription, 7th edn. Philadelphia: Baltimore; 2014.
4. Cornier MA, Desperes JP, Davis N, et al. Assessing adiposity: A scientific statement from American Heart Association. Circulation. 2011;124:1996-2019.
5. Nordhamn K, Sodergren E, Olsson E, et al. Reliability of anthropometric measures in overweight and lean subjects: consequences of correlations between anthropometric and other variables. Int J Obesity. 2000;24:652-7.
6. Dasgupta R, Pillai R, Kumar R, et al. Sugar, salt, fat, and chronic disease epidemic in India: Is there need for policy interventions? Indian J Community Med. 2015;40(2):71-4.
7. Monteiro CA, Levy RB, Claro RM, et al. Increasing consumption of ultra-processed foods and likely impact on human health: evidence from Brazil. Public Health Nutrition. 2010; 14(1): 5-13.
8. Schwab S, Xu T, Ryan K, Steinle N. Eating Behavior Disinhibition Predicts Insulin Resistance in the Old Order Amish. J Hum Nutr Food Sci. 2017;5(2):1109.
9. Singh RB, Pella D, Mechirova V, et.al. Prevalence of obesity, physical inactivity and undernutrition, a triple burden of diseases during transition in a developing economy. The Five City Study Group. Acta Cardiol. 2007;62(2):119-27.
10. Rotella CM, Dicembrini I. Measurement of body composition as a surrogate evaluation of energy balance in obese patients. World J Methodol. 2015;5(1):1-9.
11. McLean RC, Morrison DS, Shearer R, et al. Attrition and weight loss outcomes for patients with complex obesity, anxiety and depression attending a weight management programme with targeted psychological treatment. Clinical Obesity. 2016;6(2):133-42.
12. Shibata S, Tahara Y. Circadian rhythm and exercise. J Phys Fitness Sports Med. 2014;3(1):65-72.

13. van der Ploeg HP, Chey T, Korda RJ, et al. Sitting Time and All-Cause Mortality Risk in 222 497 Australian Adults. Arch Intern Med. 2012;172(6):494-500.
14. Biswas A, Paul I, Faulkner GE, et al. Sedentary time and its association with risk for disease incidence, mortality, and hospitalization in adults: A systematic review and meta-analysis. Ann Intern Med. 2015;162(2):123-32.
15. Lee JS, Bacha F, Hannon T, et al. Effects of aerobic versus resistance exercise without caloric restriction on abdominal fat, intrahepatic lipid, and insulin sensitivity in obese adolescent boys: A randomized controlled trial. Diabetes. 2012;61:2787-95.
16. Christine Hancock. The benefits of regular walking for health, well-being. C3 Collaborating for Health. 2011.
17. American College of Sports Medicine: Guidelines for Exercise Testing and Exercise Prescription, 8th edition. Lippincott Williams & Wilkins, 2010.
18. Fink B, Riddick V. Developing after school activities and nutritional programs kids love. ACSM's Health and Fitness Journal. 2013;17(4):23-7.

13.2 PREVENTING CORONARY HEART DISEASE

Mariya Prakash Jiandani

Introduction: Mortality from cardiovascular disease is on the rise due to unhealthy habits, change in lifestyle and increased stress levels. Cardiovascular diseases (CVD) are responsible for about 25% Disability adjusted life years (DALYs) lost due to NCD in South East Asian Region. With increasing numbers it is essential that a coordinated set of actions are undertaken not only at individual level but also at community level. The risk factors for coronary artery disease are in parallel with that of cancer. Targeting these at primary prevention and primordial level by change in government and school policies and inculcating healthy lifestyle and behavioral change would reduce the economic burden and suffering.

Keywords: Prevention, Cardiology, Lifestyle

INTRODUCTION

Millions of deaths are preventable every year. Leading causes of these deaths include cardiovascular disease, diabetes, chronic respiratory disease and cancer. Lifestyle changes and behavioral patterns of people have favored the onset of these chronic diseases. Coronary heart disease (CHD) is a 'Pandemic' with no known borders. It has been referred by WHO as 'Mankind's greatest epidemic striking more and more young subjects'. CVD-Stroke is another substantial cause of death and disability. The impact of chronic disease in terms of poverty, disability and family problems is serious.

NEED OF PREVENTION

India is experiencing a rapid health transition with a raising burden of non-communicable disease (NCD) in both urban and rural population.There is considerable loss in potentially productive years (age 35–64 yrs) of life. Athersoclerotic cardiovascular disease is a chronic disorder developing insidiously throughout life and progressing to an advanced stage by the time symptoms occur.[1]

Cardiovascular diseases (CVD) are responsible for about 25% Disability adjusted life years (DALYs) lost due to NCD in South East Asian Region. Of these ischemic heart disease accounts for about 40% of DALYs lost, cerebrovascular disease 19%, rheumatic heart disease 6%, inflammatory heart disease 6% and other conditions 19%.[2] The WHO has estimated that India lost 9 billion USD in national income from premature deaths due to heart disease, stroke and diabetes in the year 2005.[3]

It is estimated that there were approximately 46.9 million patients with CVD in India. The prevalence of CVD is reported to be 2–3 times higher in urban population as compared to rural.[3] Though advanced technology and improved income has reduced age associated cardiovascular mortality, cardiovascular disease still continues to be a leading cause of mortality and morbidity. Prevention is essential, as more than 50% reduction in CHD mortality relate to change in risk factors and 40% to improved treatment. There is a large scope for improvement in risk factor control in population and in individuals with high-risk.[4]

DEFINITION

Cardiovascular disease (CVD) prevention is defined as a coordinated set of actions, at the population level or targeted at an individual, that are aimed at eliminating or minimizing the impact of CVDs and their related disabilities. These are measures taken for disease prevention rather than treatment. It includes a lifetime approach to prevent CVD as both cardiovascular disease and risk are dynamic and changing with process of aging and presence of comorbidities.[5]

Prevention needs to be at the population level by promoting healthy lifestyle behavior in the community and at individual level in subjects with moderate or high-risk of CVD or patients with established CVD by tackling unhealthy lifestyle and optimizing risk factors to prevent recurrence and complications.

SCREENING FOR RISK FACTORS[5]

The active search for a disease among apparently healthy people is a fundamental aspect of prevention. Screening is identification of unrecognized disease or an unknown increased risk in individuals without symptoms by means of rapidly applied tests, examinations or other procedures in apparently healthy individuals. Epidemiologist has extended the concept to screening for 'risk factors' as these factors apparently antedate the development of actual disease.

Risk factors that alter the pathophysiology like serum cholesterol, impaired glucose tolerance, increased weight are amenable to effective interventions. Hence preventive measures can be applied before disease occurs. A risk estimation system such as SCORE can assist in clinical decision making for management, and may assist in both under and over treatment. It may also help in reinforcing individuals of the need for intensive lifestyle change.[1] The importance of risk factors in the development of CVD has received increased attention over the past decade. In addition, along with cardioprotective medications, the roles of lifestyle interventions, psychosocial factors, air pollution, dietary patterns, physical inactivity, low cardiorespiratory fitness, obesity, cardiac rehabilitation, and inflammation have been better elucidated as modulators of CVD and as targets for education, behavioral interventions, and policy approaches to improving health.[6]

The INTERHEART study examined the risk factors associated with first acute myocardial infarction (AMI) in 52 countries, including 15 152 cases and 14 820 controls. Collectively, 9 risk factors (abnormal lipids, smoking, hypertension, diabetes mellitus, abdominal obesity, psychosocial variables, consumption of fruits and vegetables, regular alcohol consumption, regular physical activity) accounted for 90% of the population attributable risk in men and 94% in women.[7]

Population can be divided as:

1. ***Apparently healthy:*** An individual with no major known coronary risk factors. CVD risk is most frequently due to multiple interacting risk factors.
2. ***Increased risk:*** An individual who has symptoms suggestive of possible coronary disease and has at least one major coronary risk factor.
3. ***Known disease:*** An individual with known cardiac, pulmonary, or metabolic disease at any age.

Risk factors are broadly classified as modifiable and non-modifiable: Since 1951 the Framingham heart study has played a major role in establishing the nature of coronary heart disease risk factors and their relative importance.

Non-modifiable Risk Factors

Age, gender, ethnicity and genetics or family history are considered as non-modifiable risk factors for CVD by virtue of inability to modify them. Prevalence of diseases like hypertension, diabetes increases with age and runs in the family. Degeneration, stiffness of vessels and increased atherogenecity, increases the risk of cardiovascular event. Men are at more risk compared to women, however after menopause the protective effect of estrogen is lost and gender bias disappears. CVD appears to be the biggest cause of death in women. Women on oral contraceptives are at increased risk of developing CVD.[8]

Family history of premature CVD in first-degree relatives, before 55 years of age in men and 65 years of age in women, is a crude but simple indicator of the risk of developing CVD.[1] It reflects both the genetic trait and the environment shared by family members.

Modifiable Risk Factors

Tobacco: Both direct tobacco and second hand smoke is a major CVD risk factor.[6,7] Cigarette smoking increases CVD risk due to several mechanisms such as induced atherogenesis, nicotine stimulated adrenergic drive raising blood pressure, altering lipoprotein levels. The degree of risk developing CHD is directly related to number of cigarettes smoked per day and is calculated as pack years.[10] Cigarette smokers die 10 years younger than non-smokers. Quitting smoking at age of 60 or 40 years increased life expectancy by 3 and 9 years, respectively.[9] For those who have had myocardial infarction, the risk of fatal recurrence may be reduced by 50% after giving up smoking.[8,9]

Even a very short period of passive smoke exposure has persistent vascular consequences, such as the mobilization of dysfunctional endothelial progenitor cells with blocked nitric oxide production.[11]

Sedentary lifestyle: People who are physically inactive have 20–30% increased risk of all-cause mortality. Sedentary lifestyle, coach potatotes and inactive recreation such as television watching, playing video games promotes obesity and is important risk factor to develop type 2 diabetes. Regular physical exercise increases the concentration of high density lipoprotein (HDL) and decreases both body weight and blood pressure, both of which are beneficial to cardiovascular health.[12]

Unhealthy diet: High consumption of saturated fats, transfatty acid and refined carbohydrates and low consumption of vegetables and fruits is linked to heart disease. High salt consumption is an important determinant of cardiovascular risk. Unhealthy diet is rising rapidly in low resource settings and low income countries. Fast availability of ready to eat food which contain high levels of transfatty acids, burgers, pizzas are one of the factors for predisposition to risk to obesity and diabetes.

Associated comorbidities: Presence of diabetes, hypertension, raised cholesterol and obesity or overweight are major risk factors of CVD. The risk of CVD is 2–3 times higher in diabetics than in non-diabetics.[13]

AHA reclassified obesity as a major modifiable risk factor for CHD. Subsequently, numerous studies have substantiated that obesity confers an independent and additive risk of all-cause and cardiovascular mortality, even in the absence of metabolic syndrome.

Obese are at higher risk of developing hypertension. Data indicates a reduction in blood pressure with reduction in weight. There is an increased risk of myocardial infarction with elevated serum cholesterols.[14]

There is vast body of evidence showing triangular relationship between habitual diet, blood cholesterol-lipoprotein levels and coronary heart disease. It is the level of low density lipoprotein (LDL) that is most directly associated with risk. VLDL is more associated with peripheral vascular disease. HDL is protective against the development of CHD.[15]

High alcohol intake more than 75g/day is an independent risk factor CHD and hypertension.[16]

Psychosocial risk factors: They act as barriers to treatment adherence and efforts to improve lifestyle, as well as to promoting health in patients and populations.

Psychological risk factors such as depression, anxiety, hostility and anger exacerbate the development of CVD through associated unhealthy behaviors. Type A personality is associated with competitive drive, restlessness, hostility and a sense of urgency and impatience. They are more prone to CHD than calmer counterparts.[17] It may also lead to unfavorable outcomes such as myocardial ischemia, ventricular arrhythmias, and increased thrombosis potential and inflammation.

Low socioeconomic status defined as low education level, low income, holding a low status job or living in a poor residential area, lack of social support(living in isolation) are at increased risk of dying prematurely with CVD.[18,19]

There is moderate evidence that work related stress (high psychological demands and job strain) are risk factors for men and conflict, crisis in family life contribute to the risk of CVD in women.[20]

Air pollution and cardiovascular risk: Numerous epidemiological studies have demonstrated consistent associations between short-term elevations in particulate matter (air pollution) and increases in nonfatal and fatal cardiovascular events, including myocardial ischemia and infarction, ventricular arrhythmia, heart failure exacerbation, and stroke.[15]

LEVELS OF PREVENTION[4,5]

Prevention can be divided into following (Fig. 13.1).

Primordial Prevention

It is a population based strategy that involves preventing the emergence and spread of CHD risk factors and lifestyles that have not yet appeared or become endemic. This approach is based on the principle that small changes in risk factor levels in total populations can achieve biggest reduction in mortality.[4]

The aim is to change the underlying risk factors by alteration of lifestyle based practices in the community as a whole rather than individual.

Primary Prevention

It includes methods to avoid occurrence of disease either through eliminating disease agents or increasing resistance to disease. The aim is to identify and treat risk factors. Examples include maintaining a healthy diet and exercise regimen, and avoiding smoking as a multifactorial risk factor modification and control in subjects who have not had a cardiovascular event.

The prevention of coronary artery disease in adults begins in childhood. Children at high-risk for cardiovascular disease can be identified through medical history (i.e. positive family history of coronary disease,

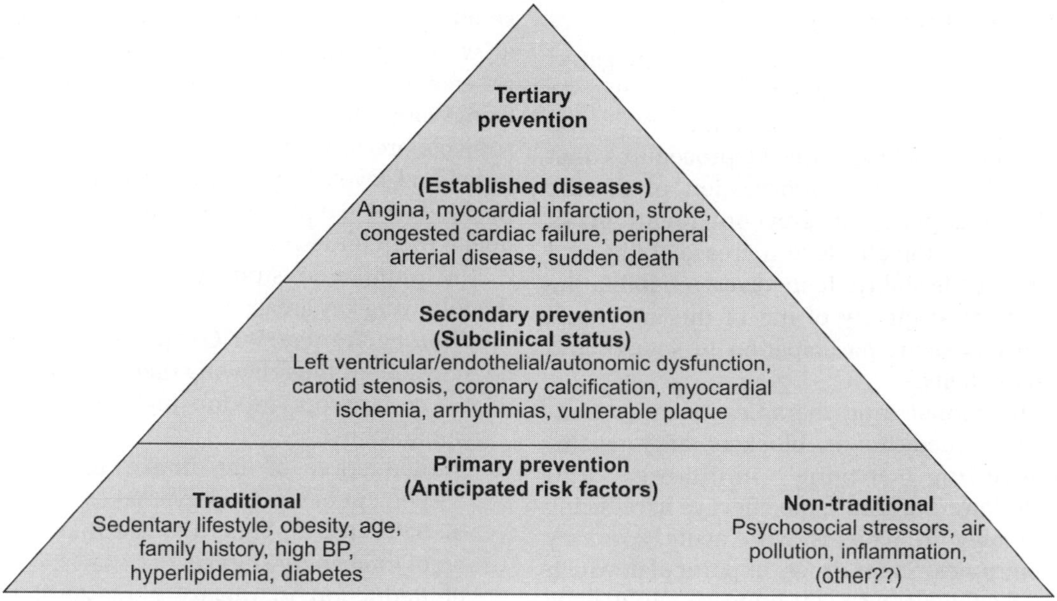

Fig. 13.1: Risk factor framework and the progression of cardiovascular disease, with types of prevention interventions. MI indicates myocardial infarction; CHF, congestive heart failure; and PAD, peripheral arterial disease

Source: **Barry A Franklin and Mary Cushman. Recent Advances in Preventive Cardiology and Lifestyle Medicine: A Themed Series** (*Circulation*. 2011;123:2274–2283)

history of tobacco use, and physical activity history), routine measurements (i.e. height, weight, and blood pressure), and selective laboratory screening (i.e. lipoprotein measurement).[21]

Offsprings of diabetic pregnancies tend to develop obesity in childhood and are at high-risk of developing type 2 diabetes at an early age. Children at high-risk should receive special counseling on diet; physical activity; smoking cessation; and, if indicated, pharmacologic therapy.

People with known risk factors and not yet developed overt symptoms or a cardiovascular event should be targeted for primary prevention and lifestyle change strategies to control risk factors. They should be screened for risk prediction of an event in 10 years (EUROSCORE) and interventions should be monitored and modified to check the reduction in the score.

Secondary Prevention

It is continuation of primary prevention. It aims at prevention of progression of disease, recurrence of cardiovascular events and disability in patients diagnosed with the underlying disease. It includes methods to detect and address an existing disease prior to the appearance of symptoms.

Patients with known cardiovascular, pulmonary or metabolic disease on cardio-protective medications with or without revascularization procedures need to be educated and protected from another event. Cardiac rehabilitation, lifestyle modification and control of risk factors in these individuals form secondary prevention. Controlling and modulating risk factors can have a profound and favorable impact on decreasing the incidence of initial and recurrent cardio-vascular events.

Tertiary Prevention

It includes methods to reduce negative impact of symptomatic disease, disability or death, through rehabilitation and treatment. Examples include surgical procedures that halt the spread or progression of disease like angioplasty or preventing end organ damage.[22] The aim is to increase ability and limiting disability. It involves rehabilitating to improve quality of life of the individual and increasing participation in society and productivity.

Individual drug therapies, such as anti-platelet medications, blockers, angiotensin-converting enzyme inhibitors, and lipid-lowering agents, are effective in reducing mortality in patients with acute coronary syndromes. Statin drugs, in particular, which markedly decrease and increase low-density lipoprotein and high-density lipoprotein cholesterol respectively, have been heralded as a potential breakthrough to prevent initial and recurrent atherosclerotic events.[23] Cardiac rehabilitation is the evidence based standard of care post CHD.

Diabetic patients if inadequately treated develop multiple chronic complications like diabetic retinopathy, neuropathy, and nephropathy resulting in deterioration of quality of life leading to irreversible disability and death.[1] Lower limb amputation are 10 times more common in diabetics than non-diabetics.

Central adiposity has long been accepted as a risk factor of type 2 Diabetes and risk is related to degree and duration of obesity.[24]

PREVENTION INTERVENTION STRATEGIES[12]

In order to prevent at different levels two approaches are considered population and high-risk (Geoffrey Rose).

Population Strategy

Population strategy aims at reducing the CVD incidence at the population level by bringing small shifts in the risk of the disease across a whole population consistently leading to greater reduction in disease burden. It brings larger benefits to the population as all subjects are targeted and offers little at the individual level. It addresses cardiovascular health over the entire life course and reduces health inequalities.[25]

The population strategy centers around the following key areas:

1. ***Dietary changes:*** WHO expert committee considered the following dietary changes to be appropriate for high incidence populations:
   - i. Reduction of fat intake to 20–30 percent of total energy intake.
   - ii. Saturated fat limited to less than 10% of total energy intake.
   - iii. Reduction of dietary cholesterol to below 100 mg per 1000 kcal/day.
   - iv. Increase consumption of vegetables, fruits, whole grains and legumes (30–45 g of fiber/day).
   - v. Reduction of salt intake to 5 g daily or less.
   - vi. Avoidance of alcohol consumption.
2. ***Smoking:*** It aims to achieve a smoke free society with implementation of public policies, legislative restrictions, fiscal measures and smoking cessation programs. Ban smoking in public places, enforcing bans on tobacco advertising, raising tax on tobacco and curbing sale of loose cigarettes are steps towards achieving a smoke free society.
3. ***Blood pressure:*** Small reduction by an average blood pressure of the whole population by a mere 2 or 3 mm Hg would produce a large reduction in the incidence of cardiovascular complication. To reduce the mean population blood pressure a multifactorial approach based on 'prudent diet', weight control and regular physical activity is required.
4. ***Physical activity:*** Encourage regular physical activity to be a part of normal

daily life. Initiatives like 'Equal Streets' and 'Yoga by the Bay' promote inculcation of physical activity. Walkathons and marathons introduce a practice of regular physical activity to stay fit.

Tools to Implement

Public Health Strategies[26]

Tobacco cessation, good nutrition, and increase physical activity are important to lower the cardiovascular risk of the population. Nationwide cooperation between local government, non-governmental organization, food industry, retail, catering, school, workplace and other stakeholders is needed to implement policies and ensure success of heart healthy programs.

Government initiatives like a) High taxes on tobacco products and banning sale of loose cigarettes, b) Restrictions on advertising, promotion and sponsorship by tobacco industry, c) Restriction on smokeless tobacco (strong evidence of harm), d) Banning smoking in public places, workplaces, restaurants, public transports, e) Telephonic and internet counseling on smoking cessation, f) Pictorial and text warning on cigarette package, g) Use of Media and educational campaigns, h) Adolescence is most vulnerable period for uptake of smoking which continues as lifelong behavior. Ban on sale of tobacco in shops near school and creating, awareness and warning of 'cigarette as a health menace' would help inculcate healthy behavior.

Healthy Environment

Every school and workplace should have a policy to promote a healthy environment, provide healthy food and daily physical activities of at least 30 minutes. Interventions to promote walking could contribute substantially towards increasing the activity levels of the most sedentary.[17]

Government mandates should be there when planning and sanctioning new constructions. Tax incentives to be provided on purchase of exercise equipment, sports participation and fitness memberships. Increased availability of parks, playgrounds and open gymnasium are important. Pricing strategies to decline use of unhealthy food like 'Fat tax' and increase in healthy food consumption by subsidizing rates would increase availability of healthy foods.[27]

Packaging strategies of color coding nutrients and labels. Indicators of transfatty acids and calories would facilitate people in choosing the right foods as consumers understand this and it has a positive impact.[28]

Education and awareness of nutritive value of foods and counseling in health care should be provided regularly. Health education should be a part of school curriculum. Movement for education on physical activity should start at kindergarten. Good neighborhood and safe environments for cycling and walking should be provided. School initiative of walk to school and community travel would inculcate healthy habits in childhood.

Promoting physical activity within the work time schedule by changing environment forming groups and putting down policies may enforce behavioral modifications. Provision of healthy nutritive meals at subsidized rates in canteen or mess should be made available.

Work environment and culture should be made 'heart friendly.' Linking salary increments and perks to improved fitness levels can motivate individuals towards a healthy lifestyle. Government can provide subsidies to companies who follow such heart healthy norms. Introduction of compulsory physical activity within the work time frame. Minimizing the use of elevators over any two floors and introducing standing work stations, no parking facilities within a specified radius promotes increased physical activity. Facility for gymnasium or sports and arranging tournaments would promote healthy recreational activities. Formulate walking groups, arrange walkathons, marathons regulary aims to sustain fitness levels.

Budgetary provisions and funds should be created for promoting such activities.

Screening

It is recommended that the risk factor screening including lipid profile may be considered in adult men >40 years old and in women >50 years of age or post-menopausal in apparently healthy individual.[1] It is crucial to create a healthy work culture. Employers should conduct regular screening for health risks and provide health related targets to employees. Regular screening camps can be arranged during festive occasions to promote awareness. Screening should be for identification of presence of risk factors, risk estimation and secondary prevention. SCORE (Systemic coronary risk estimation) charts are easy methods for screening for risk estimation.

Physiotherapist can contribute to public health strategies through health counseling and as advocates for public health strategies both at local and higher levels. They can contribute in conducting health awareness and education programs, being advocates of promoting healthy lifestyle and enabling program implementation. They can participate at school, community programs in promoting health talks, creating awareness and recommending activities and fitness programs to modify and reduce risk.

High-risk strategy: In the high-risk (individual level) approach, preventive measures are aimed at reducing the risk factor levels in those at highest risk, either individuals without CVD at the upper part of the total cardiovascular risk distribution or those with established CVD. Individuals targeted in the strategy are more likely to benefit than the population. It encompasses individual choice, family influence, cultural and ethnic grouping, workplace and health care policy.

Cardiovascular health is defined in 3 categories of ideal, intermediate, and poor on the basis of seven simple health factors and modifiable behaviors. Behavioral patterns represent the number one factor contributing to premature death, exceeding genetic predisposition, social circumstances, environmental exposure, and access to healthcare.

Identify risk: High-risk intervention can only start once those at high-risk are identified. Risk estimation is recommended in individuals having risk factors or a strong family history or if they ask for. It is recommended to repeat every 5 years and more often in those close to thresholds mandating treatment.

Counseling: Cognitive behavioral methods are effective in adopting healthy lifestyle of individuals and patients with risk regarding cardioprotective lifestyle changes. Lifestyle is usually based on long-standing behavioral patterns acquired during childhood and adolescence. It involves interaction of genetic, environmental and social factors.

Caregivers in clinical practice are in unique position to directly support their patients regarding psychosocial risk factors in individuals with high cardiovascular risk or with established disease.[29,30]

Specialized psychosocial interventions include individual or group counseling in psychosocial risk factors and coping with illness, stress management programs, meditation, breathing and yoga, relaxation, biofeedback and autogenic training.[31]

'Collaborative care' in depression which may involve a systemic assessment of depression, a non-physician care manager to perform longitudinal symptoms monitoring, treatment interventions and care coordination resulted in 48% lower risk for developing first CAD events 8 years after treatment compared to usual care.[32]

A friendly and positive approach to develop a therapeutic alliance is necessary. Active involvement of the individual, caregiver and family is required to ensure lifestyle change and medicine adherence. The individual has to be assisted to understand the relationship between behavior and health and the barriers to behavior change. Provide patient information in the form of booklets and web based material and promote cardiac rehabilitation.

Changing lifestyle habits can be difficult and a gradual change that is sustained is often permanent. Individuals may need support for a long time and repeated efforts to maintain lifestyle change may be necessary.

Realistic goals: An important step to change negative into positive behavior is to help individual set a realistic goal allowing identifying and selecting the risk factor to change. This helps in moving in small consecutive steps. There are number of factors such as cost, convenience in time, geographical area, satisfaction, motivation and interest or fear of health which may drive the individual to change behaviors.

The Life's Simple Seven (AHA 2020 Strategic Plan)

1. Quit Cigarette Smoking

Quitting smoking must be encouraged in all smokers though it is complex and difficult process. The most important predictor of sucess is motivation.

The 5 As' for smoking cessation:[1]

- ***Ask:*** Enquire if the person smokes or any form of tobbaco.
- ***Advise:*** To quit in a clear strong personalized manner.
- ***Assess:*** The individuals degree of addiction and readiness to quit.
- ***Assist:*** In preparing a plan to quit. Set a date, use social and family support, behavioral counseling and pharmacological support (nicotine replacement therapy, or bupropion).
- ***Arrange:*** A follow-up schedule to congratulate success or more intensive intervention if relapse.

2. Control Weight (Obesity)

Increased BMI, central adiposity and increased waist circumference needs to be kept in check. Waist circumference of >94 cm in men or >80 cm in women represents a threshold at which no further weight should be gained and values of >102 cm in men or >88 cm in women represents the threshold at which weight reduction should be advised. Diet, exercise and behavior modification are the mainstay therapies. Medical therapies and or bariatric surgery is recommended for patients with a BMI >35 kg/M^2.

3. Glucose Control

The recommended HbA1c is <6.5 to <7.0%. Hypoglycemia and excessive weight gain has to be avoided. Most patients with DM are obese so weight control is central component. A combination of aerobic and resistance exercise training is effective in the prevention of progression of DM and control of glycemia.

Reducing body weight by 5–7%; decreasing fat and saturated fat intake to 30% and 10% of total energy intake, respectively; increasing fiber intake to 15 g/1000 kcal; and an increase in exercise to 30 min/d or 150 mins of physical activity per week resulted in a 58% reduction in the development of diabetes mellitus in high-risk overweight subjects with impaired glucose tolerance compared with a usual-care control group over 3.2 years (Prevent Finnish Diabetes Prevention Study and Diabetes Prevention Program Research Group) whereas there was a 31% reduction with metformin (850 mg twice daily) compared with placebo.

A multifactorial approach to achieving low BP levels and low LDL and cholesterol concentrations and ideal body weight and antithrombotic therapy is beneficial in preventing CVD events in patients with DM.

4. Blood Pressure Control

Blood pressure has to be measured frequently on several occasions as necessary. Family history of hypertension and tracking of blood pressure from childhood helps in early diagnosis. Screening and follow-up is important. When required, ambulatory and home BP monitoring should be done for diagnosis and pharmacological intervention.

A hypertensive has to learn to take his own blood pressure and keep records. Aim of treatment is to maintain blood pressure below 140/90 and ideally 120/80. Control of hypertension reduces the incidence of stroke. Compliance with antihypertensive therapy reduces the morbidity and mortality from coronary, cerebrovascular, kidney and retinal disease. It can be improved through education directed to patients, families and community as the treatment is lifelong.

Lifestyle interventions include weight reduction, reduction in use of sodium to <5g/day, DASH diet and regular physical activity.

5. Keep Cholesterols Low

Increased plasma cholesterol are among the main risk factors for CVD. Hypertriglyceridemia and low HDL are independent CVD risk factors. Low HDL-C is independently associated with cardiovascular risk. An HDL-C level <40 mg/dL in men and <45 mg/dl in women may be regarded as marker of increased risk. The recommended target levels are less than 190 mg/dL for total plasma cholesterol and less than 115 mg/dL for LDL cholesterol for subjects at low to moderate risk. In patients with high and V high CVD risk the LDL levels should be less than 100 and 70 mg/dL respectively.

All patients with familial hypercholesterolemia should be considered as high-risk and treated with lipid lowering therapy (statins). Patients with acute coronary syndrome, non-hemorrhagic stroke, and occlusive arterial disease should be treated with statins.

6. Healthy Diet Plan

A 2-year study of weight loss diets, using either low-fat, Mediterranean, or low-carbohydrate strategies, reported a significant regression of carotid atherosclerosis, irrespective of the dietary intervention.[1,30]

Diet as recommended by WHO expert committee should be followed.

Adequate consumption of fruit and vegetables reduces the risk of CVD, stomach and colorectal cancer.

Reduce intake of saturated fat. Avoid margarine and bakery products (transfatty acids).

Avoid sugar sweetened soft drinks which is largest source of empty food calorie.

Mediterranean diet which consists of nutrient and high intake of fruits, vegetables, legumes, whole grain products, fish and unsaturated fatty acids esp olive oil.[1]

A systematic review found strong evidence of a causal relationship for cardioprotective dietary practices, including vegetables, nuts, and Mediterranean eating patterns, as well as associations for harmful factors, including intake of trans fatty acids and foods with a high glycemic index or load, and CHD.[18]

Modest reductions in dietary salt[6]: Increase consumption of omega-3 fatty acid consumption, especially the longer-chain fatty acids from marine sources, on cardiovascular end points.

Strategies such as 'nudging' and 'default' have been proposed as tools.

7. Increase Physical Activity

Participation in regular physical activity and aerobic exercise training are associated with decreased cardiovascular mortality. There are multiple mechanisms by which moderate to vigorous physical activity may decrease mortality rates associated with CVD (Flowchart 13.1),[26,33] including antiatherosclerotic, antithrombotic, anti-ischemic, antiarrhythmic, and psychological effects.

Cardiorespiratory fitness, expressed as metabolic equivalents (MET) is one of the strongest prognostic markers in persons

Flowchart 13.1: Mechanisms by which moderate to vigorous exercise training may reduce the risk of nonfatal and fatal cardiovascular events

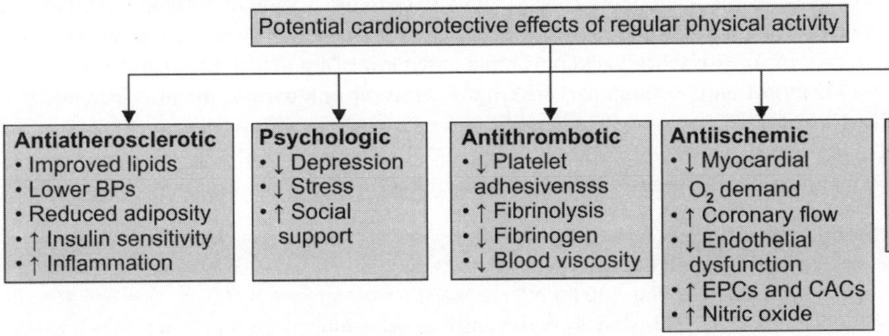

Source: Adapted from Franklin BA, McCullough PA. Cardiorespiratory fitness: an independent and additive marker of risk stratification and health outcomes. Mayo Clin Proc. 2009; 84:776–9.

with and without CHD (1 MET= 3.5 mL O_2/kg/min). In healthy men and women, each 1 MET increase in exercise capacity reduces all-cause mortality and cardiovascular events by 13% and 15%, respectively. Participants with an aerobic capacity of 7.9 metabolic equivalents had the most favorable health outcomes.[1]

Assess physical activity level. Days and minutes per day spent on average doing physical activity. Questionnaires such as IPAQ can be used to assess the level of physical activity.

Warn against inactivity and sedentary lifestyle. Help add physical activity using individual preferences.

Set personal goals and advise on appropriate types of activities and ways of progressing.

Find an activity that is enjoyable and or can be included in daily routines. Active traveling (cycling/walking), reduce screen time and chair time. Introduce rewards for every small goal achieved. Help them notice the difference and perceive benefit. Walking is a popular, familiar, convenient, and free form of exercise by which many sedentary people could gain the health benefits of moderate intensity physical activity. It is influenced by environmental and societal conditions as well as by interventions targeted at individuals.

Interventions tailored to people's needs, targeted at the most sedentary or at those most motivated to change, and delivered either at the level of the individual or household or through groups can increase walking by up to 30–60 minutes a week on average, at least in the short-term.[34]

Moderate intensity physical activity from 2.5 to 5 h/week or vigorous physical activity of 1–1.5 hrs/week–reduction in all cause and cardiovascular mortality. Multiple daily bouts of >10 minutes each on most days of the week also reduces CVD risk.[33] Table 13.1[1,35] reflects various intensitities. It is recommended to carry out moderate intensity—30 min/day, 5 days a week or 150 mins/week or vigorous intensity—15 min/day, 5 days a week or 75 mins/week. For individuals requiring lipid control-long

Table 13.1: Intensity levels

	Moderate intensity	Vigorous intensity
VO2 or heart rate reserve	40–59%	60–85%
RPE on CR 10 Borg scale	5–6	7–8
MET (absolute energy expenditure)	4.8–7.1 (young) 4.0–5.9 (middle aged) 3.2–4.7 (old) 2.0–2.9 (v.old)	7.2–10.1 6.0–8.4 4.8–6.7 3.0–4.2

Case Study 1

Mr Shah is a 44-year-old designer. He is a tobacco chewer. Since 10 years, he has job of 8–10 hours sitting and follows an irregular diet. His weight is 85 kg for a height of 160 cm. His father was diagnosed as hypertensive and had an infarct at the age of 46. He is tensed. His lipid profile shows low HDL and high trigylcerides. His blood sugar levels fasting are 112 mg/dL and postprandial is 165 mg/dL. He is the only earning member in family of 4.

1. What are his risk factors?
2. What is the level of prevention would you work at?
3. What strategies would you adopt to prevent a cardiovascular event?

Case Study 2

Miss Mitra is a 25-year-old clerk. She has BMI—30 kg/m^2. Her waist circumference is 100 cm. She has a family history of hypertension and obesity. She occasionally partys and is a social drinker. She does not smoke however her friends do.

1. What are her risk factors?
2. What level of prevention would you work at?
3. What strategies would you adopt?

duration—40 mins/day and for body weight reduction—60-90 mins/day. Resistance training should be added 2-3 sets 40-60% 1 RM at least twice a week.

Cardiac rehabilitation (CR) is a comprehensive program involving exercise training, risk factor modification, education and psychological support. It is predominantly implemented in hospitals or in community centers. Home based program has greater flexibility and options for activities. Mortality rates in elderly with CHD who undergo CR are 21 to 34% lower with a dose response relationship on the number of sessions attended.[36-39]

As suggested by Green et al, 'Coronary interventions treat a very short segment of the diseased coronary tree, whereas exercise exerts beneficial effects on endothelial function and disease progression in the entire arterial bed.'

Risk factor intervention trials: There are number of risk factor intervention trials which have proved beyond doubt that lifestyle modification and risk factor reduction in community is possible and strategies are needed not just at the local level but legislative and public health policies to curb the growing danger of CHD. Some of them are Multiple Risk Factor Intervention Trial (MRFIT) in the US, The Stanford Heart Disease Prevention Program in California, the North Karelia Project in Finland, Oslo Heart Study, Lipid Research Clinics and Interheart and Framingham Study.

It is never late to begin the change. 'Prevention is better than cure' the age old adage stands true.

REFERENCES

1. Piepoli MF, Hoes AW, Agewall S, et al. European Guidelines on Cardiovascular Disease Prevention in Clinical Practice. Eur Heart J. 2016 Aug 1;37(29):2315-81.
2. Health situation in the South East Asia region 1998-2000. World Health Organization, Regional Office for South East Asia: New Delhi, India, 2002.
3. Ajay VS, Prabhakaran D. Coronary heart disease in Indians, implications from the inter heart study. Indian J Med Res. 2010;132(5):561-6.
4. Park K. Epidemiology of chronic non-communicable diseases and conditions. Park's Textbook of Preventive Medicine, 21st edn. Banarsidas Bhanot Publishers. 2011,337-70.
5. Barry A. Franklin and Mary Cushman. Preventive Cardiology and Lifestyle Medicine. Circulation. 2011;123:2274-83.
6. Shaper AG, Pocock SJ, Walker M, et al. British Regional Heart Study: cardiovascular risk factors in middle-aged men in 24 towns. Br Med J. 1981;283:179-86.
7. Yusuf S, Hawken S, Ounpuu S, et.al Effect of potentially modifiable risk factors associated with myocardial infarction in 52 countries (the INTERHEART study): case-control study. Lancet. 2004;364:937-52.
8. Peter Croft, Philip C Hannaford. Risk factors for acute myocardial infarction in women: evidence from the Royal College of General Practitioners' oral contraception study. Br Med J. 1989;298:165-8.
9. Stone D, Shapiro S, Rosenberg L. Relation of cigarette smoking to myocardial infarction in young women. N Eng J Med. 1978;298:1273-6.
10. Centers for Disease Control and Prevention. How Tobacco Smoke Causes Disease: The Biology and Behavioural Basis for Smoking-attributable Disease 2010.
11. Heiss C, Amabile N, Lee AC, et al. Brief secondhand smoke exposure depresses endothelial progenitor cells activity and endothelial function. J Am Coll Cardiol. 2008; 51:1760-71.
12. World Health Organization. Primary Prevention of Coronary Heart Disease. Copenhagen: World Health Organization Regional Office for Europe, 1985. EURO Reports and Studies 98.
13. World Health Organization. Diabetes Mellitus: A Report of a WHO Study Group, Geneva, World Health Organization. 1985; Tech Rep. Ser. No 727.
14. Gordon T, Castelli WP. High density lipoprotein as a protective factor against coronary heart disease, the Framingham study. Am J Med. 1977;62:707-14.
15. Brook RD, Franklin B, Cascio W, et al. Air pollution and cardiovascular disease: a statement for healthcare professionals from the Expert Panel on Population and Prevention Science of the American Heart Association. Circulation. 2004;109:2655-71.
16. Community Prevention and Control of Cardiovascular Diseases. Report of WHO Expert Committee. WHO Technical Report Series 732, Geneva 1986.
17. Kittel F, Kornitzer M, Zyzanski SJ, et al. Prediction of clinical coronary heart disease by a test for the coronary-prone behaviour pattern. N Engl J Med. 1974;290:1271-5.
18. Albert MA, Glynn RJ, Buring J, et al. Impact of traditional and novel risk factors on the relationship between socioeconomic status and incident cardiovascular events. Circulation. 2006; 114:2619-26.
19. Alter DA, Franklin B, Ko DT, et.al. Socioeconomic status, functional recovery, and long-term mortality among patients surviving acute myocardial infarction. PLoS One. 2013;8:e65130.
20. Kivimäki M, Nyberg ST, Batty GD, et al. Job strain as a risk factor for coronary heart disease: a collaborative meta-analysis of individual participant data. Lancet. 2012;380:1491-7.

21. Gidding SS. Preventive pediatric cardiology. Tobacco, cholesterol, obesity, and physical activity. Pediatr Clin North Am. 1999;46(2):253-62.
22. Leavell HR, Clark CG. Preventive medicine for doctor in his community. Mc Graw Hill, New York, 1965.
23. Nissen SE, Nicholls SJ, Sipahi I, et al. Effect of very high-intensity statin therapy on regression of coronary atherosclerosis: the ASTEROID trial. JAMA. 2006;295:1556-65.
24. Hodge AM, de Courten MP, Zimmet P. Obesity and type II diabetes mellitus. In: Bjorntorp P (Ed). International Textbook of Obesity. John Wiley and Sons, Ltd. 2001, pp 352-64.
25. Rose G. The Strategy of Preventive Medicine. Oxford University Press, Oxford, 1992.
26. Franklin BA, McCullough PA. Cardiorespiratory fitness: an independent and additive marker of risk stratification and health outcomes. Mayo Clin Proc. 2009;84:776-9.
27. Hawkes C, Smith TG, Jewell J, et al. Smart food policies for obesity prevention. Lancet. 2015;385:2410-21.
28. Grunert KG, Wills JM. A review of European research on consumer response to nutrition information on food labels. J Public Health. 2007;15:385-99.
29. Albus C, Ladwig KH, Herrmann-Lingen C. Psychocardiology: clinically relevant recommendations regarding selected cardiovascular diseases. Dtsch Med Wochenschr. 2014;139:596-601.
30. Ladwig KH, Lederbogen F, Albus C, et al. Position paper on the importance of psychosocial factors in cardiology: update 2013. GerMed Sci. 2014;12:Doc09.
31. Whalley B, Thompson DR, Taylor RS. Psychological interventions for coronary heart disease: cochrane systematic review and meta-analysis. Int J Behav Med. 2014;21:109-21.
32. Huffman JC, Mastromauro CA, Beach SR, et al. Collaborative care for depression and anxiety disorders in patients with recent cardiac events: the Management of Sadness and Anxiety in Cardiology (MOSAIC) randomized clinical trial. JAMA Intern Med. 2014;174:927-35.
33. Stewart JC1, Perkins AJ, Callahan CM. Effect of Collaborative Care for Depression on Risk of Cardiovascular Events: Data from the IMPACT Randomized Controlled trial. Psychosom Med. 2014 Jan;76(1):29-37.
34. Kodama S, Aaito K, Tanaka S, et al. Cardiorespiratory fitness as a quantitative predictor of all-cause mortality and cardiovascular events in healthy men and women : a meta-analysis. JAMA. 2009;301:2024-35.
35. Ogilvie D, Foster CE, Rothnie H, et al. Interventions to promote walking: systematic review. BMJ. 2007; 334(7605):1204.
36. Howley ET. Type of activity: resistance, aerobic and leisure versus occupational physical activity. Med Sci Sports Exerc. 2001;33:S364-9.
37. Greaves CJ, Sheppard KE, Abraham C, et al. Systematic review of reviews of intervention components associated with increased effectiveness in dietary and physical activity interventions BMC Public Health. 2011;11:119.
38. Suaya JA, Stason WB, Ades PA, et al. Cardiac rehabilitation and survival in older coronary patients. J Am Coll Cardiol. 2009;54:25-33.
39. Hammil BG, Curtis LH, Schulman KA, et al. Relationship between cardiac rehabilitation and long term risk of death and myocardial infarction among elderly medicare beneficiaries. Circulation. 2010;121:63-70.

13.3 PREVENTION OF ADDICTIVE BEHAVIORS

Shubhangi Parker

INTRODUCTION

The increasing threat of alcohol and drug abuse is mammoth public health problem globally for many decades and continued to be till date. It has contributed to disease burden in health sector and deterioration in quality of life of not only of those who are direct victims of addictive behavior but also of their families and community (Hem Raj Pal and Amardeep Kumar 2005). There are various serious medical complications associated with addictive behaviors such as metabolic disorders, liver disease, cardiovascular problems, peripheral neuropathies and neuropsychiatric disorders (Srinivasan and Chandramauli 2013). Besides, the increase risk of crime, accidents and suicides, violence and drunk driving is also enormous social burden associated with addictive behavior (Ghodse H 1989). This serious public health concern along with tremendous economical burden is constantly distressing for the existing infrastructure and resources worldwide. Many efforts have been tried to combat this all-encompassing problem at national and international level for many decades with limited progress in developing countries. Addictive behaviors are understood as a biopsychosocial health problems, which needs to be handled with both medical intervention and psychosocial management (Ghodse H 1989). For such a multifaceted behavioral problem, the interventional and rehabilitative aspects also required to be likewise multidimensional in nature. Addictive behavior of alcohol and other drugs is a chaos not only for the addict but also for the family, community, workplace, and the public in general. The combating against peril of addictive behavior is more than treatment and rehabilitation of those who suffer from it. It is essentially, critical matter of public health concern to treat those who are previously affected by addictive behavior and to prevent those who are not addicted as yet but can be victim of it in future.

UNDERSTANDING ADDICTIVE BEHAVIOR

Generally any substance that modifies perception, mood, cognition, behavior or motor functions is called a psychoactive drug. This definition includes legal and illegal substances that can lead to repeated consumption and dependence.

The following psychoactive substances are known in the society:

1. Alcohol
2. Opioids (opium, heroin, morphine, ethidine, buprenorphine, codeine, etc.)
3. Cannabis ('ganja', 'bhang', 'charas')
4. Sedative—hypnotics (tranquilizers')
5. Cocaine
6. Other stimulants, including amphetamines and caffeine
7. Hallucinogens (e.g. LSD, 'acid')
8. Tobacco
9. Volatile solvents (typewriter correction and dilution fluids, kerosene, gasoline, petrol, paint-thinners, nail-polish removers, etc.) and other organic hydrocarbons (e.g. those in shoe-polish, iodex, etc.).

In India the frequent drug of addiction for decades are tobacco, alcohol, cannabis, opioids, various tranquilizers and in recent times volatile solvents and methamphetamine. Before we consider about the principles of prevention of addictive behavior it is prudent to understand why people take addictive drugs. Generally dugs are consumed to have 'feel good' outcome to get high, to get euphoric, to feel pleasure and enjoy recreational effect as well as to diminish 'feel bad' effect, i.e. to lower boredom, tension, anxiety, worries and depression. When people in general and teens in particular recognize the drug taking behavior as hazardous they will decrease the use of drugs hence efficient deaddiction prevention programs demonstrating this facet will be always supportive (Parkar and Iyer, 2000). Besides why people take drugs is not clear-cut understanding but it is multi-factorial etiology. It includes genetic vulnerability, psychological factors, personality and social factors and recently integral approach of spirituality is moreover accepted (Amodia DS et al. 2005).

Addiction is common, conventional and well-known term since time immemorial. A person having addiction can get used to, become dependent, or compulsively obsessed with chemicals or behavior like compulsive gambling. Psychological dependence is identified with many other activities as well, such as eating disorders, internet addiction and compulsive gambling. Susceptibility to addiction is more than uncomplicated perceptive, it is complex relations of genetical vulnerability, environment and chemical nature of drug (Kreek et al., 2005). In behavior science physical addiction is identified to various psychoactive drugs ranging from tobacco to alcohol and cannabis to heroin. Similarly various tranquilizers or sleeping pills mainly recognized as on the counter drugs are also used for addictive purpose. Addiction as a general term and in local conversational language is not so trendy because of derogatory expression and associated stigma associated with the term. Substance abuse and dependence are accepted medical concepts in recent times under the umbrella of addictive behaviors. A typical progress towards drug dependence begins with experimentation followed by occasional use, leading to regular use and finally dependence. Drug dependence is pathological stage when person cannot stop drugs to avoid withdrawal features (NIDA, 2014). Most individuals usually begin with use of substances like tobacco, alcohol or cannabis and then gradually learn the use of other severely addictive substances. A progression of substance use in terms of graduation from a less dependence producing and moreover socially acceptable substance to more dependence producing, illicit and harmful forms of substances. This is known as the 'Gateway Hypothesis or Theory' (Kandel D, 2002) where conventionally accepted substances like tobacco, alcohol or cannabis open the gate of access into the world of addictive substances and behavior (Lynskey MT et al. 2003). It is understood that any individual rarely starts his drug use career with hard chemicals like heroin/cocaine directly.

Though, the causes and factors associated with drug abuse are multifaceted and biopsychosocial in nature, these causes vary across diverse section of the population. While developing successful, prevention strategies the need to be attended to not only the 'drug' addictive behavior in solitary capsule but also the appropriate biopsychosocial factors such as social, cultural, ethnic, and other environmental aspects of the population segments. The various harms related to drug addiction are physical harms such as systemic HIV infection, occupational/financial harms such as absenteeism from work, financial difficulties and debt; familial/social harms such family disharmony and also stigma and discrimination. Various psychological harms like suicide and associated mental disorders complicate the treatment and progress of addictive disorders. Besides, various legal harms like arrest, legal penalties and antisocial activities constantly challenge the social security. Identifying the range of social risk and harm in public health domain and reducing it, is very critical aspect of preventive strategies in addictive behavior. As addiction being a chronic, relapsing condition consequently relapse prevention and management is a central concern in the treatment of addictive behaviors. As per the prevention strategies in traditional public health classification of disease prevention, addiction prevention drug strategies may need to consider *the agent*—the substance itself such as alcohol, tobacco, and other drugs; the host—a person and his or her biological, psychological, and social vulnerabilities to drug problems, their knowledge and attitudes that manipulate the addictive behavior and lastly the setting in which the addictive behavior happens in the community. Addiction prevention programs need to consider any of these three factors. The agent can be transformed by supply reduction strategies; the individual's craving can be managed by demand reduction strategies. Environmental strategies need to focus on the setting, i.e. the neighboring atmosphere of the addict including residential area, the school or the workplace. Environmental prevention programs can be included into both supply and demand reduction.

The prevention of addictive behavior in public health system can be understood and organized at the continuum of primary, secondary and tertiary prevention (Parkar and Iyer, 2000). The objective of primary prevention is to save individuals who have not begun to use substances from harm, thereby diminishing the incidence of new users in the general public. The objective of secondary prevention (also called *early intervention) is* to intervention with addictive persons in the early stages of addiction or management of mental health problem linked with substance abuse. The purpose of tertiary prevention is to end drug dependency and addiction and/or improve the negative effects of addiction through treatment and rehabilitation.

1. Demand reduction strategies aim to reduce the desire to use drugs and to prevent, reduce or delay the initiation of drug use in newer users.
2. Supply reduction strategies aim to disrupt the supply and availability of drug in market.
3. Harm reduction strategy aim to reduce the negative impact of drug use and drug-related activities on individuals and communities.

India has been part of various international conventions like, Single convention on Narcotic Drugs, 1961, as amended by the 1972 Protocol, Convention on Psychotropic Substances, 1971 and UN Convention against Illicit Trafficking in Narcotic Drugs and Psychotropic Substances, 1988. Government of India has developed own legislation of Narcotic Drugs and Psychotropic Substance Act (NDPS) in 1985, amended in 1988 involving all-inclusive tasks of different Ministries with focused responsibilities. The Ministry of Social Justice and Empowerment and ministry of health and family welfare looks after prevention and rehabilitation aspect of addictive behaviors. The Ministry of Health and Family Welfare provided funds to boost more than 100 drug de-addiction centers in various part of the country (December 2003: 122). Most of these centers are situated in the major hospitals and medical institutes. Being in the comprehensive medical set up these centers are primarily involved in acute and chronic medical management and rehabilitation of alcohol and drug addicts (secondary and tertiary level prevention). However these centers are also involved in quite a few primary prevention activities such as education and awareness.

DEMAND REDUCTION

The key concerns addressed in demand reduction (DR) mainly are activities related to psychosocial problems especially the social context of addictive behaviors. The DR Concept mainly entail essential public health model for efficient control of demand for illicit drugs. These factors are mostly related to peer pressure, high-risk occupations, street children, youth groups and school programs. Educating people at large such as parents and teachers and vulnerable population like adolescents students and youth is valuable strategy. However it sounds like more intellectual approach. Nonetheless appropriate and adequate information without overstatement along with social skills training can be useful. In India and globally in voluntary organizations it is appreciated that they also have performed a key role in various aspects of drug demand reduction. As the example of DR, The Ministry of Social Justice and Empowerment presently provide funds to more than 400 counseling and rehabilitation centers throughout the country (Parmanand Kulhara Debashis Basu 2005). In last couple of decades rigorous programs on awareness in school, colleges and youths organizations were conducted by both Government and voluntary organisations.

Primary Prevention

Along with various demand reduction and supply reduction activities many government and voluntary organization are also involved in primary prevention program.

- General public awareness program
- Development and allotment of print materials
- Mass media appeal and media advertisements
- Anti-drug awareness campaigns
- Awareness programs in schools and college
- Developing drug free workplaces
- Targeting specific groups like street children

Social and Resistant Skills

The addictive drugs are available in the market and neighborhood. The vulnerable population can get tempted easily due to peer pressure and social incentives. In such a situation it is vital to teach susceptible population to say no to drugs. Some social skills and coping strategies are contributory to development of resistant skills.

- ***Assertiveness training:*** Saying no to drug
- Adjustment and coping skills during vulnerable phase
- General stress management
- Parent-child conflict management
- Academic stress management
- Coping with peer pressure
- Teaching health oriented healthy lifestyles.

DRUG TREATMENT AND REHABILITATION

Various pharmacological and rehabilitative programs are basic to assist people with substance use disorders for abstinence and improve their socio-occupational functions (McGrady BS, Epstein E, 2013).

- Detoxification (mainly medical management)
- Treatment with pharmacological drugs like anticraving agents like acamprosate, deterrents like disulfiram antagonists such as naltrexone
- Pilot treatment programs for opiate abusers
- Facilitating twelve-step programs of alcohol anonymous
- Therapeutic communities
- Long-term rehabilitation programs
- Programs in jails
- Rural detoxification camps in villages
- Community based identification of cases and treatment programs.

EDUCATION TO HIGH-RISK GROUP

Education to children teachers and parents will go a long way. Awareness program to prevent addiction in school going children need to be developed critically. It is vital to provide education on addictive behavior to children, teachers and parents. Follow some easy steps while dealing with our youths and adolescents as per the guideline of the US. Department of Health and Human Services: These are:

- Converse with your child about alcohol and other drugs
- Listen to your child about drug related query
- Teach your child cope up with peer pressure
- Facilitate feelings of comfort in your child
- Be a good role model or exemplar in your own concepts and behavior related to alcohol or other drugs
- Set assertive no drug use
- Encourage healthy, creative activities
- Connect and coordinate with other parents
- Learn to identify the drug problem at earliest to seek help immediately.

RELAPSE PREVENTION STRATEGIES

It is possible to initiate abstinence for patients. However to maintain abstinence over the period is difficult. Substance use disorders are chronic and relapsing disorders. Relapse is defined as an unfolding process in which the resumption of substance use is the last event in a series of maladaptive responses to internal and external stressors (Marlatt and George, 1984). Lapse happens occasionally but individual is still able to maintain abstinence. However, in relapse individual returns back to his dependence pattern hence focus on both biological and psychosocial assets is imperative. There are various models to understand relapse. Most important perspective of relapse is craving that includes biological causes. The progression from abstinence to relapse occurs when the client is vulnerable and also exposed to a high-risk situation that threatens sobriety. The high-risk situations may be physical, psychological or social dysfunction. Relapse prevention includes learning to identify stressful life events and situations like interpersonal problems and augment coping skills to adapt and deal with problem. Besides relapse prevention also includes relaxation and yoga, review of jobs vulnerable for relapse, i.e. bartenders, self monitoring of risks, developing new interest and creative activities. The most important part of relapse prevention is active participation in sober activities that can fill in unoccupied time and also have self-disciplined social circle.

SUPPLY REDUCTION STRATEGIES

A supply reduction strategy basically involves reducing the availability of the addictive drugs in community. It is though based on the same theoretical principles of reducing availability. It is basically different for licit and illicit substances.

- ***For licit substances modus measures include***
  - Controls on availability (setting minimum age limit, licensing
  - Price controls
  - Controls on the use of alcohol and tobacco (while driving, in public spaces)
  - Strict safety standards (specification of contents and warning on health hazards)
  - Controls on marketing (advertisements and surrogate advertizing)
- ***For illicit substances measures include***
  - Public education
  - Awareness
  - Culturally significant and suitable for youths.

HARM REDUCTION STRATEGIES

Commonly harm reduction strategies involve secondary and tertiary prevention measures to prevent harm related to addictive behavior (Dr Alex Wodak AM 2011). It focuses more on quality of life of person and well being of the community. In harm reduction the vulnerability of the individual either biological or environmental is taken into consideration. Drug addiction is chronic medical illness ranging from extreme addiction to abstinence and it is complicated because of multiple factors. It is not cured with acute treatment but it is process that also involves relapse. Hence, helping patients to be safer with addictive behavior is sensible to prevent lethal morbidities and complications. It thus leads to reduce drug related common morbidities (HIV-AIDS, tuberculosis) and mortalities, accidents, antisocial activities and related crime in the society. In India we have good examples in Manipur and Nagaland, two states in the northeast region of India. People who inject drugs (PWID) and unsafe sexual practices are at high-risk for HIV AIDS. WHO included needle exchange program as Harm reduction strategy (WHO 2003). In both vulnerable population needle exchange programs was tried in North-Eastern part of India (Gregory Armstrong et al. 2014).

We need better policies, public awareness and alert society to fight against global menace of addiction.

BIBLIOGRAPHY

1. Alex Wodak AM. Demand Reduction and Harm Reduction in Working Paper Prepared for the First Meeting of the Global Commission on Drug Policies, Geneva, 2011.
2. Armstrong G, Nuken A, Medhi GK, et al. Injecting drug use in Manipur and Nagaland, Northeast India: injecting and sexual risk behaviours across age groups. Harm Reduction Journal. 2014;11:27.
3. Drug Abuse and Addiction, Drugs, Brains and Behaviour: The Science of Addiction. NIH Publication No 14-5605, 1st edn., National Institute of Drug Abuse, 2007.
4. Ghodse H. The global drug problem: international perspectives. Drug and Addictive Behaviour: A Guide to Treatment, 4th edn. Cambridge University Press. 1989:19-60.
5. Kreek MJ, Nielsen DA, Butelman ER, et al. Genetic influences on impulsivity, risk taking, stress responsivity and vulnerability to drug abuse and addiction. Nat Neurosci. 2005;8(11):1450-7.
6. Kulhara P, Basu D. Prevention of substance abuse in India. In: Lal R (Ed). Substance Use Disorders: Manual for Physicians. National Drug Dependence Treatment Centre, All India Institute of Medical Science, New Delhi. 2005:138-45.
7. Marlatt GA, George WH. Relapse prevention: introduction and overview of the model. Br J Addict. 1984;79(3):261-73.
8. McCrady BS, Epstein EE. Addictions: A Comprehensive Guidebook, 2nd edn. Oxford University Press. 2013:477-98.
9. Pal HR, Kumar A. Epidemiology of substance use. In: Lal R, Rao R, Mohan I (Eds). Substance Use Disorders: Manual for Physicians. 2005: 9-14.

10. Parkar SR, Anupama I. Prevention of drug abuse. In: Ray R (Ed). Substance Use Disorder: A Manual for Physicians. Published by Drug Dependence Treatment Centre and Department of Psychiatry, All India Institute of Medical Science, New Delhi. 2005:138-45.
11. Srinivasan K, Chandramauli KS. Health hazards of long-term alcohol, opioid and cannabis use. In: Lal R, Rao R, Mohan I (Eds). Substance Use Disorders: Manual for Physicians. 2005: 9-14.
12. Treatment and Recovery, Drugs, Brains and Behaviour: The Science of Addiction. NIH Publication No 14-5605, 1st edn., National Institute of Drug Abuse, 2007.
13. World Health Organization (2003). Harm reduction approaches to injecting substance use http://www.who.int/hiv/topics/harm reduction.

14

Health in the Context of Occupational Activities

14.1 PHYSIOTHERAPEUTIC PERSPECTIVE IN INDUSTRIAL HEALTH

Bhavana Suhas Mhatre

Abstract: Occupational health is defined as the promotion and maintenance of the highest degree of physical, mental and social wellbeing of workers in all occupations. This chapter focusses exclusively on the occupation related musculoskeletal issues along with brief review on the need of understanding issues related to Industrial health. It discusses in details about the etiological factors, assessment and management aspect of various repetitive stress/motion injuries and cumulative trauma disorders.

Work-related musculoskeletal disorders (WMSD) are category of injuries involving damage to muscles, tendons, nerve, neurovascular bundles caused by 'Misuse' or 'Overuse' and are noted for their lack of specific diagnosis. They occur over a time and are associated with strenuous and repetitive work.[1]

- These injuries takes place when the capacity of the human body cannot resist the biomechanical and physiological strain to external load. In addition to the magnitude of load, the duration and frequency of loading and recovery periods specific to the task of the job are important. The capacity to resist a load will vary according to individual characteristics, i.e. body build and size, gender, age, and general health. This capacity varies with time and the human body adapts to the loading, e.g. training effects/weakening.[2]
- WRMD are the most common causes of disability, sick leave and early retirement.
- WRMD need to be differentiated from traumatic and degenerative conditions.

Ergonomic Risk Factors for WMSD

Are the aspects of a job or a task that impose a biomechanical stress on the worker.

Ergonomics is defined as the science of designing workplaces, machines and tools with the capabilities and limitations of the human body in mind. Ergonomics aims to make sure that tasks, equipment, information and the environment suit each worker.

When work stations, machines or tools are not designed as per the principles of ergonomics they too are considered as risk factors for development of WMSD.

The following risk factors are known to cause WMSD:[3–11]

- ***Physical factors:*** Work postures either sustained or awkward postures, repetition of the same movements, forceful exertions, inadequate rest periods.

- ***Psychosocial factors:*** Work pace, autonomy, monotony, work/rest cycle, task demands, social support from colleagues and management and job uncertainty.
- ***Individual factors:*** Age, gender, professional activities, sport activities, domestic activities, recreational activities, alcohol/tobacco consumption and previous WMSD.
- ***Design of the workstation, equipments and tools:*** Height of the working surface (too high or too low), horizontal reach is long, vertical reach is above the shoulders or below knees, vibrating working surfaces, machinery, or vehicles.
- ***Physical environment of the work area:*** Cold or heat, poor lighting and ventilation, noise, floor surfaces that are uneven or slippery or lighting can create glare or shadows that may require workers to adopt awkward positions to see clearly what they are doing. High levels of noise may cause the body to tense in static body postures resulting a more rapid onset of fatigue.

Symptoms and Signs

- Pain is the most common symptom associated with WMSDs. Local pain in the muscles, ligaments and joints
- Weakness of the affected limb, weak precision and power grips
- Sensation of pins and needles or heaviness or numbness
- Intermittent swelling
- Loss of coordination and proprioception
- Loss of responsiveness, (e.g. the tendency to strike wrong key)
- Vascular disturbance, skin color changes
- Joint stiffness, muscle tightness
- Decreased sweating of the hands.

Commonly affected area of the musculoskeletal system: Low back pain followed by the neck and upper extremity and lower extremities.

The most common WRMD observed in the industrial environment include:

- ***Shoulder:*** Supraspinatus/bicipital tendinitis, bursitis.
- ***Elbow:*** Epicondylitis, cubital tunnel/radial tunnel syndrome.
- ***Wrist and hand:*** De Quervain, tenosynovitis, trigger finger, Carpal tunnel/Guyon's canal syndrome, Raynaud's syndrome, Hypothenar hammer syndrome.
- ***Hip:*** Piriformis syndrome, trochanteritis.
- ***Knee:*** Prepatellar/Infrapatellar tendonitis.
- ***Leg, foot and ankle:*** Achilles tendonitis, shin splints, varicose vein.
- ***Lumbar spine:*** Low back pain, sacroiliac (SI) joint pain, piriformis syndrome.
- ***Cervical spine:*** Tension neck syndrome, thoracic outlet syndrome.

Diagnosis of WRMD

- WMSDs may progress in stages from mild to severe, hence early diagnosis is necessary.
  - ***Early stage:*** Aching and tiredness of the affected limb occur during the work shift but disappear at night and during days off work. No reduction of work performance.
  - ***Intermediate stage:*** Aching and tiredness occur early in the work shift and persist at night. Reduced capacity for repetitive work.
  - ***Late stage:*** Aching, fatigue, and weakness persist at rest. Inability to sleep and to perform light duties.[13]
- Diagnosis of WMSDs is confirmed by performing laboratory and electronic tests that determine nerve or muscle damage. Electromyography (EMG) and nerve conduction velocity (NCV).

Magnetic Resonance Imaging (MRI)

- Detail description of all the work processes involved during the day should be sought during subjective examination. It is important to include all the relevant activities performed both at work and outside work as most of the factors can occur both at work and in leisure time activities.

- A detailed evaluation of **ergonomic risk factors** is also essential for effective injury prevention and rehabilitation process.
- Hence an indepth assessment of all the risk factors is essential.

Physical Demands of the Job

Forceful Exertions

Exerting considerable force to complete a motion will require muscles to contract strongly, e.g. a car mechanic who has to loosen nuts of an old tyre. When this strong contraction is sustained the muscle will fatigue quickly or strained. These forceful exertions can also irate tendons, joints and discs. Disorders of the nervous system, e.g. carpal tunnel syndrome may be caused due to compressive forces from the muscle contractions or inflamed tendons. Jobs that require forceful lifting/lowering, pushing/pulling, and carrying as well as those which require to apply pinch forces with the fingers like placing small items on the assembly line need to be considered as risk factors.

Frequent manual material handling is described as 'any activity requiring the use of force exerted by a person to lift, lower, push, carry or otherwise move, hold or restrain any object or person'.

Factors such as weight of the object and their placement in relation to the body, grips used to lift will denote the amount of force required. It requires more force to lift and carry a box with arms outstretched and held away from the body or to lift the same objects in a 'pinch' position than in a 'hook' position. If the weight is held farther from the body, the impact on the shoulders, arms and back increases. Muscles are at a greater mechanical disadvantage, as the load arm increases, greater torques are required from the muscles consequently result in their fatigue and injury.

Characteristics of the objects or people handled such as the shape of the object, slippery or objects that have no handles, the tools used are bulky, too large or heavy will generate forceful contractions of the muscles.

Manual handling tasks that require the hands to be lower than the knees or higher than mid torso requires the muscle to exert more force than if the starting point is at the waist level.

Low starting points require bending or squatting which add stress to the back and knee.

Permissible and safe weight to be lifted by one person (Guidelines of Occupational Health and Safety Administration (OSHA), Western Countries) is 51 pounds, within 7 inches from the front of his/her body, is at waist height, there is no twisting involved, there is a handle on the object and the load inside does not shift once lifted. If these conditions are not met then the weight should be reduced or it should be a two person lift or mechanical assistance should be provided to make it a safe lift.

Lifting and carrying a load even for a short distance and with proper mechanics can be a source for injury for back. Back injuries from overexertion are leading cause of workplace injuries. It affects many workers, is associated with high costs to industry and the individual, and can negatively influence the quality of life.

Work related low back pain and shoulder dysfunctions are prevalent in health care professionals.

Kroemer and Grandjean have indicated that fatigue inducing static effort occurs when a high level of effort is maintained for 10 seconds or more, moderate effort persists for 1 minute and slight effort that is 12% of maximal voluntary lasts for 5 minutes or more.

Repetitive Motions

Jobs that require repetition of same movement again and again. Tasks are considered to be hazardous when they involve the same joints and muscle groups over and over and when same motion too often, too quickly and for too long. Tasks requiring repetitive movements always involve other risk factors for WMSD such as fixed body position and forceful exertions.

Wrist, fingers, shoulders, elbows are more susceptible to injury. Repetitive work done with the foot, e.g. tailors or knees, climbing ladders may also result in WMSD. Some researchers classify a job as 'high repetitive' if the time to complete such a job was less than 30 seconds or 'low repetitive' if the time to complete the job was more than 30 seconds.

Inadequate Rest Periods

Pace of work determines the amount of time available for rest and recovery of the body between cycles of a particular task. The faster the pace of a task, higher is the risk for WMSD. When the worker has no control over timing and speed of work because of external factors like assembly line speed then stress level increases. With higher stress level comes muscle tension causing fatigue and again increased risk for WMSD. Controlling the pace of work externally denies the worker the flexibility to determine their own work speed. Research shows that tendons and muscles in the wrist may not be able to recover when task cycles are repeated more than 12 times per minute or repeated task cycle are less than 5 seconds in length.

Static/Awkward Postures

These postures adopted as per the demands of the job, poor workstation layout or fixed work stations. Posture maintained for any length of time without interruption will become uncomfortable and even painful as creep sets in. Sustained or prolonged postures reduces blood flow, depletes nutrients and leads to a build-up of metabolic waste. Awkward or non-neutral postures of the spine, e.g. twisting, bending or flattening the lower back can cause back pain by contributing to, overworked muscles and ligaments. Thus these tissues may become susceptible to fatigue failure, and the insidious development of musculoskeletal symptoms despite no obvious trauma (McKenzie and May 2003).

Stretching and compression of tendons and nerves occur when working with body parts held at end range of movement for example the torso bent forward, backward or twisted can place too much stress on the low back as tissues are subjected to tensile compressive as well as shearing forces making them more susceptible to injuries. Other examples of stressful body positions include reaching above shoulder level reaching behind the body, rotating the arms, bending the wrist forward, backward, or side to side and reaching forward too far out in front of the body.

To perform any control movement with the arm, muscles in the shoulder and the neck contract and stay contracted for as long as the task requires.

The contracted muscles squeeze the blood vessels, which restricts the flow of blood all the way down to the working muscles of the hand. However, this is where the blood is needed the most because of the intense muscular effort. The neck/shoulder muscles become overtired even though there is little or no movement. At the same time, the reduced blood supply to the rest of the arm accelerates fatigue in the muscles that are moving, making them prone to injury.

Awkward postures are also adopted when workstations are fixed and cannot be adjusted or they have poor layout. Work surfaces that are too high or too low, e.g. if the height of the desks, tables or other work surface when operated from a sitting position is less than or more than 30 inches, or it is not between 36 and 40 inches when operated from a standing position.

Workers are exposed to twisting movements when the work activities are done in confined areas or constrained sitting and without a swivel chair. Twisting is considered to be the most damaging movement the back as the spine is subjected to compression, torsional and shearing forces.

Jobs that require prolonged standing in a static or hard concrete surface is physiologically and mechanically stressful. Erect standing imposes a hydrostatic handicap that makes humans liable to peripheral circulatory collapse. Peak plantar (foot) pressures of 137 (kilopascals) kPa exceed the normal systolic pressure of 17 kPa, resulting in occlusion of blood flow through the foot. Standing causes back muscles to fatigue, physiological changes like peripheral pooling of blood, a decrease in stroke volume and increase in heart rate, diastolic and mean arterial pressure, peripheral resistance and thoracic impedance. A foot rail, box, or stool to raise one foot, anti fatigue mats, cushioned shoe inserts, cushioned soles/heel designed for work should be made available to the worker to reduce stress. Chairs and stools should be adjustable, should provide support for the low back and pelvis and the feet should rest on the ground. Chair adjustments controls should be easily accessed from the sitting position. The height, angle, and position of the back support relative to the seat pan of the back support should be easily adjustable and should be curved to support neutral inward curve of the low back.

The chair should roll and pivot easily and should have arms. Cushions and back supports should be used for office chairs, automobiles and truck seats if the back support is flat.

Environment Conditions

Temperature of the workplace affects the body muscles: excessive heat increases overall fatigue and produces sweat which makes it hard to hold tools requiring more force, e.g. construction workers. Excessive cold can make the hands feel numb making it hard to grip and requiring more force; every movement and position involving more effort are more likely to develop work-related neck and upper limb disorders, e.g. meat processing units.

Exposure to Vibrations

Vibration can cause damage to tendons, muscles, joints, nerves and blood vessels. Hand-arm vibrations can cause tingling and numbness, or loss of sensibility, requiring a higher clamping force and awkward body positions because vibration hand tools are harder to control. Workers can be exposed to either whole body vibration or localized vibration. Whole body vibration is experienced by truck and bus drivers.

Risk factors Related to the Worker

- ***Fitness of the worker:*** Evidence indicate that workers who are in a poor physical condition and practice unhealthy lifestyles are at a greater risk of injury.
- ***Psychosocial stress:*** Another potential occupationally related risk factor that has gained recognition is that of psychosocial factors.

  Reviews by Davis and Heaney (2000) have indicated following factors:
  - Highly demanding work
  - Poor scope for decision making/limited job control
  - Lack of social support from superiors, colleagues
  - Dissatisfaction with work
  - Insufficient gratification
  - Monotony of work
  - Workplace insecurity.

  Stress causes a direct impact on human performance. The person's effectiveness is low at high stress and as a result there is high probability of human error, the graph indicates that at no stress, the work is probably dull and unchallenging. Maximum effectiveness observed when a person is working with moderate stress.

A combination of lifestyle issues and overall environmental stress is creating tremendous pressures for individuals leading to heart attacks and mental health issues such as depression or suicides.

According to the latest data from Optum (a top provider of employee assistance to corporate) a 46% of workforce in organizations in India suffer from some form of stress, 43% have skewed body mass index, and 30% have diabetic and another 30% have hypertensive risk.

- Work style and job design is also important while evaluating a job. The concept of work style was constructed by Feuerstein et al.[12] and represents the individual responses to high work demands. In case of high work demands, workers will be less inclined to pay attention to their body posture, adjust their workplace properly and take adequate no of rest pauses and do pause exercises.

  Claire M Bernaards et al.[14] in their study defined work style as three individual responses to high work demands:
  i. Optimal body posture and proper workplace adjustment
  ii. The number and quality of breaks and
  iii. Coping with high work demands

The therapist should be able to find whether the employee is at a risk because of the working style or the job forces the employee to do the work in a certain way or both.

Physiotherapy Management[17–19,23]

- A multidisciplinary approach is essential for effective implementation of worker oriented measures taken to keep them healthy and productive and if injured restore them to maximum job functions as quickly and cost effectively.
- Management of work related musculoskeletal disorders include all three levels of prevention—**Primary, Secondary and Tertiary.**
  i. ***Primary prevention*** aims at avoiding the occurrence of a disorder by reducing or avoiding risk factors.
  ii. ***Secondary prevention:*** Early recognition of disorders and halting their progression.
  iii. ***Tertiary prevention:*** Rehabilitation of disorders already occurred and prevention of recurrence, including maintenance of fitness to work.

Primary Prevention

Aiming at eliminating or minimizing risks to health or well-being and includes:

- Risk assessment process
- Ergonomic interventions
- Organizational interventions
- Person-oriented interventions

Risk Assessment Process

- A systematic examination of all the risk factors associated with the physical demands of the job, the worker and the psychosocial factors as described above.
- Allows to identify prevention priorities.
- Ergonomic assessment, redesign and evaluation of crane cabin was carried out based on identification of risk of WMSD by detailed questionnaire from 27 crane operator. It was revealed that almost all crane operators were continuously suffering from some kind of WMSD. This study shows that intervention of ergonomics in workplace reduces the mismatch between man and machine and makes workplace comfortable for work.[15]

Measures used for assessment of physical workloads at workplace[5,20]

1. Rapid Upper Limb Assessment (RULA) (McAtamney and Corlett, 1993), was developed to evaluate the exposure of individual workers to ergonomic risk

factors associated with upper extremity MSD. The RULA ergonomic assessment tool considers biomechanical and postural load requirements of job tasks/ demands on the neck, trunk and upper extremities. A single page worksheet is used to evaluate required body posture, force, and repetition.
2. Rapid Entire Body Assessment (REBA), Hignett and McAtamney, 2000, A tool for whole body - static, dynamic, unstable or rapidly changing posture.
3. Strain Index (SI) (Moore and Garg, 1995)
4. Occupational Repetitive Actions (OCRA) Checklist (Colombini et al., 2000 and Colombini et al., 2011).
5. Threshold Limit Value® (TLV®) for Hand Activity (2001) evaluates job risk factors associated with musculoskeletal disorders of the hand and the wrist. The evaluation is based on assessment of hand activity and the level of effort for a typical posture while performing a short cycle task.

Ergonomic Interventions

- Aims to reduce physical workloads, focus is to eliminate or reduce the risks related to manual handling of loads, working in awkward postures, and repetitive work.
- Important ergonomic considerations are:
  - ***Automation or mechanization:*** Powered or mechanical transportation should be implemented, transportation or handling equipments such as conveyor belts, lift trucks, electric hoists, patient lifting devices, etc.
  - ***Workplace redesign:*** Workstations and environment should enable working in a comfortable postures. Examples are adjustment of working heights, modification of lighting.
  - ***Ergonomic work equipment and tools:*** Strain reducing work equipments should be provided, e.g. an ergonomic chairs or keyboards.
  - ***Protective equipment:*** Lumbar supports, wrist splints, masks for mine workers or in textile industry, helmet for construction workers.

Organizational Interventions

- Aims to improve work processes and work tasks by reducing exposure time to high physical load and increase recovery time.
- ***Pre-employment screening and functional capacity evaluation:*** To assess workers' safe physical capabilities in performing several different functions and comparisons are made to the worker's actual job.
- ***Work processes:*** Changing work cycle frequencies, working hours or breaks, staffing levels.
- ***Work tasks:*** Job rotations, job enlargement.
- Organizational development with regard to health and safety, e.g. improvement of leadership skills of superiors, development of team spirit, participative work (place) design, health panel/occupation-specific expert body (task force).

Person Oriented Interventions

- ***Two important interventions:***
  - Education and
  - Exercise, both are physiotherapist's domain.
- ***Education to workers, management, and the employers:***
  - Focus is to raise awareness among workers and attempting to change their working behavior.
  - Appropriate educational topics include beliefs and attitudes, expectations, activity, safe work practices, and an understanding of risk management, job and workplace design and an understanding of injury, pain and the recovery processes.
  - Training and guidance on proper working methods and practices should aim to reduce physical strain in the worker.

- In company training programs or Back/Neck schools to train workers in the adoption of good working posture, the use of correct lifting/handling techniques and strengthening exercises.
- Beliefs and attitudes are the main barriers one needs to overcome during education programs, e.g. explaining the importance of health education amongst workers regarding use of protective gear and dust control measures at workplace needs to be emphasized considering the fact that the detrimental effects of hazardous particles may be prevented. Breathing exercises especially forced expiratory techniques may facilitate.

- ***Health promotion and general fitness program:*** Screening of musculoskeletal, cardiopulmonary and neuromuscular systems should be conducted before starting exercise programs.

  Fitness exercise program should promote components of:
  - ***Health related fitness:*** Motor control, mobility, flexibility, strength and musculoskeletal and cardiopulmonary/aerobic endurance
  - ***Performance related fitness:*** Balance, coordination, power, reaction time, speed, agility
  - Postural correction exercises
  - Breathing exercises incorporating yoga techniques
  - Relaxation therapy must be a part of this program and cannot be neglected.
- Workers are encouraged to increase their general physical activity by means of active commuting, sports, and daily physical activities at work and/or during leisure time. Increasing physical activity might be effective in reducing the symptoms.
- In a study with neck and shoulder myalgia, Kadi et al. showed an increase in oxidative capacity (i.e. capillary density) and muscle functioning of the trapezius muscle resulting from strength and endurance training.[22]
- Literature reports that physical exercises with cognitive behavioral therapy (CBT) to be useful for promotion of health and wellbeing. These programs should be an integral part of work culture of both formal and informal sector.
- Physiotherapist have the expertise to design an exercise program and as a part of CBT knowledge regarding importance of safe body mechanics during exercising, activities of daily living, and at workplace should be emphasized. This CBT program should aim at changing the belief and attitude towards physical exercises and body mechanics that is control of posture and body awareness, both very important for wellness.

Secondary Prevention

Aim is to identify workers at risk of injury and monitoring their health recognition of 'red and yellow flags' (potentially serious physical or psychological/psychosocial risk factors for the development of WMSD).

- On-site evaluation of the physical demands of the job, task analysis, and the workstation evaluation using the principles of ergonomics. Evaluation conducted along with the ergonomist and other relevant team members to enable the therapist to identify potential risk factors which can be remediated with physiotherapy interventions.

  A person's working posture is a result of the requirements of the task, the design of the workspace and personal characteristics such as body size and shape and eyesight. Consideration of all three components is needed in posture analysis and workspace design.[6]

  Physical demands of the job and task analysis: Exposure to repetitive work either light or heavy and manual materials handling done in static or awkward posture for long hours without adequate rest pauses are identified.

- Pause exercises, can be incorporated at regular intervals to relieve fatigue or musculoskeletal discomfort related to fixed work postures and repetitive motion. They are specific set of:

  Warm up exercises used at the beginning of the work day to prepare the muscles and joints of the worker for their work tasks.

  Stretching program to restores circulation and oxygen to muscles after sustained periods of work. The muscle can be stretched to gain flexibility before work or they can be stretched to 'breathe' during the work.
- Targeted occupational health preventive check-ups of employees with pre-existing conditions/earlier disorders or exposures with regard to particular risks in the place of work.

Tertiary Prevention

- A rapid and safe return to work is the primary objective.
- Actions are taken to support return-to-work and modifying the workplace to accommodate any residual injury.
- ***Work conditioning and work hardening*** are components of Return to Work (RTW) programs.
- ***Injury care:*** Begins immediately after the injury and continues till pain and healing is stabilized. Early intervention during this phase will enable the worker to begin the process of functional intervention.

  Early intervention also includes precise physical therapy diagnosis (function orientated diagnosis) and appropriate physiotherapy interventions along with the medical interventions by the physician.

  Physiotherapy management aims at identifying the stage of tissue healing, structural source for the patient's dysfunction, dominant pain mechanisms and precautions and contraindications to be followed during assessment and interventions aimed at healing of the injured tissues. This will assist the injured worker in a safe, functional and rapid return to workplace.
- ***Post injury care phase:*** Post healing of the tissues incorporation of the functional tests in to the rehabilitation process is vital, e.g. Functional Capacity Assessment (FCA) or tests that takes in to account specific job requirements.

  FCA is a process of measuring recording and analyzing a person's ability to safely perform a number of job related functions. Post injury care phase they are used to guide the rehabilitation as the tissues are not ready to take the stress of entire day's work.
- ***Return to work programs:***
  - These retraining the worker post injury care phase address injured worker's needs between acute care and return to work.
  - Establishes the current status, FCA assessments are used to find the needs of the injured worker and match the rehabilitation process to those needs.
- ***Components of RTW-Work conditioning and work hardening:***
  - ***Work conditioning[21] (APTA):*** Is a work related intensive goal oriented treatment program specifically designed to restore an individual's systemic, neuromusculoskeletal (motor control, flexibility, movement, strength, endurance) and cardiopulmonary functions.

    The objective is to restore client's physical capacity and function so the client can return to work.
  - ***Work hardening[21] (APTA):*** Is a highly structured, goal-oriented, individualized treatment program designed to return the person to work.

Work hardening programs are interdisciplinary in nature, use of real or simulated work activities designed to restore physical, behavioral, and vocational functions.

Work hardening addresses the issue of productivity, safety, physical tolerances and work behaviors.

Enhancing quality of life is the key goal for tertiary prevention. Participation in these RTW programs will enable the injured worker to achieve specific capabilities necessary functional capabilities and maximum productivity at work place.

A Brief Review on Physiotherapeutic Perspective in Industrial Health

Occupational health is defined as the promotion and maintenance of the highest degree of physical, mental and social wellbeing of workers in all occupations.

Case Study 1

Sheela, a 31-year-old female, is working in a stone painting unit in the rural India. She is a widow with two girls of age 12 and 10 years.

Her chief complaints are pain and stiffness in the cervical region and a feeling of heaviness in the forearm since 6 months. She reports her symptoms have started affecting her ability to work.

She paints mainly show pieces made out of stone, e.g. wall hangings, photo frames, flower vases, etc.

All the work is done on the floor sitting cross legged. Small articles are taken in non-dominant hand and painted with the dominant hand. Duration of work is 8–10 hours and can extend up to 12 hours depending on the orders received and time deadlines. Painting activities are carried out for a minimum of 30 to 2 hours at a stretch.

Postures adopted during the activity are neck flexion, kyphotic back, arm in forward flexion and abduction and repetitive pronation and wrist in flexion–extension.

1. Identify the risk factors associated with Sheela's work.
2. Plan strategies to address her risk factors
3. What measures are needed to improve her physical capability.

Case Study 2

Ramesh, a 50-year-old, working as a ward boy in a 1000 bed tertiary care government hospital in a city since 25 years. His duty hours include 8 hours. He is married and has two children. Both his children are working in a office.

He comes with a chief complaint of pain in the low back which aggravates when he has to lift weights, or assist patients for their transfer activities. He has this back pain on and off for last 5 years.

He has taken medicines for the same and has found relief in the past. His duties since last five years are in the Orthopaedic ward. Prior to this he has been working in various operation theaters of the hospital. His other duty includes sweeping and mopping the floor, giving bed pan to the patients, taking the patients clothes for laundry in a wheeled cart but across the road.

He also has to get food from the pantry for the ward patients. He uses patient's trolley to get the food which is also across the road. The time required wheeling the cart or trolley across the road is approximately 15 minutes.

His co-worker is not on duty most of the time and when he is on duty 50% of the time he is busy attending to his relatives and friends in the hospital.

He has complained several times to the higher authorities regarding his co-worker, but no action has been taken till now.

Ramesh, also works as a attendant to patients at home, post his duty hours. This is approximately 10–12 hours of work.

1. State with rationale whether Ramesh's low back pain is work related or a degenerative condition
2. State job demands and personal risk factors for Ramesh
3. What measures are required at workplace to address his problem.

A multidisciplinary activity aiming at:

1. Protection and promotion of the health of workers by preventing and controlling occupational diseases and accidents and by eliminating occupational factors and conditions hazardous to health and safety at work.
2. Development and promotion of healthy and safe work, work environments and work organizations.
3. Enhancement of physical, mental and social well-being of workers and support for the development and maintenance of their working capacity, as well as professional and social development at work.
4. Enablement of workers to conduct socially and economically productive lives and to contribute positively to sustainable development.[1,2, 25,26]

Need for Occupational Health and Safety

- ***Workforce of the country is the main backbone of economy:*** Providing safe and healthy working conditions is not only in the interest of the workers but also for employers, government and the public. The most successful economies have demonstrated that workplaces designed according to good principles of occupational health, safety and ergonomics are also the most sustainable and productive.[25,26]
- ***Huge workforce involved:*** Approximately 45% of the world's population and 58% of the population over 10 years of age belongs to the global workforce, i.e. 60–70% of the adult male and 30–60% of the adult female population of the world. An estimated 70–115 million children are part of Indian work force. The percentage is even higher when informal work are taken into account.[25,27,28]
- ***Exposure to hazardous work conditions:*** Approximately 30–50% of the global work-force spends one-third of their adult life exposed to hazardous conditions at work. This neglect mainly observed in developing countries is due to competing social, economic, and political challenges.[25]
- ***An increase in female population at workplace:*** Makes them susceptible to Musculoskeletal injuries as the tasks and equipment used are normally designed for men. Also double burden of work at home and workplace, low salaries and less decision making make them vulnerable to stress. When exposed to occupational hazards, women of reproductive age are susceptible to specific adverse effects on reproduction, like abortions and malformations of the foetus from exposure to toxic materials.[29]
- Even in advanced economies, a large proportion of work sites is not regularly inspected for occupational health and safety.[27]

Occupational Health Scenario in India

- India is one of the largest and most important developing countries of the world. 72% of the total population resides in rural area where illiteracy, poverty and access to health and their facilities are scarce.[29]
- Little attention is paid towards control of environmental and occupational hazards in the country. Occupational health is not integrated with primary health care and is a mandate of Ministry of Labor and not Ministry of Health.[30]
- Occupational health includes child labor, poor industrial legislation, vast informal sector, less attention to industrial hygiene and poor surveillance data.[29]
- The major legal provisions is the Factories Act and Mines Act (1948) which deals with occupational health and safety as well as welfare of workers employed in a factory. However, more than 90% of the Indian labor force does not work in factories,

hence; they fall outside the purview of the Act.[31]

- A study conducted in urban city of India reported high incidence of Silicosis in Indian flour mills workers working with grinding stone containing silica.[32] A similar study conducted in rural India on flour mill and construction workers also indicated high incidence of silicosis.[33]

  Adult carpet weavers in Mirzapur also reported respiratory problems as major occupational risk, the causal factors are carpet dust particles.[34]
- Globalization and rapid industrial growth in the past few years have added further to complexities of occupational health related conditions in our country. India at present has to deal with the risk factors associated with the traditional sectors like agriculture as well as those with modern industrial exposure. Child labor in the agriculture sector accounts for 80% of child laborers in India.[28]
- Factors that aggravate worker's health hazards-lack of education, unawareness of hazards in one's occupation, general backwardness in sanitation, poor nutrition and climatic proneness to epidemics.[35]
- Unemployment issues-workers are prepared to accept any job, irrespective of the dangers involved. Even the educated apply for class IV jobs. Cheap and easily replaceable labor is available so employers see no need for improving occupational safety and health.[30,35]
- Labor unions are mostly controlled by full-time politicians who consider health a political issue, especially when their party controls the country's government.[35,36]

Occupational Health—Developed and Developing Countries[25-29]

- A wide variation is seen in economic structures, occupational structures, working conditions, work environment, and the health status of workers in different countries and in different sectors of economies.
- There are also special occupational settings and types of enterprises, where work and workplace deviate substantially from the norm.
- Accidents and physical and chemical agents are the main problems in manufacturing industries, while pesticides and organic dusts, heavy physical work, biological factors and accidents are the occupational burdens of agricultural workers.
- The overall occupational accident and disease rates are found to be slowly declining in most industrialized countries but are increasing in developing and industrializing countries as indicated by the recent data from the ILO and WHO.
- Occupational exposure to crystalline silica (silica) dust occurs in many industrial operations worldwide. The reduction of silica dust exposure levels in most developed countries during the last century resulted in dramatic decreases in morbidity and mortality from silicosis and silica dust associated tuberculosis (TB).
- The most common Occupational disorders in the developed countries are musculoskeletal disorders and stress whereas India and other developing countries continue to be exposed to occupational lung disease such as silicosis, asbestosis, coal workers' pneumoconiosis, byssinosis, pesticide poisoning, noise induced hearing loss and musculoskeletal disorders.
- In industrialized nations, like USA and Western Europe where the employment in the agricultural sector is between 4 and 12% as against 58% in India. International Labor Office (ILO) and International Ergonomic Association (IEA) in 2012 documented agriculture as one of the most hazardous sectors in both the developing and the developed worlds.

- The proportion of employment in manufacturing and service sector is much lower in India compared to other developing nations.
- Urban India: Attempts are being made to reduce ergonomic risk factors at workplace and prevention of injuries, e.g.
  - Provision of wheeled bins to dispose garbage and modern waste management vehicles which can tilt the container of the truck so lifting to empty the bin's is avoided.
  - Conveyor belts are present at the airport too and ergonomically designed workstations in corporate offices.
  - Provisions of on site physical fitness centers to promote wellness are seen in multinational companies.

Occupational Safety and Health Programmes and Policies for India, Need of the Hour[25–27]

- Systematic monitoring of health events in working populations through occupational disease and injury surveillance is essential to assess the nature, magnitude and pattern of occupational diseases and injuries. The surveillance data will be useful in determining control strategies and research priorities, and for evaluating the effectiveness of any interventions.
- Occupational and industrial accidents are all caused by preventable factors which could be eliminated by implementing already known and available measures and methods. This is demonstrated by continuously reduced accident rates in industrialized countries. The application of preventive strategies therefore offers significant human and economic benefits, e.g. construction workers to change their attitude towards the use of helmets which they consider it as cumbersome. Understanding and minimizing the exposure of farmers and their families to pesticides in the developing world requires an understanding of farmers' knowledge, values, and beliefs of the contribution of the agricultural sector.
- The National Health Policy of India 1983 and 2002 has outlined the urgent need to prevent and treat diseases and injuries arising due to occupational hazards in both the organized and unorganized sectors.[37]
- Occupational safety and health for the 12th five-year plan (2012–2017) is an action-focused legislative and pragmatic intervention to transform the existing state of OSH in both formal and informal sectors of economic activity through proactive approaches and implementation of the National Policy.
- Efforts must be focused above all on primary prevention and protection at the workplace level. Occupational lung diseases and cancers are not curative and involves a lot of burden to the families especially a worker is from the informal sector.
- Compensation, rehabilitation and curative services must be made available to workers who suffer occupational injuries, accidents and work related diseases. Action must be taken to minimize the consequences of occupational hazards.
- There is a need to make policy makers, employers, administrators and employees aware of our effective contribution based on scientific knowledge in prevention, curative and rehabilitation of occupational health. Inclusion of physiotherapy services in this worker oriented multidisciplinary approach should be mandatory in both traditional and modern technological advanced sector in rural as well as urban areas.

Scope for Physical Therapy Practice in Occupational Health

- As a member of multidisciplinary team Physical therapist has an important role in proactively preventing and promoting health and well-being of the worker to be productive at workplace and if injured restoring them to their maximum job function as quickly and as cost effectively as possible.

- Physical therapist's diagnostic skills, clinical reasoning ability and knowledge of functional anatomy, physiology, tissue healing, bio-mechanics enable them to provide services to assist the workers and employers in injury/disease prevention and their management. Early diagnosis and timely intervention will facilitate return to work and prevent long-term disability and work loss.
- Participating in epidemiological research as well as clinical research especially in the areas of work related respiratory diseases and musculoskeletal disorders.
- There is paucity of Physiotherapy research especially in prevention and management of Occupational lung diseases in India.

REFERENCES

1. Isabel LN. Introduction to musculoskeletal disorders. EU-Occupational Safety and Health Agency website.
2. Esa-PT. Pathophysiological mechanisms of musculoskeletal disorders. EU-Occupational Safety and Health Agency website.
3. Marras WS. Occupational low back disorder causation and control. Ergonomics. 2000;43(7):880-902.
4. Davis KG, Heaney CA. The relationship between psychosocial work characteristics and low back pain: underlying methodological issues. Clinical Biomechanics.2000;15:389-406.
5. Prabir M, Saurabh S. Ergonomic risk factors in some craft sectors of Jaipur. HFESA Journal Ergonomics Australia. 2010;24(1):4-14.
6. Reginaldo KF. Static work: design for standing and seated workers. ebm.ufabc.edu.br/wp-content/uploads/2014/06/Cap4StaticWork.pdf.
7. Risk factors. Environmental Health and safety, Iowa State University. https://www.ehs.iastate.edu/occupational/ergonomics/risk-factors
8. Danuta L. Risk factors for musculoskeletal disorders-working postures. EU-Occupational Safety and Health Agency website.
9. Metka T. Risk factors for musculoskeletal disorders in manual handling of loads. EU-Occupational Safety and Health Agency website.
10. Vivorica P, Aurelia. Risk factors for musculoskeletal disorders development hand, arm tasks, repetitive work. EU-Occupational Safety and Health Agency website.
11. Swennke Van den H. Psychosocial risk factors for musculoskeletal disorders. EU-Occupational safety and Health Agency website.
12. Feuerstein M, Shaw WS, Nicholas RA, Huang GD. From cofounders to suspected risk factors: Psychosocial factors at work related upper extremity disorders. J Electromyogr Kinesio. 2004,14 (1):171-8.
13. Canadian Centre for Occupational Health and Safety website. https://www.ccohs.ca/
14. Claire MB, Geertje AM, Vincent H. The (cost) effectiveness of a lifestyle physical activity intervention on the recovery from neck and upper limb and symptoms in computer operators. BMC Musculoskeletal Disorders. 2006;7:80.

15. Kushwaha DK, Kane PV. Ergonomic assessment and workstation design of shipping crane cabin in steel industry. Int J Ind Erg. 2016;11(52):29-39.
16. Anagha NC, Suhana G. A comparative assessment of the impact of different occupations on workers static musculoskeletal fitness. Int J Ind Erg. 2007,13(3):271-8.
17. Michaelis M, Karajannis N, Hofmann F. IPP-aMSE "Identification and prioritization of relevant prevention strategies for work-related musculoskeletal disorders(MSDs)." www.dguv.de/medien/content/prevention/project/msd/review/ap_4_e.pdf.
18. Lieven E. Strategies to tackle musculoskeletal disorders at work. EU-Occupational Safety and Health Agency website.
19. Rik Op Deb. Strategies to tackle musculoskeletal disorders at work training. EU-Occupational Safety and Health Agency website.
20. Rolf E. Assessment of physical workloads to prevent work related MSDs. EU-Occupational safety and Health Agency website.
21. Guideline: Occupational Health Physical Therapy: Advanced work Rehabilitation Guidelines. Rescinded as APTA guidelines in 2011 May, adopted by Orthopaedic Section BOD, 2011 July 11.
22. Kadi F, Ahlgren C, Waling K, Sundelin G, Thornell L. The effects of different training programs on the trapezius muscle of women with work-related neck and shoulder myalgia. Acta Neuropathol. 2000;100(3):253-8.
23. The physiotherapist's role in occupational rehabilitation. Australian Physiotherapy Association, Position Statement, 2012.
24. Glenda LK, 1949. Industrial therapy (1st ed). Mosby, St. Louis, 1995.
25. Global strategy on occupational health for all: The way to health at work. Recommendation of the second meeting of the WHO Collaborating Centers in Occupational Health, 11-14 October 1994, Beijing, China.
26. Benjamin OA. Fundamental Principles of Occupational Health and Safety. ILO, Geneva, second edition, 2008.
27. Hogstedt C, Pieris B. Occupational Safety and Health in Developing Countries: Review of strategies, case studies and a bibliography.
28. Mathews R, Reis C, Iacopino V. Child labor: A matter of health and human rights. J Ambul Care Manage. 2003;26:181-2
29. Habibullah NS, Tiwari R. Occupational health research in India. Industrial Health. 2004;42: 141-8.
30. Tripathy JP. Occupational health hazard in India: need for surveillance and research. Current Science. 2014;106(5):668-9.
31. Murlidhar V, Murlidhar VJ, Kanhere V. Byssinosis in a Bombay textile mill. Natl Med J India. 1995;8:204-7.
32. Amita A, Aparna I, Debasis S, Neeti K et al. Incidence of silicosis in flour mill workers. Indian J Occup Environ Med. 2011;15(3):104-8.
33. Madhavi LG, Sarla K, Gouroju S, Effect of construction and flour mill air pollution in rural area. Int J Intg Med Sci. 2015;2(2):70-7.
34. Das PK, Shukla KP, Ory FG. An Occupational health program for adults and children in the carpet weaving Industry, Mirzapur, India: a case study in the informal sector. Soc Sci Med. 1992;35:1293-302.
35. Vilanitam JV. A historical and socioeconomic analysis of occupational safety and health in India. Int J Health Serv. 1980;10(2):233-49.
36. Agnihotram RV. An overview of occupational health research in India. Indian J Occup Environ Med. 2005;9(1):10-4.
37. National Policy on Safety, Health and Environment at Workplace, Government of India, Ministry of Labour and Employment. www.ilo.org/asia/WCMS_182422/lang--en/index.htm

14.2 PREVENTIVE PHYSIOTHERAPY IN SPORTS

Akhoury Gourang Sinha

Abstract: The success of the physiotherapist attached with the team should be judged not on the basis of how often he treats the injuries but how much less injuries his team had suffered.

Injuries are the inherent risk of sports participation. The incidence of sports injuries can be reduced by incorporating the principles of injury prevention. Physiotherapists play a very important role in all three levels of prevention. The secondary and tertiary stages of prevention of sports injuries essentially require physiotherapy. Of late the skills and knowledge of physiotherapists is increasingly being used to design and implement primary level prevention. This chapter includes a detailed discussion on the impact of sports injuries, risk factors of sports injuries and strategies for injury prevention. The specific role of physiotherapists at each level of prevention is also discussed at length.

Preamble: This chapter elaborates on risk factors responsible for sports injuries and discusses all the three levels of prevention (primary, secondary and tertiary).

INTRODUCTION

Sport participation is considered an important component of socioeconomic development of a country. The execution of a mega sporting event helps in developing infrastructure, generates employment, secure inflow of foreign capital, generates players and athletes, and thus contributes significantly to the economic development of a country.[1] Emergence of sports as a significant social and economic activity is a recent phenomenon in India. Winning few medals in last two Olympics has added fuel to the national desire of making India a major sporting nation. At the same time, the emergence of sedentary lifestyle as a major risk factor in the genesis of several diseases has brought back the measures promoting physical activity into limelight. Sports participation is now viewed as an important public health strategy that encourage mass participation in physical activity for reducing the incidence of lifestyle induced communicable diseases such as cardiovascular disease, diabetes, obesity, and depression. It is believed that regular physical activity reduces the risk of premature mortality.[2] People participate in sports not only for medals and glory but also for preservation of health and fitness. However, it is interesting to note that active sports person is also the one who is more likely to visit hospitals than his sedentary counterpart.[3] Injuries are the inherent risk of participation in sports.

Injuries to musculoskeletal system are a common occurrence in sports. About 20–30% injury rates are reported during competitions and little higher during training. Epidemiological studies indicated that every 6th of injuries seen by a physician is sustained during sporting activity in Scandinavia.[4] Among children, every 3rd hospital-treated injury is the result of sports participation. During 1997 and 1998, there were an estimated 3.7 million sports and recreation-related emergency department visits annually in the United States, representing approximately 11% of all injury related emergency department visits. The medical charges for these visits were estimated at 500 million US$ annually.[4]

Obtaining similar data in the Indian context is a difficult task. However we have observed alarming high prevalence rate of injuries in several games.[5-8] We reported a prevalence rate of 17% of shoulder impingement syndrome in swimmers in Delhi,[9] 79.03% prevalence of wrist injury in gymnasts,[10] 40%

point prevalence and 81% yearly prevalence of low back pain in female athlete of Patiala.[11] During 14 months of preparatory training before 1982 Asiad games, Ahuja and Ghosh[12] reported the loss of approximately 50 days of training by each athlete while convalescing from sports injury. It would not be incorrect to state that if exercise is medicine, then injury is its side effect.

SPECTRUM OF SPORTS INJURY

The spectrum of sports injuries can be divided into 3 major groups—minor acute injuries, major acute injuries and overuse injuries. Minor acute injuries such as sprain, strain, contusion, laceration, abrasion are quite common. These injuries produce minor discomfort but can seriously interrupt the training and performance. The incidence of major acute injuries such as fracture dislocation, major ligament ruptures, and damage to internal organs are few. These injuries require intensive treatment, longer healing time and significantly curtail the persons involvement in the sports. The residual complications of these major injuries may compel an athlete toward permanent retirement from the sports. Approximately 50% of all sports injuries are secondary to overuse[13] which develop insidiously. Overuse injuries result from repetitive microtrauma that leads to local tissue damage in the form of cellular and extracellular degeneration, and are most likely to occur when an athlete changes the mode, intensity, or duration of training. Management of overuse injuries requires significant modification in the training methods, schedule and intensity.

EFFECT OF SPORTS INJURY

Excellence in sports requires a perfect harmony between joints, muscles, nervous system and cardiopulmonary system. Therefore, even a small imbalance can drastically alter the result of performance. Medals are won or lost by a fraction of a second margin. Therefore, sports persons are often disabled by problems which are often considered trivial by a common man. Sports injuries also have social and psychological dimensions (Table 14.1). Injuries are one of the main reasons for inconsistent performance and premature termination of sporting career. Injury during tournament or at the time of selection is a disaster to a profession athlete that prevents him from enjoying the benefits of long hard training. In a team, sports injury of a key team player during match may convert a win to loss. For a common man who uses sports as a medium for recreation and fitness, injury is a demotivating factor that reduces adherence to regular activity. At junior level of play, injury this is one of the reasons for parents not sending their wards to playing fields. In order to enjoy and avail the benefits of sports, it is important to keep the sporting environment safe and players free from injury. Sports conducted in safe environment not only protect the players from injury but also ensure lifelong adherence to active physical lifestyle. Therefore, injury prevention has now emerged as an important aspect of modern sports.

Physiotherapy has become an essential part of the sports medicine team.[14] Sports physiotherapy can be defined as skillful selection and application of various techniques of physiotherapy on sports persons with the

Table 14.1: Detrimental effects of sports injury

Physical suffering
Loss of training
Inconsistency in performance
Reinjury
Ouster from team
Financial loss
Bad effect on moral and motivation
Non-adherence to training schedule

aim of enhancing and prolonging the quality length of career in the sports. Until few years ago, physiotherapy was mainly used for the treatment and rehabilitation of sports injuries with the goal of facilitating rapid resolution of symptoms. In the recent years, the interest has shifted towards development of strategies that help to prevent the occurrence of injuries. For a competitive athlete, resolution of acute features such as pain, swelling, etc. is not the goal of sports medicine practitioner; rather the focus is shifted towards restoration of form and function after resolution of symptoms.[15] Physiotherapy plays an important role both in treatment as well as prevention of sports injuries. The purpose of this chapter is to highlight the specific role of physiotherapy in the prevention of sports injuries.

INJURY PREVENTION

The incidence and severity of sports injuries can be minimized to a great extent by incorporating the principles of injury prevention. Injury prevention in sports is a complex process involving several interrelated multidisciplinary steps to mitigate the cumulative effects of intrinsic and extrinsic factors.

Prevention can be organized into three levels of primary, secondary, and tertiary prevention.[3] **Primary prevention** aims at avoidance of injury and involves the measures taken before the occurrence of injury. If primary prevention measures are successful, a player will not sustain injury in the first place. However, once the injury has taken place **secondary prevention** measures that minimize the impact of injury in the form of appropriate early identification, and intervention treatment assumes significance. The objectives of **tertiary prevention** are restoration of function and prevention of recurrence of injury. Secondary and tertiary prevention are important for reducing the recurrence of injuries and have greater involvement of physiotherapist.[16] In order to realize the important role of physiotherapists in each stage of prevention, an understanding of risk factors of injuries and methods utilized for injury prevention is necessary.

Risk Factors of Sports Injuries

Injury is the disruption of the structural integrity of tissue. The sports injury is the result of interaction between applied force and the structural strength of the body. An external force far beyond the structural strength of tissue will no doubt disrupt the structural integrity of the tissue. On the other hand, application of even normal force can produce injury if the structural strength of the tissue is low. The risk factors of sports injury can be broadly classified under two broad categories—intrinsic and extrinsic. Intrinsic factors are the physical and psychological characteristics that make a player vulnerable to injury whereas the factors that increase the chance of exposure to higher forces are known as extrinsic risk factors.[13,16] When intrinsic and extrinsic risk factors act simultaneously, the athlete is at far greater risk of injury than when risk factors are present in isolation. Table 14.2 enlists the risk factors of sports injury. A cursory analysis of this table reveals that many of these risk factors are amenable to physiotherapy methods. Some risk factors such as age, gender, history of previous injury, nature of sports, etc. cannot be modified and thus can be termed as non-modifiable factors. However, it is possible to mitigate the effects of several factors by organized intervention. These factors can be termed as modifiable factors.

Intrinsic Risk Factors

The major role of physiotherapy in prevention of sports injury is the identification of intrinsic risk factors and designing and implementing a preventive program directed at modifying the risk factors.[16] Reduced flexibility, local or general muscular weakness, imbalance of

Table 14.2: Risk factors of sports injury

	Intrinsic	Extrinsic
Modifiable	Inflexibility Muscle weakness Muscle tightness Malalignment instability Imperfect neuromuscular coordination Lack of fitness Psychological make up	Poor execution of technique • Training error – Excessive distance – Fast progression – High intensity – Hill work – Poor technique – Monotonous/asymmetrical training – Fatigue Poor quality of equipment
Non-modifiable	Previous injury Age Gender Maturity Female with menstrual irregularity Morphological profile	Nature of game Sports specific skills Nature of sports Environmental factors: environment heat, humidity, cold altitude, ground

muscular strength, joint laxity, proprioceptive deficits, biomechanical malalignment, previous injury are the known risk factors of sports injuries. Gender, age, psychological makeup of the athlete is also implicated in the causation of sport injury.

Alteration in normal joint range of motion: Two pattern of joint range of motion alteration implicated in the causation of sports injuries are reduced range (hypomobility) and increased range (hypermobility). Reduction in the range of motion is a known consequence of injury. It can also evolve as adaptive shortening associated with practice of a specific movement pattern. Forcing a joint to move beyond the available range produces macro/micro trauma. The decreased extensibility of connective tissue mechanically hinders the amount of joint excursion and decrease the efficacy of the movement pattern. Athletes with decreased ROM are more likely to suffer from musculotendinous unit tears than their flexible counterparts.

Increased range of joint motion or joint laxity reflects the attenuation of joint stabilizing structures. It is known risk factor for injuries to spine and shoulder. It can develop as a consequence of traumatic attenuation of stabilizing structures such as ligaments and capsule, either due to a single traumatic event or due to practice of a specific sports activity. Genetics may also play a role in the genesis of hyper mobility. Athletes of certain sports such as gymnastics, dancing, etc. demonstrate relatively larger range of motion in certain joints. Joint laxity makes the joint unstable and can be potential factors for injury to the same joint or injury of the distant part of kinetic chain. Instability often interrupts the fine synergistic contraction of the muscle and exposes the tendino-capsulo-ligamentous structure to excessive stress and overuse.

Alteration in Muscle Function

Production of functional and non-stressful movement pattern requires an appropriate synergistic coactivation of stabilizers and prime movers muscles. A change in the strength of one muscle alters the length and strength of other muscles and reduces the efficiency of movement. Like alteration in joint range of motion, muscle imbalance can also emerge as a consequence of trauma or practice of specific sports activity. Overemphasis on one pattern of movement in training can generate imbalances if the athlete does not perform strengthening exercise of muscle involved in opposite pattern. The unbalanced development of strength across joints is the known factor for several acute and overuses injuries. Disuse following injury and immobilization is also a known reason of reduction of strength of specific muscles. A weak muscle has poor ability to absorb the force of impact and practice of specific skill in presence of a weak muscle virtually increases the change of overuse injury. A reduction in the isometric strength of muscle reduces the stability of joint and predisposes to overuse injury. On the other hand, increase in the dynamic strength is implicated in the acute injury.[16] Besides increase and decrease in force producing ability of muscle faulty recruitment of muscle or ***poor*** muscle control have also emerged as risk factors for development of subtle functional malalignment and overuse injury.[17] Inability to dissociate hip extension from pelvic motion due to poor motor control of abductor, gluteus, hamstring and hip external rotator increases the anterior tilt in running giving rise to increased length and tension of hamstring and abdominals[16] which could lead to strain of these muscles. Poor control of vastus medialis and external rotator of shoulder contributes to development of patellofemoral pain and shoulder impingement syndrome respectively.

Balance Deficits

Ligament injured joints often display deficit in proprioception. Reduced proprioception is known cause of ankle sprain. When stress is applied to ligament, a specific pattern of neural activity is initiated for activating those muscles that are in anatomical and biomechanical position to oppose the applied forces. The lack of proprioceptive inputs reduces the amount of protective muscular activation and gives rise to reduction in functional stability, deviation in the biomechanical axis of joint motion from its ideal path and alters the contact area of the articular surface. This would lead to abnormal compression and shear stress on the articular structures (cartilage) and eventually progress to degenerative changes in the joint.

Malalignment

Deviation in the alignment of various segments of the body such as flat foot, cavus foot, leg length discrepancy, bow leg, knock knee and scoliosis alters the distribution of applied force within the kinetic chain produces concentration of force to some specific area and makes them vulnerable to overuse injury. Hyperpronated or flat foot increases ground reaction forces on the medial aspect of foot and is held as predisposing factor for medial tibial stress syndrome, tibialis posterior, achilles tendonitis and stress fracture. On the other hand, hypopronated foot or cavus or rigid foot increases ground reaction force to the lateral side and acts as a predisposing factor for trochanteric bursitis, ITB friction syndrome, stress fracture and metatarsalgia.[13,18]

Previous Injury

Inadequately treated previous injury is a strong risk factor for majority of the sports injuries.[13,15,16] Treatment of sports injuries is directed at the restoration of anatomical continuity of the injured structure by bridging the gap with new tissue. Structural strength of repaired new tissue takes a long time even after complete resolution of symptoms to achieve near normal strength. Therefore, in the initial stages, their stress withstanding capacity is lower. In many circumstances, it may not reach the original value even after complete treatment and rehabilitation. If the athlete participates in athletic activity at the same intensity before the injury, the chance of disruption of tissue increases many fold. Further, during the period of healing, an athlete develops several impairments in the musculoskeletal and cardiopulmonary systems. Certain impairments are inevitable consequence of the injury and its treatment, whereas others are produced due to detraining and loss of mechanical stimulus of movement. Sports participation in presence of these impairments is risky.

Age

Adolescent, children and elderly carry higher risk of injury due to physiological changes of growth. The adolescent athlete is more susceptible to injury than the prepubescent athlete because circulating androgens promote the fast development of muscle mass and enhance movement velocity and power. Adolescent athletes also have reduced flexibility due to a physiological lag in the lengthening of musculotendinous structure as compared to the longitudinal lengthening of the bone.

Gender

The anatomical and physiological difference between male and female such as wider pelvis, inward slanting thigh, shorter limb length, wider carrying angle, more mobile joints, less muscle mass (25% < male), lower hematocrit, smaller heart and lungs and less reduced oxygen carrying capacity are suggested as probable reasons for increased vulnerability of female athletes to injury.[18] However, research does not entirely support this. In fact, when the training load and sporting activities are similar, there appears to be no difference in the rate of injuries between male and female.[19] However, the low bone density due to less estrogen level as seen in menstrual irregularity does increase the chance of stress fracture in female athletes.

Psychological Makeup of Players

Over assertiveness, aggressiveness and engagement in high-risk taking behavior appears to increase the risk of injury to the player and also to the fellow players. Inability to cope up with stress of social life makes the player vulnerable to injuries. It is reported that player who has sustained a major loss such as demise of beloved one had higher incidence of sports injury. Many a time, injury is also used as an excuse for not participation in physical training and at times, it becomes difficult to identify whether the complaint of pain during activity is malingering or the early symptoms of overuse injury.

Extrinsic Factors

The situations which includes to increase the chance of exposure to higher forces can be termed as extrinsic risk factors. Training errors, environment, playing surface, equipment and the manner in which preparation of the activities are undertaken are some of the known extrinsic risk factors. Besides, the nature of sports is, in itself, a biggest non-modifiable extrinsic risk factor.

Errors in Training

The manner in which the training of sports is undertaken is most important extrinsic risk factor of both acute and overuses injuries. Training error can be broadly divided into four categories—neglect of safe training habit, rapid progression in the intensity, excessive mileage (loading) and inadequate recovery.[13,18] Players pay much attention to the technical and tactical training but neglect safe training habit such as warm up, cool down, stretching and proper conditioning. Prior to rigorous technical and tactical training, it is important to ensure the player has learnt the correct execution of specific skills and his body is well adapted to withstand the stress of sports. Improper conditioning is one of the principal causes of sports injuries. An athlete who maintains proper muscular balance and strength, cardiovascular conditioning, and flexibility is less likely to sustain an injury than an athlete who does not maintain good levels of conditioning year round.[20] Subjecting a poorly conditioned and novice player to a sudden progression in the volume and/or intensity of workout is the sure way of making him/her injured. Second component of training errors is the inappropriate progression of intensity or distance, sudden increase in the intensity or mileage, distance, excessive downhill running, number of overs bowled, number of throws, etc. increase the chance of injury many fold. This often happens to a novice player and also to an athlete after return from an injury. Recovery from stress of training is essential to gain full training benefits and prevent injuries. Recovery refers to post event activities directed to relieve the neuromuscular and psychological stress following a strenuous activity. In order to derive complete advantage of the strenuous training regimen, the recovery from the stress of training is of paramount importance as the adaptation takes place during the period of recovery. Excessive volumes of intense training and competition when associated with inadequate recovery can potentially cause symptoms of overreaching, overtraining, fatigue and results in the suppression of performance and overuse injuries. The very stimuli that are used to bring improvement in performance can become the cause of reduced performance.

Nature of Sports

Several sports skills such as throwing, bowling, swimming, weightlifting, to name a few, impose heavy loads on the body which itself may be a causative factor of injury and when these are not performed correctly, the risk of injuries increases many folds. Pars interarticularis fracture and subsequent spondylolysis and listhesis are common in fast bowlers in cricket mostly due to risky bowling techniques.[16] Besides, the aims and rules of games also dictate the pattern of injuries. Higher scoring for risky skills does contribute to increased injury rate in a given sports. Famous bodyline series of cricket is an example of how the rule of the game be utilized to win the game without considering the safety requirement of the opponents. In team sports, certain positions are more prone to injuries, e.g., the deep fielder in cricket experience shoulder problems in contrast to forward short leg players who are more exposed to high velocity contact injuries of head and face.

Ground or Playing Surface

The role of ground on which game is played in inciting sport injuries is well-recognized. Play on slippery surface increases the possibilities of fall. Training on hard surface such as concrete and asphalt can increase the impact loading and predispose to overuse injuries. On the other hand, running on very compliant—soft surface increases the cost of running and induce early fatigue contributing to increased risk of making errors and injury. Artificial turf provides different harness, friction and resilience in comparison to natural grass and therefore the injury profile of these surfaces differs significantly. Inclination of surface also affects the injury. Both uphill and downhill running increase the chance of injuries to quadriceps muscle due to more muscular efforts required for controlling the movement. Running on cambered track increases stress on the inner leg and predisposes it to ankle and knee injury. When there is an abrupt change of quality and type of running surface, the injury risk raises many folds. Inadvertent collision with installations in sports fields such as metal goal post, fence, etc. can also inflict injury.

Shoe

Shoe in sports serves three purposes: shock absorption (reduce the impact force, control of foot motion and protection from untoward trauma). The requirement of all these three components is different for different sports. Games with predominance of agility skill requires better foot control whereas games involving prolonged impact loading requires more shock absorption. Shoes also serve to mitigate the friction of the field. Use of inappropriate shoes during training and competition not only contributes to injuries but also affects the skills and performance. A running shoe loses its efficacy to absorb impact after 400 km by 30–50%. Excessive perspiration or running on wet surface accelerates the wear and tear of the shoes. Failure to timely replace shoes may contribute to overuse injuries.

Equipment

Poorly designed equipment, especially if combined with faulty technique, significantly increase the risk of overuse injury. The improper size, material, string tension, grip sizes of the racquet are known factors for elbow overuse injuries in racquets sports.

Protective Equipment

Failure to wear protective equipment inadvertently or willingly as a mark of courage may cause fatal injuries. Poor quality of protecting equipment is also a factor as it does not absorb the excessive force. These kinds equipment, many a times, provide false sense of security that encourages the players to indulge in risk taking behavior. At times, these kinds equipment are misused to inflict injury on the other players. For example, helmets can be used as battering ram in tackling and blocking in rugby and football.

Adverse Climatic Condition

Sports conducted in adverse climatic conditions are known to produce higher incidence of injuries. Cold and hot environments influence the metabolic rate and vascular supply to the soft tissue and limit their ability to work efficiently for longer duration. It may change the playing style as well. For example, stride length shortens in cold conditions which put excessive strain on the decelerating muscles, hams and hip stabilizing muscles. Heat injuries (exhaustion, collapse) are known to occur in endurance sports if conducted in hot and humid climate.

Injury Prevention Methods

Sports injury is the result of a complex and intricate interaction of extrinsic and intrinsic factors. Therefore, the implementation of principles of injury prevention requires efforts from all stakeholders such as players, coaches, support staff, medical doctors, physiotherapists, organizers and promoters of sports and sporting federation. The injury prevention methods are directed at reducing the magnitude and duration of applied external force and increasing the force withstanding capacity of the body. For example, increasing the range of a stiff joint and strengthening a weak muscle through organized exercise helps to increase the capacity of body to withstand the higher loads. On the other hand, application of brace or protective device reduces the impact of external forces acting on the body. Several preventive methods are recommended and applied by sports participants for reducing the risk of injury. Preparticipation examination, warm up, strengthening, eccentric work, stretching, proprioceptive training, neuro-muscular training, shoe, insole, tape brace, protective equipment, modification of training schedules, technique analysis and modification of technique, and recovery methods are some methods commonly advocated for prevention of injuries as well as for performance enhancement. In addition, the role of organizing competition and training in safe environmental condition, emphasis on strict enforcement of rules to avoid foul play and unruly behaviors and at times modifying the rules of games become critical.

Prevention methods can be described as active measures and passive measures.[2] Active measures are the choice of individual which requires voluntary efforts of players. Engagement in safe training habits such as warm up, cool down, stretching, taking proper treatment of injury prior to returning to sports are the examples of active measure. Being the individual's choice, active measures can be successful only if players understand the importance of these measures. The correction of intrinsic risk factors largely requires active measures.

Passive measures are mandatory conditions set up by rules that must be fulfilled prior to sports participation. Wearing protective equipment during play is the example of passive measures. Implementation of passive measures means strict enforcement of rules. Passive measures are usually more successful in preventing injuries than active measures; the amelioration of the extrinsic risk factors relies heavily on passive methods of constructing and rigorously implementing safety rules. A comprehensive injury prevention program requires both the measures.

Specific Role of Physiotherapy in Different Level of Prevention

Van Mechelen[21] in 1992 proposed a model to develop preventive strategies within a given sporting team. This model has following four steps, as mentioned below.

1. Establishing the extent of the injury problem through epidemiological research
2. Identifying the factors and mechanisms of sports injuries
3. Introducing a preventive measure
4. Assessing its effectiveness by repeating step one.

A physiotherapist plays a valuable role in each of these stages of organized injury prevention strategy. A sports person often performs despite preexisting injuries. In London Olympics, of all the visits for physiotherapy, 45.5% were for the treatment of preexisting injuries, which reflects the significant level of persisting musculoskeletal problems among athletes entering major sport events.[22] In practical terms, this means that for individual player methods of prevention of all three levels may be applied together for management of different injuries. This makes the task of physiotherapists more challenging. For efficient results, a player requires a constant physiotherapy support throughout his/her playing career. The specific role of physiotherapist in each level of prevention is listed in Table 14.3.

Primary Level Prevention

The main role of physiotherapists in the primary level prevention is detection of intrinsic risk factors and their amelioration through remedial program and making the players realize the importance of indulgence in safe training habits, balanced training, using appropriate safety appliances and respecting the principle of individuality, progressive overload and recovery. The specific duties of physiotherapists at this phase includes preparticipation examination to identify the existing deficits in range, muscle function, balance and fitness, design and implement remedial program for correction of identified deficits, design awareness and sensitization program about

Table 14.3: Role of physiotherapy in each level of prevention

Level of prevention	Broad aim	Objective	Methods
Primary (player without injury)	Avoidance of injury	Identification and modification of risk factors	Preparticipation examination, remedial program inculcating safe training habits, awareness and sensitization injury surveillance and epidemiological research
Secondary (injured player)	Treatment of injury	Early identification and intensive management	PRICE, electrotherapy, exercise therapy, manual therapy, patient education
Tertiary (recovering player)	Reduce and/ or correct an existing disability	Restoration of abilities of players, prevention of reinjury	Rehabilitation, reconditioning, protective equipment, movement analysis and technique modification

the importance of injury prevention and need to incorporate principles of injury prevention in overall training program, guidance on warm up, stretching and cool down and depending on the need and nature of sports design and implement recovery program.

Preparticipation Evaluation

The Preparticipation Physical Exam (PPE) is the first step to keep sports participation healthy. It is the basis upon which preventive strategies are built up. The goals of PPE are identification of medical and orthopedic problems that may predispose an athlete at risk for injury, reinjury or illness, identify correctable problems that may impair the athlete's ability to perform and assess fitness level for specific sports. Ideally, preparticipation examination should be carried out by a team of medical doctors, physiotherapists, exercise physiologist, and coach. However, in Indian context, this ideal situation is seldom achieved. Therefore, a single practitioner associated with team should have a basic knowledge of the principles of PPE so that if required the athlete may be referred to appropriate professionals. The components of PPE include detailed history, clinical screening, and detailed evaluation of components to fitness (flexibility, strength, balance, agility, speed, cardiopulmonary endurance and body composition). Primary inquiries in the history must focus on previous musculoskeletal injury, training profiles and aspiration of player, sudden cardiac death (SCD) in family members, previous concussions, exercise-induced respiratory symptoms, the female athlete triad, missing organs, vaccination etc. The essential information may be collected by self-administered questionnaire. If the history suggests certain cardiorespiratory pathology, then a more detailed physical examination of associated areas is suggested.[19,23]

Musculoskeletal screening includes examination of range of motion of all joints, clinical examination of key muscles, and key joints and looking for biomechanical deviations. The inclusion of functional tests and fitness specific examination further broaden the scope of PPE. It is recommended that PPE should be conducted 6 weeks before the start of sports season.[23] This 6 week window provides an opportunity to correct any risk factors before the start of session.

Remedial Program

A history of previous injury to the joint or muscle with signs of reduced proprioception, residual inability to execute high velocity concentric/eccentric muscle work, reduced flexibility, tenderness, fibrous adhesion or adverse neural tension tests require the physiotherapist to get into its traditional role of musculoskeletal rehabilitation and utilize all the procedures available in his repertories. Emphasis should be on an active exercise approach with priority on the use of therapist independent techniques. Deficits in structural or functional instability should be given due attention. Similarly, specific deficiency of fitness components needs to be addressed through remedial conditioning program. The detected biomechanical abnormalities must be corrected using appropriate shoe insert, orthosis, taping, and by balancing the flexibility, strength and coordination by exercises. Many authorities call this stage as prehabilitation.[23]

Inculcating Safe Training Habits

Warm up, stretching, cool down, periodization of training and recovery are the important component of safe training. It is important to educate the players about the importance of these practices. Physiotherapists are the best positioned members of the team for this task. It is shown that having a physiotherapist teach the soccer players how to warm up, and stretch before after match, tapping the ankle and use of shin guard have reduced the incidence of injuries by 75%.[24] Most important step for intrinsic risk elimination is the balanced training program respecting the principles of progressive overload, specificity and individuality. Each individual has different capacity of training and recovery which should be acknowledged during overloading. Increase in training load should correspond to the induced adaptations. A good training is the balance between stress and recovery which can be achieved using the principles of periodization of training. In order to keep the training load balanced the entire session should be broken in three main phases—conditioning, technical and tactical training and recovery. Conditioning phase focuses on first developing fitness then the sporting skills. Competition phase concentrates entirely on technical and tactical training and excellence in performance. Recovery phase focuses on recuperation of athlete and correction of existing or imminent impairments. The concept of periodization should also be followed on monthly, weekly and on daily basis. At daily level, microcycle of periodization involves warm up stretching–training–cool down and recovery. In each week, the participants should have fixed days for fitness, skill training, higher intensity work out and recovery. Physiotherapists have no role in designing the training schedule of players, it is the responsibility of coaches. But physiotherapists can effectively educate the players about the importance of periodization and facilitate the reorganization of training schedule according to the capacity of the players. This step requires a close cooperation and faith between coach and physiotherapist. Importance of periodization in the prevention of overuse injuries cannot be overemphasized.

Recovery

For a competitive athlete, recovery attains as important a role in as skill acquisition, strength, speed and endurance training. It is one of the prime concerns of every professional group dealing with physical exercises. Recovery methods are expected to bring about an early reversal of altered homeostasis and a feel good factor on the psyche of the athlete. Athletes employ a number of methods to expedite recovery. These procedures range from simple rest to diversified psychological techniques, nutritional supplementation, medication, application of physical agents and specific exercises. While the psychological recovery and nutritional, recovery are the specialization area of sports psychological and sports nutritionist, the domain of physical recovery would greatly benefit from the knowledge and skills of sports physiotherapists. The physical procedures for speeding recovery from exercise can be grouped under two broad categories- 'active recovery' and 'passive recovery'. The modifications of passive recovery include massage, cold shower, hot shower, sauna, steam bath, underwater massage. Of late, some electrotherapy modalities like electrical stimulation, TENS and LASER have also been explored as tools of recovery.[25] Many of these methods require the skill of expertize of physiotherapists therefore active involvement of physiotherapists in facilitating recovery would help athlete to maintain optimal performance while remaining free from injury. One of the reasons for the use of drugs in sports is to mask fatigue while retaining alertness with increasing training loads. The properly administered recovery method provides the athlete with the opportunity to combat the rigorousness of training without sustaining injury.

Awareness Sensitization

Implementation of injury prevention strategies at grass root level can only succeed when the players, coaches and organizers have knowledge and faith in them. Sensitizing them about the need of prevention and making them aware about the possible causation and methods of prevention is vital.

Injury Surveillance and Epidemiological Research

Epidemiological studies are required to obtain information on the magnitude, severity and distribution of injuries and help identify the potential factor predisposing to injury. These studies are also needed to determine the effectiveness of preventative measures.[26] Being the member of medical team that comes in direct contact with player almost on daily basis, physiotherapist can contribute significantly to the task of injury surveillance which forms the basis of epidemiological research. Systematic documentation of the occurrence and outcomes of injuries is necessary to design specific preventive strategy. Many countries have established system of injury surveillance where the injury data of players are collected. Analysis of such data provides the basis for rule modification and other prevention strategies. Such approach is largely missing in Indian context. Many risk factors go unnoticed and culminate over the years to increase the risk of injury during important tournaments. A physiotherapist can play valuable role in establishing a system to monitor injuries and exposure within the team.

Secondary Level of Prevention

Secondary level prevention essentially requires physiotherapist's involvement. It is now accepted that about 80% of sports injuries require only physiotherapy treatment and even the injuries requiring surgical interventions essentially require pre- and postoperative physiotherapy for safe and early return to play. Besides facilitating repair on the injured tissue, physiotherapists at this stage should also work to minimize the secondary impairments and blunt the effect of detraining.

Facilitates Healing and Repair

Repair of an injury is a natural process. The different methods of treatment work to reduce the impact of those factors that may impede the process of healing. The ultimate result of healing is bringing the gap created by the injury by scar—a fibrous tissue strong enough to withstand the higher loads of athletic activities. Majority of soft tissue injuries are treated conservatively. Occasionally, when the loss of tissue is substantial, surgical procedures are also required to restore the anatomical continuity. The pathological management of any athletic injury consists of three distinct phases, i.e. damage control, facilitation of repair and reconditioning of the recovered lesion.[16]

The initial period after the injury when the pain, discomfort and disability are maximal is referred as phase of damage control. The pathological process of inflammation is in full swing and the focus of management revolves around control of damage evoked by the inflammation and prevention of the extension of lesion. The methods employed in this phase are termed as PRICE (Protection, Rest, Ice, Compression and Elevation) along with anti-inflammatory medications. These initial treatments can be rendered by anybody and in fact all the persons dealing with sports should be familiar with the first aid of injuries. The facilitation of repair phase is the time period when the actual biological repair of the injured tissue takes place. The stage constitutes the matrix and cellular proliferation phase of healing and lasts for between 72 hours to 6 weeks. Physiotherapy at this stage is aimed at reducing the swelling, facilitating the nutrition and oxygenation of the injured site and restoring the normal movement pattern while minimizing further deterioration (muscle atrophy, proprioceptive loss, etc.) and avoiding reinflammation.

The physiotherapy methods employed in this stage can be grouped under four broad heading i.e. manual therapy, electrotherapy, exercise therapy and patient education. manual therapy methods like joint mobilization, soft tissue manipulation, etc. seek to restore the mobility of the injured area, whereas the various electrotherapy modalities (ultrasound, SWD, MWD, ultrasound, various electrical stimulation currents, cryokinetics) are used for facilitating the biological repair and smoothing the process of range and strength restoration. Exercise therapy remains the main stay of long-term treatment and prevention of sports injuries. It addresses the goal of minimizing muscle wasting, restoring the movement pattern, and developing the strength and coordination. It is important to understand that in the absence of active exercises, the benefit obtained by manual therapy and electrotherapy modalities will not be retained for a long time. An informed player demonstrates better compliance of the instructions. Therefore, educating the injured player on the causes of injuries, methods of avoiding reinjury, rationale behind rest, importance of change of training schedule, technique, etc. should be considered as important as any other intervention.

Minimize the Impact of Detraining

Higher performance ability and physique of athlete are the results of short-term and long-term adaptations produced due to physical training. These adaptations are transient and reversible in nature. The maintenance of fitness requires regular participation in training. Sports injuries disrupts the normal training schedule of players and give rise to decline in parameter of flexibility, strength, balance and cardiopulmonary endurance which culminates into deterioration of sports skill and performance. It is important to blunt the impact of detraining by instituting alternative exercise schedule that does not disrupt the healing process.

Tertiary Level of Prevention

The tertiary level of prevention is the prediction and treatment of possible complications during the post-injury phase. Measures in this level constitute an individual level of prevention specific to the need of player. Besides rehabilitation, the involvement of physiotherapists in this stage of prevention should also extend to movement analysis, technique modification and epidemiological research. The implementation of this phase essentially requires close cooperation between physiotherapist and the coaching staff.

Rehabilitation

In context of health care delivery, rehabilitation is described as the process of minimizing the impact of impairment and disability and restoring the previous level of function. Every athletic injury produces impairments that persist long after the healing of injury and limit the functional capability of athlete. These impairments must be addressed in a systematic manner. Sports rehabilitation involves the judicious use of therapeutic exercises and modalities. This phase is mainly exercise oriented where the injured tissue is subjected to gradual loading and the specific attention is paid to correct deficits in range, strength, proprioception, agility, aerobic and anaerobic fitness and restoration of sports specific skills. The objectives are to maximize the loading tolerance of the repaired tissue and condition the body in general prior to returning to the competitive sports situation.

Movement Analysis and the Technique Modification

Restoration of sports skills is the last and ultimate goal of rehabilitation program that should be started once the strength, range and balance reaches a sufficient level. Execution of these skills in presence of impairment has the potential to produce a compensatory deviation that not only reduces the efficacy of movement but makes the player vulnerable to reinjury. It is important to identify these deviations through kinetic and kinematic analysis of sports skills. Once the deviations are detected, they can be corrected by neuromuscular training.

Case Study 1: National Level Marathon Runner

Mr X–A national level long distance runner-came to sports physiotherapy OPD of punjabi university with complaint of pain in right shin interfering with training since 2–3 months. Pain in shin appeared everyday when he would reach certain speed and increased in intensity with progression of training and soon he was incapacitated to train further. On examination the only positive findings were painful resisted contraction of TA, EHL, ED muscles with normal range of motion and no localized tenderness. He was treated with ultrasound, heat, massage, progressive strengthening of involved muscle. He himself was taking over the counter medicine of NSAID group. Within 10 days of treatment his symptoms were relieved and he returned to play. He came again after 7 days with recurrence. Same treatment was given and he returned back to play. He was advised this time to increase the training intensity and duration slowly which he could not follow. His only interest was to get relief from pain so that he can resume training with full intensity. The same cycle of exaggeration and remission was repeated 4 times in the season. He went on to participate in national championship where he had broken national record and won gold. However the remission and relapse of pain during training persisted for 4 month after event. He was referred to a premier tertiary hospital where he was thoroughly investigated using X-Ray MRI, NMR, hematology etc. All investigation were suggestive of chronic inflammation of involved muscle belly. He was advised rest and slow return to training. Now he could not concentrate on game. Frequent pain had interrupted his training his performance got reduced and he could not succeed in the selection trails of next season and was compelled to take forced retirement from game. A retrospective analysis of this case forced us to think that the main reason for his condition was inadequate rest and early return to play due to wrong belief and peer's pressure. Inconsistence selection policy and absence of player's protection program have contributed to strengthening of the wrong believes. This case highlights the importance of recovery and periodization and gradual progression of training loads after injury. It also suggests that temporary reduction of symptoms does not always contribute to long-term success of the players.

Case Study 2: International Level Archer

Ms Y–An international archer-met with a road traffic accident while returning from national high altitude acclimatization camp that left her right shoulder fractured and dislocated. She was treated operatively at a premier tertiary care hospital. After two months, she came to sports physiotherapy OPD of punjabi university Patiala for postoperative physiotherapy. Range of motion of shoulder was grossly limited in all directions and strength of muscles around shoulder was poor, functionally she was not able to hold the bow. She was treated with active and passive mobilization exercises. The muscle strengthening program consisted of a progression of isometric exercise, isotonic concentric exercise and eccentric exercises within the limits of pain and range. The goal was to achieve normal range of motion in all directions and pain free eccentric contractions of all the muscles especially external rotators. Four months postphysiotherapy, 70% range was achieved in all the directions and she could hold the bow and shoot within short ranges. With no rest pain and no functional difficulty in day-to-day activity she and her coach wanted to resume full practice so that she could participate in the selection trails for next session. However, I wanted to achieve complete restoration of external rotation range before she could be send back to practice. After 15th days she just stopped coming to physiotherapy center. Letter I came to know that she resumed full practice and after a week developed pain which increased in intensity with each day of practice and one day she was unable to hold the bow. She was diagnosed with complete rupture of supraspinatus tendon for which she had to undergo operative repair. Now she is no more into active play. This case again highlights the danger of early return to play without undergoing complete restoration of physical fitness parameters.

SUMMARY

Injuries are the inherent risk of sports participation. All physical activity has an inherent risk of injury; however certain player specific characteristics and environment increases the risk of injury many fold. The incidence of sports injuries can be reduced by incorporating the principles of injury prevention. Injury prevention in sport has numerous benefits. These include greater health of the individual, longevity in the activity and reduced costs to the individual, the sport, the health care system, and society. An obvious benefit is the potential for better performance. Physiotherapists play a very important role in all three levels of prevention. The secondary and tertiary stages of prevention of sports injuries essentially require physiotherapy. Of late, the skills and knowledge of physiotherapists is increasingly being used to design and implement primary level prevention. The success of the physiotherapist attached with the team should be judged not on the basis of how often he/she treats the injuries but how much less injuries the team had suffered.

REFERENCES

1. Gratton C. The economic importance of modern sport. Sport in Society. 1998;1(1):101-7.
2. Bahr R, Engebretsen L. Why is injury prevention in sports important? In: Bahr R, Engebretsen L (Eds). Sports Injury Prevention: Olympic Handbook of Sports Medicine. Wiley-Blackwell. 2009:1-6.
3. Meeuwisse W, Bahr R. A systematic approach to sports injury prevention, In: Bahr R, Engebretsen L (Eds), Sports Injury Prevention: Olympic Handbook of Sports Medicine. Wiley-Blackwell, 2009:7.
4. Bahr R, van Mechelen W, Kannus P. Prevention of sports injuries, In: M Kjaer et al. (Eds), Textbook of Sports Medicine, Basic Science and Clinical Aspects of Sports Injury and Physical Activity. Blackwell Science, Oxford, 2003:299–314.
5. Sinha AG, Kang GS, Sandhu JS. Prevalence of shoulder impingement syndrome: A cross-sectional study of male cricket players. J Sports Traumatol and Allied Sports Sci. 1999;1:48-58.
6 Kaur J, Sinha AGK. Prevalence of ankle sprain and service utilization among players of Punjab. International Journal of Therapies and Rehabilitation Research. 2015;4(1):16-24.
7. Sethy GB, Sinha AGK. Injury pattern in Indian elite men field hockey players–pre Olympic 2012. Sports research. 2013;2(4):33-42.
8. Mehta J, Sinha AGK. Prevalence of functional ankle instability and its association with risk factors in basketball players of Punjab. International Journal of Physical Education, Sports and Health. 2015;1(6): 03-07.
9. Bansal S, Sinha AGK, Sandhu JS. Shoulder impingement syndrome among competitive swimmers in India—prevalence, evaluation and risk factors. J Exerc Sci Fit. 2007;5(2):102-8.
10. Kaur Satnam, Sinha AGK. Prevalence and associated risk factors of wrist pain in Indian gymnasts. Sports Research. 2012;1(1);pp 19-32. (RNI title code PUNENGO 1366, published by sports authority of India NS NIS Patiala).
11. Atwal I, Sinha AGK. Prevalence and risk factors of low back pain among female athlete. International Journal of Fitness and Exercise Sciences. 2012,6-16.
12. Ahuja A, Ghosh AK. Pre-Asiad' 82 injuries in elite Indian athletes. Brit J Sports Med. 1985;19(1):24-6.
13. Wilder RP, Sethi S. Overuse injuries: tendinopathies, stress fractures, compartment syndrome, and shin splints. Clin Sports Med. 2004;23(1):55-81.
14. Hahn A. Sports medicine, sports science: the multidisciplinary road to sports success, J Sci Med Sport. 2004;7:275–7.
15. Frontera WR. Epidemiology of sports injuries: Implications for rehabilitation. In: Frontera (Ed), Rehabilitation of Sports Injuries: Scientific Basis Volume X of the Encyclopaedia of Sports Medicine. Blackwell Science, 2003:3-9.

16. Allingham C. Principles of Management. Zuluaga, M (Ed). In: Sports Physiotherapy-Applied Science and Practice. Churchill Livingstone, Melbourne. 1995.
17. Kibler WB, Chandler TJ. Functional rehabilitation and teturn to training and competition. In: Frontera (Ed). Rehabilitation of Sports Injuries: Scientific Basis Volume X of the Encyclopaedia of Sports Medicine, Blackwell Science. 2003:288-300.
19. Vicenzino B, Vicenzino D. Considerations in injury prevention, In: Zulanga M (Ed) Sports Physiotherapy: Churchill Livingstone, Melbourne. 1995.
20. Borsa PA, Lephart SM. Conditioning and Training. Freddie H Fu, David A, MD Stone (Eds). Sports Injuries: Mechanisms, Prevention, Treatment, 2nd edn. Lippincott, Williams and Wilkins, 1994.
21. van Mechelen W, Hlobil H, Kemper HC. Incidence, severity, a etiology and prevention of sports injuries. A Review of Concepts Sports Med. 1992;14(2);82-99.
22. Grant ME, Steffen K, Glasgow P, et al. The role of sports physiotherapy at the London 2012 Olympic Games. Br J Sports Med. 2014;48(1):63–70, doi:10.1136/bjsports-2013-093169.
23. Somogyi DM, Shrier I. Customizing the Preparticipation Evaluation. In: Freddie H Fu, David A, Stone MD (Eds), Sports Injuries: Mechanisms, Prevention, Treatment, 2nd edn. Lippincott, Williams and Wilkins, 1994.
24. Ekstrand J, Gillquist J, Liljedahl SO. Prevention of soccer injuries. Supervision by doctor and physiotherapist. Am J Sports Med. 1983;11(3):116–20.
25. Sinha AGK. Role of physiotherapy in recovery following exhaustive exercises. Sports research. 2013;2(2).
26. Holder Y, Peden M, Krug E, et al. Injury surveillance guidelines. World Health Organization, Geneva; 2001.

Index

Page numbers followed by *f* refer to figure and *t* refer to table.

D

E

F

T